# SCIENCE AND SOCCER

## Developing Elite Performers

Now in a fully revised and updated third edition, *Science and Soccer* is still the most comprehensive and accessible introduction to the science behind the world's most popular sport. Offering important guidance on how science translates into practice, the book examines every key facet of the sport, with a particular focus on the development of elite performers. The topics covered include:

- anatomy, physiology, psychology, sociology and biomechanics;
- principles of training;
- nutrition;
- physical and mental preparation;
- playing surfaces and equipment;
- decision making and skill acquisition;
- coaching and coach education;
- performance analysis;
- talent identification and youth development.

*Science and Soccer* is a unique resource for students and academics working in sports science. It is essential reading for all professional support staff working in the game, including coaches at all levels, physiotherapists, conditioning specialists, performance analysts, club doctors and sport psychologists.

**A. Mark Williams** is Professor and Head of Sport Sciences at Brunel University, London. He has published extensively in the areas related to skill acquisition, expert performance, talent identification and development and performance analysis.

# SCIENCE AND SOCCER

## Developing Elite Performers

### Third Edition

**EDITED BY A. MARK WILLIAMS**

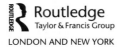 Routledge
Taylor & Francis Group

LONDON AND NEW YORK

First published 2013
by Routledge
2 Park Square, Milton Park, Abingdon, Oxon OX14 4RN

Simultaneously published in the USA and Canada
by Routledge
711 Third Avenue, New York, NY 10017

*Routledge is an imprint of the Taylor & Francis Group, an informa business*

*British Library Cataloguing in Publication Data*
A catalogue record for this book is available from the British Library

*Library of Congress Cataloging-in-Publication Data*
Science and soccer : developing elite performers / edited
by Mark Williams. – 3rd ed.
p. cm.
1. Soccer. 2. Sports sciences. I. Williams, A. M. (A. Mark), 1965–
GV943.S36 2013
796.334–dc23
2012024568

ISBN: 978–0–415–67210–8 (hbk)
ISBN: 978–0–415–67211–5 (pbk)
ISBN: 978–0–203–13186–2 (ebk)

Typeset in Eras
by Keystroke, Station Road, Codsall, Wolverhampton

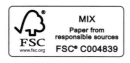

MIX
Paper from
responsible sources
FSC® C004839
www.fsc.org

Printed and bound in Great Britain by
TJInternational Ltd, Padstow, Cornwall

# CONTENTS

# CONTRIBUTORS

**H. Andersson**
Örebro University, Swedish Football Association

**C. Argus**
Australian Institute of Sport

**J. Bangsbo**
University of Copenhagen

**C. Boyd**
Manchester Metropolitan University

**D. Burgess**
Liverpool Football Club

**C. Carling**
University of Central Lancashire and Lille Football Club

**M. Coelho e Silva**
University of Ghent

**M. Court**
Manchester United Football Club

**C. Cushion**
Loughborough University

**B. Drust**
Liverpool John Moores University

**A.J. Figueiredo**
University of Coimbra

**P.R. Ford**
Liverpool John Moores University

**V. Goosey-Tolfrey**
Loughborough University

**W. Gregson**
Liverpool John Moores University

**S. Halson**
Australian Institute of Sport

**C. Harwood**
Loughborough University

**W. Helsen**
University of Leuven

**F.M. Iaia**
Manchester United Football Club

**P. Krustrup**
University of Exeter

**A. Lees**
Liverpool John Moores University

**M. Littlewood**
Liverpool John Moores University

**D. MacLaren**
Liverpool John Moores University

**R.M. Malina**
Templeton State University

**J. Morton**
Liverpool John Moores University

**I. Mujika**
University of Bilbao

**M. Nesti**
Liverpool John Moores University

**M. Pain**
Loughborough University

**R.M. Philippaerts**
University of Ghent

**H. Relvas**
Liverpool John Moores University

**D. Richardson**
Liverpool John Moores University

**D. Scott**
United States Soccer Federation

**A.J. Strudwick**
Manchester United Football Club

**R. Vaeyens**
University of Ghent

**C. Visscher**
University of Groningen

**M. Weston**
University of Teesside

**A.M. Williams**
Brunel University

# PREFACE

Soccer remains the world's most popular form of sport and an integral part of the social and cultural fabric of society in many countries. In recent decades, there has been a remarkable expansion of sports science both as an academic discipline and as a field of applied practice. A number of institutions across the globe now deliver formal academic programmes of study specifically related to soccer. Such academic programmes are supported by increasingly productive research groups, who help to update relevant knowledge of how performance can be improved in soccer, as well as how the sport can impact on society more broadly. In the applied field, many professional clubs and national associations now routinely employ support teams involving practitioners from the various sub-disciplines of sports science including physiology, psychology, biomechanics, performance analysis, sociology and coaching science. The historical development of sports science and its relationship with soccer were documented in the introduction to a previous edition of this book a decade ago (see Reilly and Williams, 2003); in the intervening years this association has continued to thrive, with existing links being consolidated and new and innovative partnerships cultivated.

The third edition of this book presents another step in the process of updating knowledge and reflecting on how improved scientific understanding can translate into a meaningful impact in soccer. The content of the book remains multi-disciplinary in scope, although the overall focus has narrowed somewhat to concentrate more specifically on how science can help to develop elite performers in the sport. This more focused approach reflects the fact that the field has grown markedly since publication of the last edition, and consequently, some attempt at delineating the scope of the book was deemed essential in order to convey sufficient depth and clarity in regard to the topics presented. The narrower focus on expert performance reflects a growing awareness in the academic (Farrow, Baker and MacMahon, 2009; Hodges and Williams, 2012; Kaufman, 2012) and popular literature (Coyle, 2009; Gladwell, 2008; Sayed, 2009) of factors that influence the development of expertise in many domains of human activity. The focus on performance is not intended to underestimate the broader impact that the sport can have on culture and society through, for example, its role in facilitating improvements in health and well-being.

The book is divided into six parts. The focus in the first part is on the biological sciences. MacLaren and Morton discuss the nutritional requirements of elite soccer players and how these differ before, during and after training and match-play. In the following chapter, Bangsbo and Iaia outline some of the key considerations when ensuring that players are optimally prepared physically for performance. These authors outline different training activities that may be used to improve aerobic and anaerobic fitness, as well as specific muscle function, at various stages in the season. The next chapter, by Drust and Gregson, provides a complementary overview of how the different components of fitness may be measured using standard field- and laboratory-based measures. Some guidelines are presented as to when during the season such tests should be employed. Mujika, Halson, Argus and Krustrup then review methods that may help players to recover following training and matches. A number of passive and active recovery strategies are presented, with no strong evidence to support use of one approach over another. In the final chapter in this part, Gregson and Drust discuss how environmental stressors, including temperature, altitude and variations in circadian rhythms, impact upon performance in soccer.

In the second part, the focus shifts to the behavioural and social sciences. Williams and Ford identify the skills, processes and mechanisms underpinning the superior ability of elite players to 'read the game'. The key components of anticipation and decision making are highlighted and implications for applied practice are discussed. Ford and Williams then consider the factors that influence effective learning and raise the possibility of a theory–practice divide by comparing existing coaching behaviours with empirical work from the skill-acquisition literature. Next, Richardson, Relvas and Littlewood consider some of the social and cultural factors that impact on elite player development and progression, such as the relative age effect, place of birth, player migration patterns and the important transition period between youth and senior professional level. Finally, Pain and Harwood review contemporary research focusing on stress, coping and other mental attributes such as resilience and toughness. The authors conclude with some suggestions as to how sport psychologists, parents and coaches can help to provide an appropriate support network.

In the third part, the focus shifts towards performance analysis, biomechanics and coaching. Carling and Court review the methods available for undertaking match and motion analysis. A review is provided of key performance indicators in soccer, and contemporary empirical work focusing on the tactical, strategic and physical components of elite performance is highlighted. Next, Cushion reviews contemporary research from the coaching sciences and discusses its application. He highlights empirical work on coach behaviours and discusses the potential implications of this work for coaching and coach education. The role of biomechanics in developing elite performers is reviewed in the chapter by Lees. The author provides an overview of methods available for analysing soccer skills such as kicking, the throw-in and goalkeeping. He illustrates how biomechanical measurement techniques provide objective methods for quantifying and improving the performance of elite players in soccer.

A cross-disciplinary emphasis is adopted in Part IV, which provides an overview of research on different population groups in soccer. The vast majority of researchers have focused on elite male soccer players and, unfortunately, there is far less published work involving alternative population groups. Scott and Andersson outline the physical demands of the women's game and discuss the implications for training, as well as the nutritional requirements of elite female players. Boyd and Goosey-Tolfrey then consider the demands placed upon soccer players with cerebral palsy and those with visual impairments. These authors outline some of the assessments they have undertaken with these players and present a case study of their work with the England Cerebral Palsy team at the 2007 World Championships. Weston and Helsen consider the specific demands of match officials, who clearly can have a significant influence on the outcome of matches involving elite players. The authors consider the physical and perceptual–cognitive demands of officiating in soccer and present implications for the preparation and development of elite referees and assistant referees. A common theme emerging from chapters in this part is the need for more systematic programmes of work with these and other populations so that each group's specific training and development needs can be met.

In the next part, two chapters are presented on the theme of talent identification and development. Vaeyens, Coelho e Silva, Visscher, Philippaerts and Williams consider some of the practical and conceptual issues underpinning the early identification of young players. The authors argue the need for cross-disciplinary and longitudinal approaches to examine how elite players are best identified and developed. Malina, Coelho e Silva and Figueiredo highlight how issues related to growth and maturity impact on performance and whether players may be included or excluded from elite development programmes. The authors conclude with some implications for current practice.

In the final part, the aim is to illustrate more explicitly how some of the principles of science presented in the earlier sections of the book are currently being applied in professional clubs. Strudwick illustrates how science underpins his work with professional players at the highest level of the game, with a particular focus on the physical conditioning and preparation of players. He highlights some of the challenges involved when working at the elite level, as well as how science can have a positive impact on the preparation and development of players. Next, Nesti draws on his experiences working as a sport psychologist at several clubs in the Premier League in England. He uses vignettes to illustrate some of the challenges faced by players in dealing with the mental demands of the game and considers how the psychological needs of players should be addressed. Finally, Burgess and Drust reflect upon their experiences of developing a physiologically based sports science support strategy in the professional game. The authors highlight key areas for consideration through the use of a detailed, case-study approach. These final chapters nicely illustrate the translational impact of sports science at the very highest level of the game.

In closing, I would like to acknowledge the sad passing of the editor of the original edition of this book, as well as my co-editor on the last edition. Professor Thomas Reilly passed away after a long and brave battle with cancer, in June 2009. His visionary leadership of this field and the phenomenal body of published scientific work that he leaves behind will continue to have a significant impact for many generations to come. He inspired many people and paved the way for future generations of scientists and practitioners interested in promoting greater understanding and application of science in soccer. We will forever be in his debt.

A.M. Williams
Brunel University

**REFERENCES**

Coyle, D. (2009). *The Talent Code*. New York: Bantam.
Farrow, D., Baker, J. and MacMahon, C. (2009). *Developing Elite Sports Performers: Lessons from Theory and Practice*. London: Routledge.

Gladwell, M. (2008). *Outliers*. London: Allen Lane.

Hodges, N.J., and Williams, A.M. (2012). *Skill Acquisition in Sport: Research, Theory and Practice* (2nd edn). London: Routledge.

Kaufman, S.B. (ed.) (2012). *Beyond 'Talent or Practice?': The Complexity of Greatness*. New York: Oxford University Press.

Reilly, T., and Williams, A.M. (eds) (2003). *Science and Soccer* (2nd edn). London: Routledge.

Sayed, M. (2009). *Bounce*. New York: HarperCollins.

# PART I
# BIOLOGICAL SCIENCES

# CHAPTER 1

## NUTRITION

D. MacLaren and J. Morton

### INTRODUCTION

Soccer consists of an intermittent activity profile, incorporating periods of intense exercise interspersed with lower levels of activity over 90 min. The estimated energy requirements for a game involving both casual recreational and top-class professional players are between 21 and 73 kJ min$^{-1}$ (5–17 kcal min$^{-1}$). For a 70-kg player, the result could be the loss of approximately 100–200 g of carbohydrate. Since the body's stores of carbohydrate are limited (approximately 300–400 g), this loss is significant. If muscle stores of carbohydrate are not adequately replenished, subsequent performance will be impaired. The carbohydrate intake of elite soccer players is often inadequate and so the concentration of carbohydrate in active muscle may become low.

The energy demands of soccer are such that there is likely to be a significant production of heat within the body. Even in cold conditions, considerable amounts of sweat are lost in an attempt to dissipate this heat, thereby resulting in a degree of dehydration. A mild degree of dehydration impairs skilled performance and affects strength, stamina and speed and thus, an adequate fluid intake is necessary to offset the effects of dehydration.

Although the major causes of fatigue for soccer players are the depletion of muscle and liver glycogen stores as well as dehydration, players should be aware that muscle is composed of protein and water, and that following training there is the need to recover muscle structure by stimulating protein synthesis (which is diminished during the exercise bout). Furthermore, players are forever looking for nutritional supplements to help improve their performance and aid recovery. Supplements which are relevant to soccer players include caffeine, creatine and β-alanine.

In this chapter the nutritional requirements of soccer players are considered in terms of carbohydrates, fluid intake and protein. In addition, reference will be made to selected ergogenic aids. Where possible, references are made to research in soccer and recommendations are stated for use before, during and after training or competition. The reader is directed elsewhere for a more complete understanding of the basic biochemistry of sport and metabolism (see MacLaren and Morton 2011).

## CARBOHYDRATE REQUIREMENTS

Carbohydrates (CHO) are the main energy source for moderate to high-intensity exercise and are therefore the most important energy source for soccer match play and training. The CHO intake for soccer players should vary according to the specific training and competitive goals of that particular day. Based on this premise of a *periodised* approach to CHO intake, an overview of recommended daily CHO intake within a typical week of the soccer player's training and match schedule is shown in Table 1.1. The scientific rationale underpinning these recommendations is discussed in the following sections. It should be noted that these guidelines may be further modified according to individual players' training and competition goals as well as their preferred food choices.

Table 1.1 Summary of suggested CHO intake for soccer players according to specific time-points of the weekly training and playing schedule. Recommended intakes are expressed as $g.kg^{-1}$ of the athlete's body mass. HGI, high glycemic index; LGI, low glycemic index.

| Specific situation | Suggested CHO intake | Additional comments |
|---|---|---|
| Day before game | 6–10 $g.kg^{-1}$ | HGI CHO foods and drinks to augment glycogen stores for competition on the following day. |
| Breakfast on match day | 1–3 $g.kg^{-1}$ | LGI CHO foods and drinks consumed. For a 3 pm kick-off, this meal should be consumed between 8 and 9 am. |
| Pre-match meal | 1–3 $g.kg^{-1}$ | LGI CHO foods and drinks consumed. This meal should be consumed 3–4 h prior to kick-off. For mid-day kick-offs, this meal would effectively be breakfast. |
| During match | 30–60 $g.h^{-1}$ | HGI CHO in the form of 6% CHO drinks or sports gels. Players could take advantages of breaks in play to consume small but regular CHO intake to avoid gut discomfort. Additionally, the half-time break should be used for refuelling according to the player's preferred approach. Players should practise fuelling strategies during training in order to develop individually suited strategies. |
| Post-match | 1.2 $g.kg^{-1} h^{-1}$ | HGI CHO foods and drinks consumed for several hours post-match so as to promote glycogen re-synthesis. |
| Day after game | 6–10 $g.kg^{-1}$ | HGI CHO foods and drinks consumed so as to promote glycogen re-synthesis. |
| General training day | 4–6 $g.kg^{-1}$ | Combination of LGI and HGI CHO foods and drinks consumed to ensure adequate CHO availability for training and recovery purposes, depending on the specific energy demands of the particular training day as well as individual training goals. For players wishing to lose body fat, <4 $g.kg^{-1}$ would prove beneficial (in conjunction with increased protein intake e.g. 2 $g.kg^{-1}$) and LGI choices should be emphasised. |

4

## Muscle glycogen utilisation

The importance of muscle glycogen availability for soccer performance was recognised as early as the 1970s. Saltin (1973) examined the effects of commencing a soccer game with normal or low glycogen stores on players' subsequent activity profiles and distances covered. The distance covered during the second half was observed to be higher for the normal versus low glycogen store (5.9 vs. 4.1 km, respectively). In the low condition, glycogen was nearly depleted at half time (Figure 1.1) and significantly more time was spent walking (50 vs. 27%) and less time spent sprinting (15 vs. 24%), as compared with the normal condition. Since this initial observation, a number of other researchers have confirmed the presence of significant glycogen depletion during soccer match play (Jacobs et al. 1982) or simulated game activity (Nicholas et al. 1999; Foskett et al. 2008).

The most informative investigation examining muscle glycogen utilisation in soccer was from Krustrup et al. (2006). These authors observed that muscle glycogen over the course of 3 friendly games was $449 \pm 23$ mmol.kg$^{-1}$ dw at the start and decreased to $225 \pm 23$ mmol.kg$^{-1}$ dw immediately after the match (Figure 1.2). These observations highlight that certain players started the game with what would be considered sub-optimal muscle glycogen availability (likely due to inappropriate dietary practices in the days leading up to competition). Although post-game glycogen values in whole muscle suggest sufficient glycogen available to continue exercising, analysis of individual muscle fibre types revealed that 50% of fibres could be classified as *empty* or *almost empty* (see Figure 1.3). This pattern of depletion or near

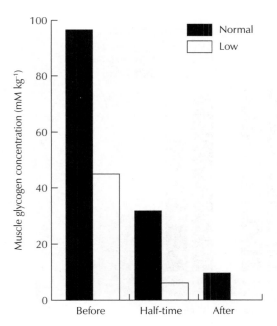

**Figure 1.1** Muscle glycogen utilisation during a soccer game when commenced with either normal or low muscle glycogen stores.

*Source*: Data taken from Saltin (1973).

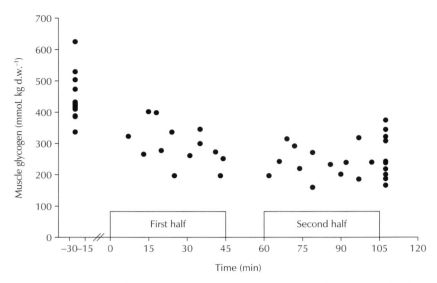

**Figure 1.2** Muscle glycogen at rest and at various stages throughout the first and second half of a 90-min soccer match as well as immediately after the game. Each dot represents individual values.

*Source*: Adapted from Krustrup *et al.* (2006: fig. 1).

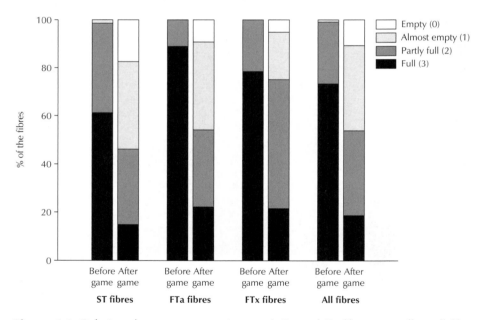

**Figure 1.3** Relative glycogen content in type I, IIa and IIx fibres as well as all fibres before and after a soccer game.

*Source*: Adapted from Krustrup *et al.* (2006: fig. 2).

depletion was evident in type IIa and IIx fibres, the fibres responsible for sprinting and high-intensity activity. The finding of glycogen depletion in these muscle fibres is likely a contributing factor underpinning the progressive decline in the amount of high-intensity running and sprinting that occurs throughout the course of a game (Mohr et al. 2003). These findings highlight the potential role of muscle glycogen depletion as a key factor contributing to nutritional-related causes of soccer-specific fatigue.

## Importance of CHO loading the day(s) before the game

It is apparent that one of the main nutritional goals for soccer players is to ensure that they commence the game with elevated muscle glycogen stores. The classic super-compensation approach to CHO loading is not applicable to professional soccer players, owing to the requirement of continual daily training as well as often playing 3 games within 7–8 days. Fortunately, more moderate super-compensation protocols were later developed which essentially focused on a reduction in training volume and a concomitant increase in CHO intake in the days leading up to competition. It is now recognised that trained athletes can CHO load and achieve high glycogen levels with as little as 1 day of a CHO rich diet and no activity (Bussau et al. 2002).

Soccer players are recommended to consume a diet high in CHO for 1–2 days before competition and certainly in the day preceding a match (see Table 1.1). In order to maximise glycogen synthesis, it is appropriate to consume high glycaemic index (HGI) as opposed to low glycaemic index (LGI) foods. A more detailed exposé on the Glycaemic Index (GI) can be seen in MacLaren and Close (2009). Burke et al. (1993) observed that glycogen synthesis over a 24-h period is approximately 50% greater when HGI as opposed to LGI carbohydrates are consumed. Such a nutritional approach coupled with the reduced energy demands associated with training the day before the game (where coaches often schedule more tactical-related training sessions) should optimise muscle glycogen availability. This approach to CHO loading has been shown to increase exercise capacity during intermittent running (Bangsbo et al. 1992). It is noteworthy that many soccer players often do not appreciate the importance of adequately fuelling up in the days prior to competition and are more concerned with the evening meal the night prior to the game or the pre-match meal per se. For this reason, it is important to educate players and coaches on the importance of nutrition for the day preceding competition.

## Pre-match meals

Nutritional strategies for match day are largely dependent on the location and timing of the match. For example, for a regular 3 pm Saturday kick-off nutritional preparation on match day would consist of a light breakfast and the main pre-match meal consumed around 11.15 am. Alternatively, for an evening kick-off between 7.45 and 8 pm, match day nutrition would be extended and the pre-match meal should be consumed at around 4–4.30 pm. Finally, at the opposite end of the spectrum is the lunch-time kick-off (usually between 12 and 1 pm), and in this situation match day nutrition would be limited, with breakfast effectively serving as the pre-match meal. Regardless of the timing of the game, it is always advised that the pre-match meal be reasonably high in CHO content and consumed 3–4 hours prior to kick off so as to allow sufficient time for digestion and avoid gastrointestinal problems such as nausea and feelings of gut fullness. It is important that the stomach be reasonably empty at the time of commencing the match so that digestion and absorption of food do not compete with the exercising muscles for blood supply. Furthermore, consumption of high fibre and high fat foods (even those associated with protein sources such as red meat and cheese) should be avoided, given that they slow down the rate of gastric emptying.

The interpretation of scientific data on the effects of pre-exercise CHO ingestion on exercise performance is complicated by variations in methodology between studies such as amount, timing and type (i.e. HGI versus LGI) of CHO provided as well as exercise mode (e.g. running or cycling) and choice of performance test (i.e. capacity or performance test). Nevertheless, the general consensus from studies in this area is that pre-exercise CHO provision improves performance or capacity, as compared with commencing exercise in fasted conditions (see Hawley and Burke 1997). However, considering that virtually all players will consume some form of pre-match meal, as opposed to commencing games fasted, it is perhaps more important to consider the effects of quantity and type of CHO consumed in pre-competition meals. In relation to the former, Sherman et al. (1991) observed that time trial performance after 90 min of steady state exercise at 70% $\dot{V}O_{2max}$ was greater when 150 g of CHO was consumed before exercise, as compared with 75 g of CHO, both of which were greater than no meal. The enhanced performance was associated with maintenance of blood glucose concentration late during exercise, which is important because liver glucose production and muscle glucose uptake and oxidation become more important when muscle glycogen concentrations decline. A previous study by the same group also demonstrated that pre-exercise feeding of 312 g CHO consumed at 4 hours pre-exercise was more effective in augmenting exercise capacity, as compared to 156 and 46 g (Sherman et al. 1989). In the case of the soccer player, such high intakes of CHO with the pre-match meal may not be practical. In our experience of working with professional soccer players, breakfast and pre-match meals on match day usually range between 100 and 250 g CHO (1.5–3 g.kg$^{-1}$ body weight) and, as such, augmenting CHO intake beyond players' habitual intake may lead to gastrointestinal problems. Furthermore, assuming that players have glycogen loaded appropriately in the day(s) preceding competition, augmenting CHO availability in the pre-match meals to such high levels may not be warranted.

The effect of the GI of the pre-exercise meal on metabolic responses during exercise and subsequent performance is a hot topic for sports nutrition researchers (Donaldson et al. 2010). Findings suggest that LGI CHO feeding in the hours prior to exercise confers a metabolic advantage over HGI by inducing a smaller insulin response in the postprandial period. In this way, there is an increased free fatty acid (FFA) availability and lipid oxidation during exercise, coupled with a more stable plasma glucose concentration. The result of these metabolic changes could be a sparing of muscle glycogen utilisation during exercise, which of course would be advantageous for the soccer player, given the link between glycogen availability and fatigue. In this regard, Wee et al. (2005) observed that provision of an HGI breakfast of 2.5 g CHO.kg$^{-1}$ body mass 3 hours before a 30 min run at 70% $\dot{V}O_{2max}$ attenuated fatty acid availability during exercise and increased CHO oxidation, whereas an LGI meal favoured lipid oxidation. Additionally, glucose concentration during exercise was more stable during exercise with the LGI meal.

# 8

More recently, researchers (Little *et al.* 2009, 2010) investigated the effects of the GI of the pre-match meal during soccer-specific exercise. No effect of GI on substrate oxidation rates was observed, though both CHO conditions increased performance, as compared with fasted conditions. In reviewing the collective literature concerning the GI of the pre-exercise meal, an important limitation is the lack of experimental trials that have provided CHO intake *during* the exercise protocol itself. Such studies are important, as this is common practice for soccer players during match play. In this regard, Burke *et al.* (1998) observed that consuming CHO during prolonged continuous exercise negates the metabolic effects of altering the GI of the pre-exercise meal. However, it is important to note that soccer players' access to energy intake during games is limited to unscheduled breaks (e.g., breaks in play due to injuries) and half time. For this reason, it is probably more beneficial to emphasise LGI CHO choices at pre-match meals, especially in situations where players have not CHO loaded appropriately and thus glycogen availability may not be optimal. Finally, many players have customary pre-match meals and are often superstitious about their pre-game preparations. For such individuals, it may be beneficial to consume their preferred meal (regardless of whether it is LGI or HGI), though the basic principles of ensuring adequate CHO provision and low fat and fibre should always remain.

## Provision of CHO within 60 min before the game

The intake of CHO should probably be avoided within the 30–60 min period prior to kick-off, owing to the possibility of experiencing *rebound hypoglycaemia* and thus low blood glucose within the first 20 min of exercise. Certain individuals are particularly sensitive to rebound hypoglycaemia and the response can be induced by as little as 20 g of CHO, equivalent to approximately 350 ml of a 6% CHO sports drink. To minimise the risks of hypoglycaemia, it is sufficient to consume CHO within 5–10 min prior to kick off (i.e., in the last stages of the warm-up or in the changing room). When CHO is consumed within this timescale, the exercise-induced (i.e., warm-up) increase in catecholamines is thought to blunt the insulin response and therefore minimise the effect of rebound hypoglycaemia (Jeukendrup and Killer 2010).

## Provision of CHO during the game

In addition to commencing the match with adequate muscle glycogen availability, there is evidence that provision of additional CHO during the game improves performance such as exercise capacity (Nicholas *et al.* 1995; Foskett *et al.* 2008), as well as ability to perform technical skills such as passing and shooting (Ali *et al.* 2007). The mechanisms underpinning enhanced performance with exogenous CHO provision may be due to factors such as prevention of hypoglycaemia, since blood glucose values <3.5 mmol.L$^{-1}$ have been observed during soccer match play (Krustrup *et al.* 2006). The maintenance of high CHO oxidation rates, glycogen sparing, and effects on the central nervous system are important considerations.

Nicholas *et al.* (1999) observed that muscle glycogen utilisation during 90 min of intermittent shuttle running was reduced when CHO was ingested during exercise, especially in type II fibres. The same group later observed that glycogen sparing is not evident when exercise is commenced with elevated pre-exercise glycogen stores, as would be expected following the

CHO loading strategies that soccer players are advised to adopt (Foskett *et al.* 2008). Nevertheless, these authors observed that intermittent running capacity was greater with CHO, as compared with placebo ingestion (158 vs 131 min), despite no differences in mixed muscle glycogen utilisation. The enhanced exercise capacity may have been due to the maintenance of plasma glucose availability and high rates of CHO oxidation required to sustain exercise. The ingestion of CHO during exercise augments plasma glucose availability and maintains its oxidation rates during soccer-specific exercise (Clarke *et al.* 2008).

In relation to the quantity of CHO that should be consumed during exercise, researchers have shown that peak glucose oxidation rates from exogenous sources are approximately 1 g.min$^{-1}$ and thus an intake of 30–60 g per hour has been advised (Jeukedrup 2010). Players would be required to consume 500–1000 ml per hour of conventional 6% CHO sports drinks, though given the restricted access to fluid intake during soccer this intake is unlikely. Given that there are no differences between exogenous CHO oxidation rates when provided in the form of liquid or sports gels (Pfeiffer *et al.* 2010), it may be prudent to provide access to both energy sources during exercise and at half time so as to cater for individual players' preferences and promote CHO intake. The provision of gels would be especially applicable to those players who prefer water for hydration purposes, as opposed to sports drinks. Soccer players should experiment with different strategies during training so as to devise individualised approaches for match play that maximise performance and minimise gut discomfort. In relation to the latter, we have shown that provision of 6% CHO drinks in repeated small amounts at 15-min intervals reduces sensations of gut fullness, as compared with ingesting an equivalent total volume of fluid and CHO when administered as two larger boluses pre-game and at half time (Clarke *et al.* 2008).

Jeukedrup and colleagues (2010) reported that adding fructose to glucose can enhance exogenous CHO rates to >1.5 g.min$^{-1}$. However, such feeding strategies are more appropriate for prolonged endurance exercise, as opposed to soccer, given the duration and intermittent activity profile of the game and also that saturation of gut glucose transporters would be unlikely. There is also growing evidence that *mouth rinsing* with CHO beverages can improve performance, likely through the central nervous system via receptors in the mouth and oral space (Jeukendrup and Chambers 2010). However, the performance-enhancing effects of mouth rinsing are not apparent when a pre-exercise meal is ingested (Rollo and Williams 2010), and so whether this approach offers any advantage to the soccer player who consumes a pre-match meal requires further research.

### Post-match muscle glycogen re-synthesis

The major goal for carbohydrate intake after competition is to replenish both muscle and liver glycogen stores. This factor is especially important in those instances where there is a further fixture in the coming days; such is the case for top players, who routinely play midweek European Champions league games 3–4 days after their domestic league game. If carbohydrate intake is not sufficient during this time, then muscle glycogen levels are unlikely to be fully restored. To maximise rates of muscle glycogen re-synthesis, it is crucial that CHO intake is consumed within minutes of the game ending, as this is the time when the glycogen-synthesising enzymes are most active. Delaying CHO intake until 2 hours post-exercise, as

10

opposed to consuming within the first 2 hours post-exercise can reduce the absolute amount of glycogen re-synthesised by 50% over a 4-hour period (Ivy et al. 1988). It is important that the CHO consumed in the first few hours is HGI and in fact, consuming HGI over a 24-hour period post-exercise induces greater muscle glycogen re-synthesis, as compared to LGI (Burke et al. 1993). In terms of quantities of CHO intake, it is generally advised (Jentjens and Jeukendrup 2003) that muscle glycogen re-synthesis plateaus at intakes corresponding to 1.2 $g.kg^{-1}$ body mass per hour. A 75-kg player would therefore be advised to consume 90 g of CHO per hour in the few hours after the game ends. Whether or not the CHO is provided in solid or liquid form is immaterial and should be left to the player's preference. In practice, therefore, a selection of high CHO snacks and drinks should be readily available in the changing room post-game (see Table 1.1). Additionally, these meals should contain moderate protein intake so as to support post-exercise protein synthesis. In those instances where CHO availability is less than 1.2 $g.kg^{-1}$, the addition of small amounts of protein (e.g. 20 g) can accentuate glycogen re-synthesis (Betts and Williams 2010).

It is noteworthy that addition of creatine to CHO feeding in the days after glycogen-depleting exercise has been shown to augment glycogen levels (Robinson et al. 1999). This approach to post-game feeding may be particularly applicable during times of intense fixture schedules. Finally, in situations where muscle damage has occurred, due to lengthening contractions, muscle glycogen re-synthesis can be impaired even when high CHO intakes are consumed (Costill et al. 1990). For those players who experience regular symptoms of muscle damage post-game, consuming additional macronutrients (e.g., protein) and micronutrients (e.g., antioxidants) in an attempt to reduce the severity of muscle damage may prove beneficial. In addition to muscle glycogen re-synthesis, it is important to incorporate strategies which promote restoration of liver glycogen. For this purpose, fructose is more effective than glucose (Decombaz et al. 2011) and thus, the provision of fructose-rich foods (e.g. fresh fruit juice) in the changing room after the match is recommended.

## CHO requirements for training

Traditional guidelines for athletes during training often focus on ensuring a high daily CHO intake that entails 60–70% of the athlete's daily energy intake. However, the terminology used to describe daily CHO requirements is now changing and Burke et al. (2011) suggest that describing a high CHO diet as a *percentage* of energy intake is a nebulous term that is poorly correlated to the actual amount of CHO consumed and the fuel requirements of the athlete's training and competition demands. These authors suggest that it is more appropriate to discuss CHO requirements in terms of the *availability* required to meet the actual energy demands associated with the training and competition schedule. Such an approach makes practical sense for the soccer player, given that the energy requirements vary according to the daily, weekly and monthly training goals and fixture schedules. In contrast to a *one size fits all* approach, it is advised that CHO intake is specific to the individual player's needs. Nevertheless, given the duration and intensity of a typical soccer training session, it can be estimated that a daily intake of 4–6 $g.kg^{-1}$ body mass is sufficient to ensure adequate CHO availability for training and recovery purposes. For those days other than pre-game CHO loading and post-game recovery, where HGI choices should be emphasised, consuming the majority of CHO as LGI sources would prove beneficial for helping to promote lipid oxidation and maintain low body fat levels (Morton *et al.* 2010).

There is a growing body of literature suggesting that *deliberately* commencing training sessions with *reduced* CHO availability provides an enhanced stimulus to induce oxidative adaptations of skeletal muscle. This approach to training has become known as the *train-low:compete-high* model, surmising that carefully selected training sessions be performed with low CHO availability but that competition is always commenced with high CHO availability. In a recent study in our laboratory, we observed that commencing 50% of training sessions with reduced muscle glycogen stores enhanced oxidative enzyme activity of both the gastrocnemius and vastus lateralis muscles (Morton *et al.* 2009). However, consuming additional CHO in the form of 6% sports drinks offset this enhanced adaptation, despite the reduced muscle glycogen prior to training. Clearly, both endogenous (i.e., glycogen) and exogenous (i.e., blood glucose) CHO availability can modulate the molecular signalling pathways that mediate mitochondrial biogenesis (see Hawley and Burke 2010). It is possible that deliberately restricting CHO availability during certain periods of the week may provide an enhanced training stimulus for the soccer player, though further research is warranted. There may be certain side-effects associated with this approach, such as impaired training intensity (Yeo *et al.* 2008), loss of lean mass (Howarth *et al.* 2010) and reduced immune function (Gleeson 2007). Soccer players should therefore work closely with sports nutrition professionals before implementing this approach. It is of course important to ensure that high CHO intakes are consumed in the day(s) prior to and after games so as to support glycogen loading and re-synthesis, respectively. A potential strategy to incorporate the train-low:compete-high model into practice would be to reduce the CHO intake on training days to <4 g.kg$^{-1}$ (but to ensure loading takes place on the pre-match and match days). The train-low:compete-high approach to training would be particularly applicable for those players simultaneously aiming to lose body fat, owing to the role of CHO intake in regulating lipid metabolism (Morton *et al.* 2010), but maximise match day performance. On those days where low CHO availability is implemented, it is important to increase protein intake (e.g., 2 g.kg$^{-1}$) so as to minimise protein oxidation and loss of lean mass, as well as to promote training-induced increases in protein synthesis.

## FLUID REQUIREMENTS

Given the intense energy demands of soccer match play, metabolic heat production can increase rectal and muscle temperature to >39°C (Mohr *et al.* 2004). The main biological mechanism for losing heat during exercise is through evaporation of sweat. Sweat losses of 2 L have been observed during both match play and training (Maughan *et al.* 2007), even when ambient temperature is <10°C. For a 75-kg player, this sweat loss equates to >2% dehydration and, if appropriate fluid intake is not consumed, performance can be impaired. Dehydration of this magnitude has been shown to reduce repeated sprint capacity (Mohr *et al.* 2010) as well as soccer dribbling performance (McGregor *et al.* 1999). For more comprehensive discussions on the effects of dehydration on performance, the reader is directed to Judelson *et al.* (2007). Potential mechanisms underpinning dehydration-induced decrements in physical and mental performance include increased core temperature, cardiovascular strain, muscle glycogen utilisation and impaired brain function (Gonzalez-Alonso 2007).

12

From observations of players during training and match play, sweat loss and dehydration appear to be lower in temperate (<10°C) as compared with warm environments (25–35°C) (Kurdak et al. 2010). To compensate for the warmer conditions, however, players voluntarily consume significantly more fluid during training. The development of fatigue during match play is more pronounced during high ambient temperatures (Mohr et al. 2010). Regardless of ambient temperature, players routinely drink less than they sweat during both training and match play (Kurdak et al. 2010; Maughan et al. 2007; Mohr et al. 2010), a finding that has been termed *involuntary dehydration*. In addition to fluid loss per se, sweat contains electrolytes such as sodium, chloride, potassium, calcium and magnesium. Loss of sodium is the most significant for athletes, and soccer players can lose between 2 and 13 g during training or match play (Kurdak et al. 2010; Maughan et al. 2007). The importance of high salt loses is underscored by observations linking them to exercise-related muscle cramps (Bergeron 2003) and, for this reason, it is important to identify players who are *salty sweaters*, so as to develop individually tailored hydration strategies.

It is difficult to provide fixed prescriptive fluid recommendations for soccer players, due to player differences in workload, heat acclimatisation, training status and match-to-match variations in ambient temperatures. Nevertheless, in order to offset the negative effects of dehydration on performance, the American College of Sports Medicine advises fluid ingestion at a rate that limits body-mass loss to <2% of pre-exercise values (Sawka et al. 2007). Players should not, however, aim to drink so as to gain mass during exercise, as this can lead to water intoxification, a condition known as hyponatremia (a serum sodium concentration <135 mmol.L$^{-1}$), which in extreme cases is fatal (Almond et al. 2005). In developing individualised hydration strategies, it is important to perform *regular* estimations of pre-exercise hydration status in order to identify those players who may need particular attention. Within the field setting of training grounds or on match days, assessment of pre-exercise urine osmolality and colour provides reasonably inexpensive and informative measures. Osmolality values <700 mOsmol.kg$^{-1}$ are suggestive of euhydration, as is a urine colour that is pale yellow.

Urine indices of hydration are sensitive to changes in posture, food intake and body water content and, for these reasons, a urine sample passed upon waking is often advised as the criterion sample. However, values indicative of dehydration at this time (e.g., 7 am) may not mean that the player is dehydrated upon commencing training at 10:30 am, assuming that appropriate fluid intake has been consumed upon waking and with breakfast. The same can be said for match day, in that samples suggestive of dehydration collected prior to the pre-match meal may not mean players are dehydrated at kick-off. Where practical, players should therefore be assessed at both the former and latter time points so as to initially identify players who are causes for concern and to verify that any subsequent hydration strategies implemented are effective to ensure euhydration prior to competition. Soccer players studied prior to an evening kick-off have exhibited pre-game osmolality values >900 mOsmol.kg$^{-1}$ (Maughan et al. 2007), despite the fact that they would have had the morning and afternoon to hydrate. Such values are indicative of 2% dehydration and effectively mean that players are commencing the game dehydrated, thereby running the risk of impaired physical and mental performance.

It is recommended that 5–7 ml.kg$^{-1}$ of fluid is consumed at least 4 hours prior to the game (Sawka et al. 2007). Additionally, if the individual does not produce urine or the urine remains dark coloured, a further 3–5 ml.kg–[1] could be consumed about 2 hours before kick-off. Drinking within this time schedule should allow for fluid absorption and enable urine output to return to normal levels. Consumption of sports drinks at this time, as opposed to water, is beneficial, given that they contain not only electrolytes but also additional CHO. For training days, fluid intake should be consumed upon waking (before travelling to training) and with breakfast, which soccer players usually consume at the training ground.

In order to promote a drinking strategy which prevents weight losses >2%, players should routinely weigh themselves nude before and after exercise to ascertain if their habitual drinking patterns are effective. Players should have individually labelled drinks bottles so that support staff can monitor habitual fluid intake, and furthermore, any urine passed during exercise should be accounted for when calculating sweat loss. Cold beverages (10°C as opposed to 37 or 50°C) are beneficial to attenuate the rise in body temperature during exercise (Lee and Shirreffs 2007), and sports drinks are considered superior than water, due to the provision of electrolytes and CHO. Sports drinks should be in the range of 4–8% CHO (administered as glucose polymers), as both high CHO concentration and osmolality can delay gastric emptying (Vist and Maughan 1995). It is important that players practise with different fluid intake strategies during training so as to develop individually suited approaches that maximise gastric emptying, fluid absorption and CHO delivery, and yet are suited for taste and do not cause gastrointenstinal discomfort during match play.

On training days (as opposed to match days), players may wish to consume water or low-calorie sports drinks only, given that CHO ingestion during exercise may attenuate skeletal muscle adaptations to training (Morton et al. 2009). This factor is especially applicable to those players who are adhering to the train-low:compete-high model. Finally, there is no need for aggressive rehydration strategies post-training or match play, as the normal schedule would allow for appropriate rehydration within several hours post-exercise. Nevertheless, those players identified as salty sweaters may benefit from the addition of sodium to drinks or foods or the provision of salty snacks, so as to promote fluid retention.

## PROTEIN REQUIREMENTS

A consequence of exercise is that muscle protein breakdown occurs and protein synthesis is reduced (Beelen et al. 2010). In the recovery period following such exercise, these processes are reversed – hence the importance of appropriate recovery between training sessions. Since muscle protein breakdown results in loss of muscle tissue, it is important to determine whether this process can be slowed or even reversed by appropriate nutritional strategies. An indicator of the protein requirements of the body is that of nitrogen balance. Nitrogen balance is a measure of whether the body is gaining or losing protein. The body is in nitrogen balance when the amount of protein taken in the food eaten is equal to that lost in faeces, urine and sweat. A positive nitrogen balance infers that more protein is ingested than is lost, whereas a negative nitrogen balance occurs when more is lost than taken in the diet. It is on this basis that various government agencies and the World Health Organisation make their recommendations for protein intake based on gender, age and activity. Current recommendations are that sedentary adults should consume around 0.8g.kg–[1] body mass per day of protein in order to achieve nitrogen balance, whereas athletes engaged in resistance training should take about 2.0 g.kg–[1]

14

body mass per day, and endurance trained athletes around 1.5 to 1.8 g.kg–1 per day (Lemon 1995). This enhanced protein requirement arises because the turnover is greater when exercise is undertaken, especially resistance exercise.

In order to achieve a protein intake of 2 g.kg–1 per day for an 80-kg player, ingestion of 160 g of protein is required. Since most meat and fish (good sources of protein) on average contain about 25 g of protein per 100 g, the player would need to eat around 500 g (this could be 5 chicken breasts!!). There are, of course, other sources of protein which can be consumed, such as eggs, milk, yoghurt, nuts, beans etc. Athletes often wish to know if they should take more protein than is recommended (i.e., is more better). In answer to the question, findings have been equivocal. However, based on consensual findings, it would be prudent to consider 1.5 to 2.0 g.kg body mass per day for soccer players, depending on the severity of the training programme.

The data presented in Figure 1.4 show why athletes need to ingest more protein during times of intense training. These data demonstrate that additional protein intake in the period before and during a training programme could prevent negative nitrogen balance until the body adapts to the training regime (which may take up to 2 weeks). After this period the protein intake may be lowered. In this study, where participants consumed 1g.kg–1 body mass per day of protein, followed by a period of training, they went into negative nitrogen balance for a period of around 14 days before becoming 'balanced'. This finding clearly highlights the need for a greater protein intake in order to achieve nitrogen balance when engaged in exercise,

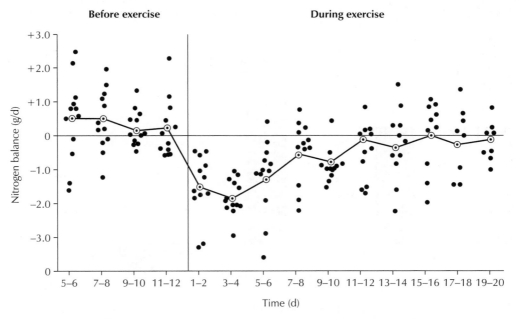

**Figure 1.4** Effect of endurance training regimen on nitrogen balance when ingesting 1g.kg body mass of protein a day.

*Source*: After Gontzea *et al*. (1974).

but also that the body does in time adapt to the training. In other words, there is a substantial net protein breakdown, as compared with protein synthesis, in the early stages of a training intervention when insufficient protein is provided. However, the stimulus of exercise in evoking greater protein synthesis (probably via increases in DNA transcription and translation into new structural proteins) takes some time before nitrogen balance is reached. Imagine that this happens during pre-season training when players arrive after a 6-week holiday period. Under such circumstances it may be advisable for such players to consider increasing their protein intake (at least for the first 2 weeks or so) to around 2 to 2.5 g.kg$^{-1}$ per day (Forslund *et al.* 1999).

## Importance of protein intake before and after training

The relationship between protein synthesis, protein breakdown and net protein balance is illustrated in Figure 1.5. After an overnight (i.e., 12-hour) fast, there is net overall protein loss from muscle (note the 'balance' is negative – greater breakdown than synthesis). Following resistance exercise after the overnight fast, there is an even greater net loss of protein. This effect would happen if a player failed to eat some protein for breakfast before morning training. Clearly, this is not desirable, and so players are strongly encouraged to eat or drink some form of protein for breakfast. Foods such as yoghurt, milk, eggs and cold meats (e.g., ham, smoked salmon, sardines etc.) are recommended.

Recently, researchers have shown that a number of dietary factors can attenuate the breakdown of muscle protein following exercise and promote protein synthesis. These include

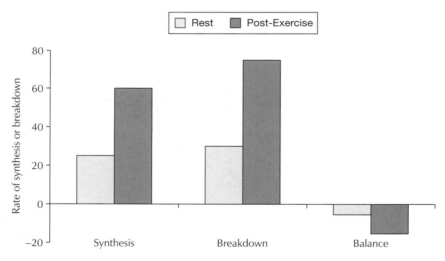

**Figure 1.5** Rates of protein synthesis, breakdown and net protein balance at rest (after an overnight fast) and 4 hours after resistance exercise. Note that there is no net recovery of protein within this 4-hour time period.

*Source*: Adapted from Phillips *et al.* (1999).

**D. MacLaren and J. Morton**

(a) ingestion of carbohydrates and either protein or amino acids before exercise; (b) ingestion of carbohydrates during exercise; and (c) ingestion of carbohydrates and protein or amino acids after exercise. For more detail see MacLaren (2008).

For protein synthesis to happen, amino acids are required in a muscle cell, where they provide the building blocks for repairing and rebuilding the muscle. In addition, there is a need for an increase in circulating anabolic hormones such as insulin and testosterone. The latter increases as a consequence of exercise (particularly high-intensity bouts), whereas the former increases if carbohydrate and/or amino acids are ingested. So, an increase in blood amino acid levels invariably results in greater uptake into muscles and a stimulation of protein synthesis. In part, some of this stimulation is as a result of elevated insulin levels brought about by some amino acids (called insulinogenic amino acids – because they stimulate the release of insulin) and by carbohydrate ingested. The muscle is most responsive to protein synthesis activation by amino acids immediately after exercise. Researchers have shown that as much as a 25% to 300% greater rate of protein synthesis occurs after training when amino acids and carbohydrate are ingested immediately, as opposed to 2 or 3 hours later (Ivy and Portman 2004). In fact, researchers have repeatedly shown that delaying protein feeding after exercise by 2–3 hours can result in a net loss of protein in the short term (Rasmussen et al. 2000). Furthermore, ingesting essential amino acids an hour before training has been shown to promote net muscle protein balance, as compared with ingestion 1 hour after the training (Tipton et al. 2001).

It has also been reported that the combination of protein and carbohydrate ingestion causes a significantly higher rate of protein synthesis than carbohydrate alone (Beelen et al. 2010). This is to be expected, since the combination not only evokes a higher insulin concentration but also that the availability of the amino acids (not found in carbohydrates) leads to incorporation of the amino acids into protein.

We would recommend that soccer players should ingest 15–20 g of protein (or 6–9 g of essential amino acids) an hour before training or a match and then repeat the amount within an hour of completion of training or a match. It is probably more suitable to drink a protein-based supplement in the hour before training, due to the ease of gastric emptying, whereas consuming protein-containing foods after training is suitable (preferably if easily digested forms such as milk, eggs, yoghurt and white meat, for example). For those players who find it difficult to eat in the hour after a match, a whey protein drink could be provided.

## Type of protein supplements

Protein supplements include whey, soya and casein. The overall quality of the protein in terms of biological value, net protein utilisation rate and chemical score is highest for whey and soya proteins and lowest for casein. In terms of some key amino acids required (i.e., branched chain amino acids and glutamine), soya contains them all, whereas whey protein is somewhat lacking in glutamine. Many trained athletes avoid soya protein because it contains plant hormones called isoflavones, which are purported to have an oestrogenic effect (though this does not mean that lowered testosterone is a consequence). For those athletes who are lactose intolerant, however, soya protein has become the protein supplement of choice, although it should be remembered that whey protein isolate has had almost all its lactose removed and may be considered an alternative source.

A few researchers have reported the beneficial effects of whey protein, as compared with casein, in terms of short-term protein synthesis, since whey protein is easily digested and elevates blood amino acids faster than the slower-digested casein (Boirie *et al.* 1997). Advantages of casein may accrue when ingested before sleep at night, where the slow release may aid recovery whilst sleeping. Tang *et al.* (2009) explored the benefits of whey vs. casein vs. soy proteins at rest and after exercise. The observations were that whey protein resulted in significantly elevated blood and muscle amino acids and an increase in muscle protein synthesis, as compared with casein and soy proteins (Figure 1.6).

We would recommend that taking approximately 15 g of whey proteins (or 6–10 g of essential amino acids) an hour before training or a match, and another dose within an hour after is advisable to help promote protein synthesis and thereby recovery of muscle. However, the choice for a bed-time protein on days of heavy training (or after an evening match) would be 20 g of casein or about 200 g of cottage cheese (which contains around 20 g casein).

## ERGOGENIC AIDS

Nutritional ergogenic aids are supplements that a player would consider ingesting in order to help improve performance or capacity. There is a plethora of products available that purport to have ergogenic properties, and it is beyond the scope of this chapter to examine them in any detail. The reader is recommended to consult recent reviews (MacLaren 2011; Chester 2011; Bishop 2010; Mujika and Burke 2010) for more detail. However, based on available evidence, Table 1.2 summarises three supplements that are considered particularly relevant for soccer performance.

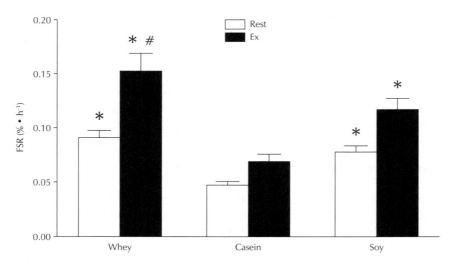

**Figure 1.6** Mixed muscle protein fractional synthetic rate (FSR) after ingestion of whey hydrolysate, casein or soy protein at rest and after resistance exercise.

*Source*: Tang *et al.* (2009).

*Notes*: * significantly different from casein for same condition, $p < 0.05$; # significantly different from soy for each condition, $p < 0.05$.

18

**Table 1.2** Overview of potential ergogenic aids which are relevant to soccer performance.

| Ergogenic aid | Recommended dosage | Proposed physiological effects |
|---|---|---|
| Caffeine | 2–4 mg.kg$^{-1}$ body mass 60 min before competition or training. | Improves function of the central nervous system (CNS), which can therefore improve reaction times and reduce perception of effort. Improves power output during single and repeated sprints. Enhances lipolysis, increases fat oxidation and spares muscle glycogen utilisation. |
| Creatine | 4–5 days of loading dose consisting of 20 g (4 x 5 g daily) followed by maintenance doses of 3–5 g per day. Should also be consumed with HGI carbohydrates to promote muscle uptake. | Increases the phosphocreatine store (PCr) of skeletal muscles which enhances the capacity to generate ATP through the ATP-PCr system. Enhances power output during single and repeated sprints and promotes PCr re-synthesis between repeated sprints. |
| | | Augments gains in fat-free mass, strength and power when used with an appropriate resistance training programme. |
| β-alanine | 3–6 g per day administered in equal doses (e.g., 3–6 x 1 g). | Increases carnosine content in skeletal muscle, which is one of the main intracellular buffers which can protect against metabolic acidosis that is induced by high-intensity exercise. Improves performance during single and repeated high-intensity exercise tasks. |

## SUMMARY

Although carbohydrate stores are limited, it is the most important energy source for soccer training and match play. There is substantial evidence relating depletion of carbohydrate reserves in the muscle or liver to fatigue. Players should therefore ensure that they are loaded with carbohydrate in the day(s) before a match, as well as consuming additional carbohydrate before and during the game itself. We recommend that the pre-match meal be based on LGI carbohydrates, whereas the post-match recovery meal should emphasise HGI carbohydrates. In addition, protein intake is of significance for players in the hour before and after training or a match so as to promote protein synthesis. Players should also incorporate protein in all their daily meals and snacks. Of equal importance is consuming appropriate fluid intake before and during training or match such that the negative performance effects associated with dehydration do not occur. Finally, consideration may be given to exploring the use of nutritional ergogenic aids such as caffeine, creatine and β-alanine so as to maximise physical, mental and technical performance on match day.

# REFERENCES

Ali, A., Williams, C., Nicholas, C.W. *et al*. (2007). The influence of carbohydrate electrolyte ingestion on soccer skill performance. *Medicine and Science in Sports and Exercise*, 39, 1969–1976.

Almond, C.S., Shin, A.Y., Fortescue, E.B. *et al*. (2005). Hyponatremia among runners in the Boston Marathon. *New England Journal of Medicine*, 352, 1550–1556.

Bangsbo, J., Norregaard, L. and Thorsoe, F. (1992). The effect of carbohydrate diet on intermittent exercise performance. *International Journal of Sports Medicine*, 13, 152–157.

Beelen, M., Burke, L.M., Gibala, M.J. and van Loon, L.J.C. (2010). Nutritional strategies to promote post-exercise recovery. *International Journal of Sports Nutrition and Exercise Metabolism*, 20, 515–532.

Bergeron, M.F. (2003). Heat cramps: fluid and electrolyte challenges during tennis in the heat. *Journal of Science and Medicine in Sport*, 6, 19–27.

Betts, J. and Williams, C. (2010). Short term recovery from exercise: exploring the potential for protein ingestion to accentuate the benefits of carbohydrate supplements. *Sports Medicine*, 40, 941–959.

Bishop, D. (2010). Dietary supplements and team sport performance. *Sports Medicine*, 40, 995–1017.

Boirie, Y., Dangin, M., Gachon, P., Vasson, M.P., Maubois, J.L. and Beaufrere, B. (1997). Slow and fast dietary proteins differently modulate postprandial protein accretion. *Proceedings of the National Academy of Sciences of the United States of America*, 94, 14930–14935.

Burke, L.M., Claassen, A., Hawley, J.A. *et al*. (1998). Carbohydrate intake during prolonged cycling minimises effect of glycemic index of pre-exercise meal. *Journal of Applied Physiology*, 85, 2220–2226.

Burke, L.M., Collier, G.R. and Hargreaves, M. (1993). Muscle glycogen storage after prolonged exercise: effect of the glycemic index of carbohydrate feedings. *Journal of Applied Physiology*, 75, 1019–1023.

Burke, L.M., Hawley, J.A., Wong, S.H. *et al*. (2011). Carbohydrates for training and competition. *Journal of Sports Science*, 29 (Suppl.), S17–S27.

Bussau, V.A., Fairchild, T.J., Rao, A. *et al*. (2002). Carbohydrate loading in human muscle: an improved 1 day protocol. *European Journal of Applied Physiology*, 87, 290–295.

Chester, N. (2011) Caffeine. In D. Mottram (ed.), *Drugs in Sport*. Oxford: Routledge.

Clarke, N.D., Drust, B., MacLaren, D.P. *et al*. (2008). Fluid provision and metabolic responses to soccer-specific exercise. *European Journal of Applied Physiology*, 104, 1069–1077.

Costill, D.L., Pascoe, D.D., Fink, W.J. *et al*. (1990). Impaired muscle glycogen resynthesis after eccentric exercise. *Journal of Applied Physiology*, 69, 46–50.

Decombaz, J., Jentjens, R., Ith, M. *et al*. (2011). Fructose and galactose enhance post-exercise human liver glycogen synthesis. *Medicine and Science in Sports and Exercise*, 43 (10), 1964–1971.

Donaldson, C.M., Perry, T.L. and Rose, M.C. (2010). Glycemic index and endurance performance. *International Journal of Sport Nutrition and Exercise Metabolism*, 20, 154–165.

Forslund, A.H., El-Khoury, A.E., Olsson, R.M., Sjodin, A.M., Hambraeus, L. and Young, V.R. (1999) Effect of protein intake and physical activity on 24-h pattern and rate of macronutrient utilization. *American Journal of Physiology*, 276, E964–976.

**D. MacLaren and J. Morton**

Foskett, A., Williams, C., Boobis, L. *et al*. (2008). Carbohydrate availability and muscle energy metabolism during intermittent running. *Medicine and Science in Sports and Exercise*, 40, 96–103.

Gleeson, M. (2007). Immune function in sport and exercise. *Journal of Applied Physiology*, 103, 693–699.

Gontzea, I., Sutzescu, P. and Dumitrache, S. (1974). The influence of muscle activity on nitrogen balance and the need of man for proteins. *Nutrition Report International*, 10, 35–43.

Gonzalez-Alonso, J. (2007). Hyperthermia impairs brain, heart and muscle function in exercising humans. *Sports Medicine*, 37, 371–373.

Hawley, J.A. and Burke, L.M. (1997). Effect of meal frequency and timing on physical performance. *British Journal of Nutrition*, 77, S91–S103.

Hawley, J.A. and Burke, L.M. (2010). Carbohydrate availability and training adaptation: effects on cell metabolism. *Exercise and Sport Science Review*, 38, 152–160.

Howarth, K. R., Phillips, S. M., MacDonald, M. J. *et al*. (2010). Effect of glycogen availability on human skeletal muscle protein turnover during exercise and recovery. *Journal of Applied Physiology*, 109, 431–438.

Ivy, J. and Portman, R. (2004) *Nutrient Timing*. North Bergen, USA: Basic Health Publications.

Ivy, J.L., Katz, A.L., Cutler, C.L. *et al*. (1988). Muscle glycogen synthesis after exercise: effect of time of carbohydrate ingestion. *Journal of Applied Physiology*, 65, 1480–1485.

Jacobs, I., Westlin, N., Karlsson, J. *et al*. (1982). Muscle glycogen and elite soccer players. *European Journal of Applied Physiology*, 48, 297–302.

Jentjens, R. and Jeukendrup, A.E. (2003). Determinants of post-exercise glycogen synthesis during short-term recovery. *Sports Medicine*, 33, 117–144.

Jeukendrup, A. (2010). Carbohydrate and exercise performance: the role of multiple transporters. *Current Opinion in Clinical Nutrition and Metabolism Care*, 13, 452–457.

Jeukendrup, A. and Chambers, E.S. (2010). Oral carbohydrate and exercise performance. *Current Opinion in Clinical Nutrition and Metabolism Care*, 13, 447–451.

Jeukendrup, A. and Killer, S.C. (2010). The myths surrounding pre-exercise carbohydrate feeding. *Annals of Nutrition and Metabolism*, 57, S18-S25.

Judelson, D.A., Maresh, C.M., Anderson, J.M. *et al*. (2007). Hydration and muscular performance: does fluid balance affect strength, power and high-intensity endurance? *Sports Medicine*, 37, 907–921.

Krustrup, P., Mohr, M., Steensberg, A. *et al*. (2006). Muscle and blood metabolites during a soccer game: implications for sprint performance. *Medicine and Science in Sports and Exercise*, 38, 1165–1174.

Kurdak, S.S., Shirreffs, S.M., Maughan, R.J. *et al*. (2010). Hydration and sweating responses to hot weather football competition. *Scandinavian Journal of Medicine and Science in Sports*, 20 (S3), 133–139.

Lee, J.K. and Shirreffs, S.M. (2007). The influence of drink temperature on thermoregulatory responses during prolonged exercise in a moderate environment. *Journal of Sports Science*, 25, 975–985.

Lemon, P.W. (1995) Do athletes need more dietary protein and amino acids? *International Journal of Sport Nutrition*, 5, Suppl., S39–61.

Little, J.P., Chilibeck, P.D., Ciona, D. *et al*. (2009). The effects of low and high glycemic index foods on metabolism high-intensity intermittent exercise. *International Journal of Sports Physiology and Performance*, 4, 367–380.

Little, J.P., Chilibeck, P.D., Ciona, D. *et al.* (2010). Effect of low and high glycemic index meals on metabolism and performance during high-intensity intermittent exercise. *International Journal of Sports Nutrition and Exercise Metabolism*, 20, 447–456.

MacLaren, D. (2011). Supplements for high-intensity exercise. In D. Mottram (ed.), *Drugs in Sport*. Oxford: Routledge.

MacLaren, D.P.M. (2008). Protein, carbohydrates, and muscle recovery. *Journal of the UK Strength and Conditioning Association*, 10, 4–7.

MacLaren, D.P.M. and Close, G.L. (2009). Glycemic index and glycemic load: relevance for athletes in training. *UK Strength and Conditioning Association*, 13, 7–12.

MacLaren, D. and Morton, J. (2011). *Biochemistry for Sport and Exercise Metabolism*. London: John Wiley.

Maughan, R.J., Watson, P., Evans, G.H. *et al.* (2007). Water balance and salt losses in competitive football. *International Journal of Sports Nutrition and Exercise Metabolism*, 17, 583–594.

McGregor, S.J., Nicholas, C.W., Lakomy, H.K. *et al.* (1999). The influence of intermittent high intensity shuttle running and fluid ingestion on the performance of a soccer skill. *Journal of Sports Science*, 17, 895–903.

Mohr, M., Krustrup, P. and Bangsbo, J. (2003). Match performance of high-standard soccer players with special reference to development of fatigue. *Journal of Sports Science*, 21, 519–528.

Mohr, M., Krustrup, P., Nybo, L. *et al.* (2004). Muscle temperature and sprint performance during soccer matches: beneficial effect of re-warm-up at half-time. *Scandinavian Journal of Medicine and Science in Sports*, 14, 156–162.

Mohr, M., Mujika, I., Santisteban, J. *et al.* (2010). Examination of fatigue development in elite soccer in a hot environment: a multi-experimental approach. *Scandinavian Journal of Medicine and Science in Sports*, 20 (S3), 125–132.

Morton, J.P., Croft, L., Bartlett, J.D. *et al.* (2009). Reduced carbohydrate availability does not modulate training-induced heat shock protein adaptations but does up-regulate oxidative enzyme activity in human skeletal muscle. *Journal of Applied Physiology*, 106, 1513–1521.

Morton, J.P., Sutton, L., Robertson, C. *et al.* (2010). Making the weight: a case-study from professional boxing. *International Journal of Sports Nutrition and Exercise Metabolism*, 20, 80–85.

Mujika, I. and Burke, L.M. (2010). Nutrition in team sports. *Annals of Nutrition and Metabolism*, 57 (Suppl. 2), 26–35.

Nicholas, C.W., Tsintzas, K., Boobis, L. *et al.* (1999). Carbohydrate-electrolyte ingestion during intermittent high-intensity running. *Medicine and Science in Sports and Exercise*, 31, 1280–1286.

Nicholas, C.W., Williams, C., Lakomy, H.K. *et al.* (1995). Influence of ingesting a carbohydrate electrolyte solution on endurance capacity during intermittent high-intensity shuttle running. *Journal of Sports Science*, 13, 283–290.

Pfeiffer, B., Stellingwerff, T., Zaltas, E. *et al.* (2010). CHO oxidation from a CHO gel compared with a drink during exercise. *Medicine and Science in Sports and Exercise*, 42, 2038–2045.

Phillips, S.M., Tipton, K.D., Ferrando, A.A. and Wolfe, R.R. (1999). Resistance training reduces the acute exercise-induced increase in muscle protein turnover. *American Journal of Physiology: Endocrinology and Metabolism*, 276, E118–E1241.

# 22

Rasmussen, B.B., Tipton, K.D., Miller, S.L., Wolf, S.E. and Wolfe, R.R. (2000). An oral essential amino acid-carbohydrate supplement enhances muscle protein anabolism after resistance exercise. *Journal of Applied Physiology*, 88, 386–392.

Robinson, T.M., Sewell, D.A., Hultman, E. *et al.* (1999). Role of submaximal exercise in promoting creatine and glycogen accumulation in human skeletal muscle. *Journal of Applied Physiology*, 87, 598–604.

Rollo, I. and Williams, C. (2010). Influence of ingesting a carbohydrate electrolyte solution before and during a 1 hour run in fed endurance trained runners. *Journal of Sports Science*, 28, 593–601.

Saltin, B. (1973). Metabolic fundamentals in exercise. *Medicine and Science in Sports and Exercise*, 5, 137–146.

Sawka, M., Burke, L.M., Eichner, E.R. *et al.* (2007). Exercise and fluid replacement. *Medicine and Science in Sports and Exercise*, 39, 377–390.

Sherman, W.M., Brodowicz, G., Wright, D.A. *et al.* (1989). Effects of 4 h preexercise carbohydrate feedings on cycling performance. *Medicine and Science in Sports and Exercise*, 21, 598–604.

Sherman, W.M., Peden, M.C. and Wright, D.A. (1991). Carbohydrate feedings 1 h before exercise improves cycling performance. *American Journal of Clinical Nutrition*, 54, 866–870.

Tang, J.E., Moore, D.R., Kujbida, G.W., Tarnopolsky, M.A. and Phillips, S.M. (2009). Ingestion of whey hydrolysate, casein, or soy protein isolate: effects on mixed muscle protein synthesis at rest and following resistance exercise in young men. *Journal of Applied Physiology*, 107, 987–992.

Tipton, K.D., Rasmussen, B.B., Miller, S.L., Wolf, S.E., Owens-Stovall, S.K., Petrini, B.E. and Wolfe, R.R. (2001). Timing of amino acid–carbohydrate ingestion alters anabolic response of muscle to resistance exercise. *American Journal of Physiology*, 281, E197–206.

Vist, G.E. and Maughan, R.J. (1995). The effect of osmolality and carbohydrate content on the rate of gastric emptying of liquids in man. *Journal of Physiology*, 486, 523–531.

Wee, L-S., Williams, C., Tsintzas, K. *et al.* (2005). Ingestion of a high glycemic index meal increases muscle glycogen storage at rest but augments its utilization during subsequent exercise. *Journal of Applied Physiology*, 99, 707–714.

Yeo, W.K., Paton, C.D., Garnham, A.P. *et al.* (2008). Skeletal muscle adaptation and performance responses to once a day versus twice every second day endurance training regimens. *Journal of Applied Physiology*, 105, 1462–1470.

# CHAPTER 2

## PRINCIPLES OF FITNESS TRAINING

J. Bangsbo and F. M. Iaia

### INTRODUCTION

Soccer players need a high physical capacity to cope with the demands of the game and to allow technical skills to be utilized throughout a match. Fitness training is therefore an important part of the overall development programme for players. In soccer, as in other sports, the exercise performed should resemble the sport (i.e., match play) as closely as possible; it is therefore crucial to understand the requirements of the game. In this chapter, after a short description of the physical demands of the game, we discuss training methods and present the various categories of fitness training in soccer, with examples of drills. In addition, the physiological adaptations that occur through exposure to the various types of training and how fitness training can be prioritized throughout the year are described. The reader is directed elsewhere for further discussion of the practical aspects of fitness training and for suggestions in relation to activities that can be used in soccer (Bangsbo, 1994a, 2008).

### PHYSICAL DEMANDS

Soccer is an intermittent sport characterized by ~1200 acyclical and unpredictable changes in activity (one every 3–5 s on average) involving, among others, 30–40 accelerations (Mohr, Krustrup, and Bangsbo, 2003), more than 700 turns (Bloomfield, Polman, and O'Donoghue, 2007), 30–40 tackles and jumps (Mohr et al., 2003) as well as other intense actions such as kicking, dribbling and tackling (Bangsbo, 1994b). All these efforts exacerbate the physical strain imposed on the body and contribute to making the game highly demanding physically for players.

The use of computerized and semi-automatic, video-based time–motion analysis systems has revealed that during a game top class soccer players perform 2–3 km of high-intensity running (>15 km/h) and ~0.8 km at sprinting speed (>20 km/h) (Bangsbo, Norregaard, and Thorso, 1991; Bradley et al., 2009; Di Salvo et al., 2007; Di Salvo, Gregson, Atkinson, Tordoff, and Drust, 2009; Mohr et al., 2003; Rampinini, Coutts, Castagna, Sassi, and Impellizzeri, 2007a; Rampinini, Impellizzeri, Castagna, Coutts, and Wisloff, 2009). These values are approximately 28 and 58% higher when compared with what is performed by moderate-level professional players (Mohr et al., 2003). In addition, less successful teams exhibit larger decrements in the total sprint distance run throughout the match (Di Salvo et al., 2009), suggesting that the ability to perform repeated intense activities over the duration of a game is of great importance.

24

Nevertheless, despite the importance of maintaining workload, it has been demonstrated that the amount of high-intensity running declines towards the end of a match (Mohr et al., 2003), with this type of activity being 20–40% lower in the last third of the second half, as compared with the first 15 min of the game (Bradley et al., 2009; Di Salvo et al., 2009; Mohr et al., 2003). Moreover, the decrement in high-intensity running is more evident when a greater amount of activity is performed in the first half (Rampinini et al., 2007a). In the 5 min following the most demanding 5-min period of a game, the distance covered at high intensity is reduced by 6–12%, as compared with game average (Bradley et al., 2009; Di Salvo et al., 2009; Mohr et al., 2003), indicating that players experience fatigue not only towards the end of a match, but temporarily during a game (Mohr, Krustrup, and Bangsbo, 2005). Accordingly, both single and repeated-sprint test performances are impaired after a high-intensity period during, as well as at the end of, the game (Krustrup et al., 2006). Fatigue development may also have a negative impact on passing ability (Rampinini et al., 2008; Rostgaard, Iaia, Simonsen, and Bangsbo, 2008), with the deterioration in technical performance being more pronounced in the less fit players (Rampinini et al., 2008). It should be emphasized that each playing position is characterized by its own activity profile and different tactical requirements (Bangsbo et al., 1991; Bradley et al., 2009; Di Salvo et al., 2007; Di Salvo et al., 2009; Mohr et al., 2003; Rampinini et al., 2007a; Rampinini et al., 2009).

The physical demands of a soccer match can also be evaluated using physiological measurements. The recording of heart-rate and body-temperature shows that the average aerobic energy production is ~70% of maximum oxygen uptake (Bangsbo, Mohr, and Krustrup, 2006; Ekblom, 1986), indicating that the aerobic energy production is highly taxed during the game, accounting for more than 90% of total energy consumption (Bangsbo, 1994b). During a competitive match, a top-class player performs 150–250 intense actions (Mohr et al., 2003), thereby reducing the concentration of muscle creatine phosphate, which is resynthesized following rest or during a low-intensity exercise period (Bangsbo, 1994b). Glycolysis leading to lactate production will also occur to a significant extent, despite the majority of the intense exercise periods lasting less than 5 s (Buchheit, Mendez-Villanueva, Simpson, and Bourdon, 2010). In support, elevated levels of muscle and blood lactate are recorded during a game (Bangsbo, 1994c; Bangsbo, Iaia, and Krustrup, 2007; Krustrup et al., 2006), further highlighting that the anaerobic energy system is heavily stimulated during match-play.

It is evident that soccer is physically demanding and that players need a high fitness level to cope with the energy demands and a well-developed capacity to express power in single actions during a match. Therefore, it is important that players improve their ability to perform repeated maximal or near maximal efforts over prolonged periods, which can be achieved by proper fitness training.

## COMPONENTS OF FITNESS TRAINING

Fitness training has to be multifactorial in order to cover the different aspects of physical performance in soccer. Thus, the training can be divided into a number of components based on the different types of physical demands during a match, as illustrated in Figure 2.1. The terms aerobic and anaerobic training are based on the energy pathway that dominates during

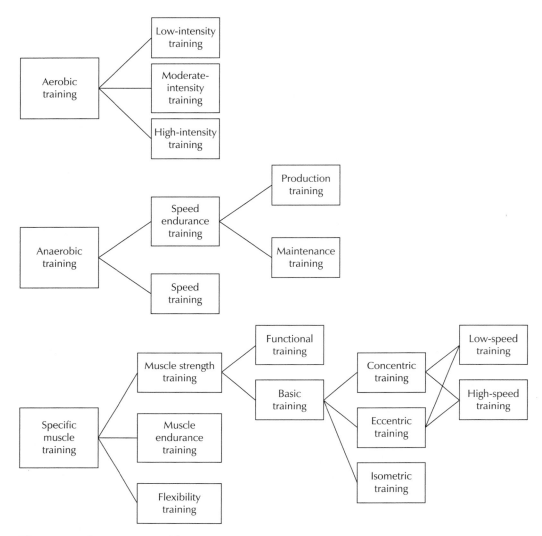

**Figure 2.1** Components of fitness training in soccer.

the activity periods of the training session. Aerobic and anaerobic training represent exercise intensities below and above the maximum oxygen uptake, respectively. However, during training practices and small-sided games, the exercise intensity for a player varies continuously, and some overlap exists between the two categories of training. The separate components within fitness training are briefly described in this chapter. These include aerobic, anaerobic and specific muscle training.

**J. Bangsbo and F.M. Iaia**

## TRAINING METHODS

Fitness training in soccer should be closely related to the activities performed in the game. Aerobic and anaerobic training can be achieved by performing games and specific drills with the ball involving changes of speed, direction and specific movement patterns typical of those performed during match play. There are several advantages to carrying out soccer-related training. The specific muscle groups utilized in soccer are trained, which means that the adaptations occur in the muscle fibres engaged during a game. A way to control the intensity during small-sided games is by manipulating variables such as field dimension and number of players involved, as well as introducing specific rules and providing verbal encouragement (Bangsbo, 2008; Rampinini et al., 2007b). A number of researchers have shown that it is possible to achieve a high exercise intensity using the ball, as demonstrated by elevated heart rates, marked blood lactate accumulations and high rate of perceived exertions (Hill-Haas, Dawson, Coutts, and Rowsell, 2009; Kelly and Drust, 2009; Rampinini et al., 2007b). In addition, significant improvements in $\dot{V}O_{2max}$ (7–9%) and running economy (3–10%) have been found after performing aerobic high-intensity training in small-sided games twice a week for 12 weeks (Chamari et al., 2005; Impellizzeri et al., 2006). Small-sided games represent a valid aerobic training stimulus.

Another advantage of performing training with the ball is that coordinative, technical and tactical skills are trained under fatiguing conditions, as during match play. A study involving the Italian Serie A league reported that players in the most successful teams cover greater total (18%) and high-intensity (16%) running distances in possession of the ball, as compared with players in less successful teams (Rampinini et al., 2009). Thus, the ability of players to exercise at high intensity when interacting with the ball may be an important determinant of success and should be developed. For example, researchers have shown that forwards often receive the ball while sprinting or turning (Williams, Williams, and Horn, 2003) and cover ~64% of the high-intensity running in ball possession (Rampinini et al., 2007a). These findings clearly indicate that for such players technical and tactical training should be performed under physically demanding conditions similar to those encountered during a competitive game. Furthermore, involvements with the ball, short passes and successful short passes decrease between the first and the second half, as well as after a very high-intensity period (Rampinini et al., 2008; Rampinini et al., 2009), which highlights the importance of experiencing a high number of contacts with the ball during training sessions involving intense exercise. Finally, training with rather than without the ball usually provides greater motivation for the players.

The specific physical game requirements of each player need to be considered in the planning process and therefore some fitness training may be performed on an individual basis. The training should be focused on improving both the player's strong and weak abilities. Nevertheless, it is important to be aware of the fact that, due to genetic differences, there will always be discrepancies in the physical capacity of players, irrespective of the training programmes employed.

## AEROBIC TRAINING

The overall aim of aerobic training is to increase the work-rate during competition and to minimize a decrease in technical performance as well as lapses in concentration induced by fatigue towards the end of a game. The specific aims of aerobic training are outlined below.

■ To improve the capacity of the cardiovascular system to transport oxygen. Thus, a larger percentage of the energy required for intense exercise can be supplied aerobically, allowing a player to work at higher exercise intensities for prolonged periods of time.

■ To improve the capacity of muscles specifically used in soccer to utilize oxygen and to oxidize fat during prolonged periods of exercise. Thereby, the limited store of muscle glycogen is spared and a player can exercise at a higher intensity towards the end of a game.

■ To improve the ability to recover after a period of high-intensity exercise. As a result, a player requires less time to recover before being able to perform in a subsequent period of high-intensity exercise.

### Components of aerobic training

Aerobic training can be divided into three overlapping components: *aerobic low-intensity training* (Aerobic$_{LO}$), *aerobic moderate-intensity training* (Aerobic$_{MO}$) and *aerobic high-intensity training* (Aerobic$_{HI}$) (see Figure 2.1). Table 2.1 illustrates principles of heart rate response for the various categories of aerobic training and takes into account the fact that training may be performed as a game, and therefore, a player's heart rate (HR) may frequently alternate during the session.

During Aerobic$_{LO}$, the players perform light physical activities, such as jogging and low-intensity games. This type of training may be carried out the day after a match or the day after a hard training session to help a player to recover to a normal physical state. Aerobic$_{LO}$ may also be used to avoid the players getting into conditions known as 'overreaching' and 'overtraining' in periods involving frequent training sessions (maybe even twice a day) and a busy schedule of competitive matches.

The purpose of Aerobic$_{MO}$ training is to elevate the capillarization and the oxidative potential in the muscle (peripheral factors). The functional outcome is optimization of the substrate

Table 2.1 Components of aerobic training.

| | Heart rate | | | | Oxygen uptake | |
|---|---|---|---|---|---|---|
| | % of HR$_{max}$ | | Beats min$^{-1}$> | | % of $\dot{V}O_{2max}$ | |
| | Mean | Range | Mean[a] | Range[a] | Mean | Range |
| Low-intensity training | 65 | 50–80 | 130 | 80–160 | 55 | 20–70 |
| Moderate-intensity training | 80 | 70–90 | 160 | 140–180 | 70 | 60–85 |
| High-intensity training | 90 | 80–100 | 180 | 160–200 | 85 | 70–100 |

Note: [a] If HR$_{max}$ is 200beats min$^{-1}$.

utilization and thereby an improvement in endurance capacity. One aim of Aerobic$_{HI}$ training is to improve central factors such as the pump capacity of the heart, which is closely related to maximum oxygen uptake ($\dot{V}O_{2max}$). The improvements obtained by Aerobic$_{HI}$ increase a player's capability to exercise repeatedly at high intensities for prolonged periods during a match. The aerobic response to training can be evaluated by measuring heart rate. For example, heart rate during aerobic high intensity should be at the least 85% of maximum heart rate, and on average around 90% at the end of each interval (Table 2.1).

## Effects of aerobic training

Aerobic training increases cardiovascular factors such as heart size, blood flow capacity and blood volume (Ekblom, 1968; Kanstrup and Ekblom, 1984; Laughlin and Armstrong, 1983). These changes improve the capacity of the cardiovascular system to transport oxygen, resulting in faster muscle and pulmonary oxygen uptake ($V^{\cdot}O_2$) kinetic (Bailey, Wilkerson, Dimenna, and Jones, 2009; Krustrup, Hellsten, and Bangsbo, 2004), as well as $\dot{V}O_{2max}$ (Ferrari et al., 2008; Impellizzeri et al., 2006; Krustrup et al., 2010). Thus, a greater amount of energy can be supplied aerobically, allowing a player to sustain intense exercise for a longer duration and to recover faster between high-intensity periods in a game.

A large number of muscular adaptations also occur with aerobic training. For example, this type of training up-regulates several mitochondrial oxidative proteins and increases the muscle glycogen content (Ross and Leveritt, 2001), which appears to be the most important substrate for energy production in soccer (Bangsbo et al., 2006). The overall effects are pronounced changes in muscle metabolism, with an increased fat oxidation (Talanian, Galloway, Heigenhauser, Bonen, and Spriet, 2007) as well as reduced glycogenolysis, glycolysis, lactate production and carbohydrate oxidation at a given exercise intensity (Henriksson and Hickner, 1996). This effect is beneficial in soccer, where an improved capacity to utilize muscle triglycerides and blood free fatty acids as substrates for oxidative metabolism could spare the limited muscle glycogen stores, allowing a player to exercise at a higher intensity towards the end of the game. Muscle capillarization is also enhanced in response to aerobic training (Jensen, Bangsbo, and Hellsten, 2004). An enriched capillary network leads to a larger area available for diffusion and shorter diffusion distance between capillaries and muscle fibres. This training effect favours the uptake of substrates, such as fatty acids, as well as release of compounds from muscle interstitium, and contributes to delaying the development of fatigue during intense exercise. In support, a higher capillary density was reported to be associated with performance improvements in a ~3-min exhaustive bout (Jensen et al., 2004) and, more recently, was shown to be an influential determinant for performance during high-intensity exercises leading to exhaustion between 30 s and ~3 min (Iaia et al., 2011). Supplementary aerobic training during the season has been shown to improve performance level even in elite players. Thus, an additional 30-min aerobic high-intensity training session per week for 12 weeks elevated the Yo-Yo intermittent recovery test (level 2) performance (Bangsbo, Iaia, and Krustrup, 2008) by 18% (Figure 2.2; Jensen, Bredsgaard-Randers, Krustrup, Bangsbo, 2009).

The optimal way to train central versus peripheral factors is not the same. Maximum oxygen uptake is most effectively enhanced by exercise intensities around 80–100% of $\dot{V}O_{2max}$

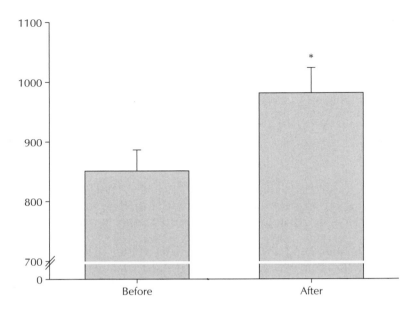

**Figure 2.2** The effect of one additional 30-min aerobic high-intensity training session a week on Yo-Yo intermittent recovery level 2 test performance.

*Note:* * Significant difference between before and after (P<0.05).

(Bassett, Jr and Howley, 2000). For muscle adaptation to occur, an extended period of training appears to be essential and, therefore, the mean intensity has once in a while to be below 80% of $\dot{V}O_{2max}$. This factor does not imply that high-intensity exercise does not elevate the number of capillaries and mitochondrial volume in the muscles engaged in training, but rather suggests that the duration of this type of training regime may be too short to obtain optimal adaptations at a local level. The dissociation between changes in $\dot{V}O_{2max}$ and muscle adaptation by means of training and detraining is illustrated by results from a study on top-class players (Bangsbo and Mizuno, 1988). The players abstained from training for 3 weeks. It was found that $\dot{V}O_{2max}$ was unaltered, whereas performance in a field test was lowered by 8% in association with a 20–30% reduction in oxidative enzymes activity.

## ANAEROBIC TRAINING

The overall aim of anaerobic training is to increase the player's potential to perform high-intensity exercise. The specific aims of anaerobic training are outlined below.

- To improve the ability to act quickly and to produce power rapidly – players reduce the time required to react and elevate sprint performance.
- To elevate the capacity to produce power and energy continuously via the anaerobic energy-producing pathways – players increase their ability to perform high-intensity exercise for longer periods of time.

30

- To improve the ability to recover after a period of high-intensity exercise, which is particularly important in soccer – players require less time before being able to perform maximally in a subsequent period of exercise and will be able to perform high-intensity exercise more frequently during a match.

## Components of anaerobic training

Anaerobic training can be divided into *speed training* and *speed endurance training* (see Figure 2.1). Anaerobic training must be performed according to an interval principle. Table 2.2 illustrates the principles of the various categories of anaerobic training.

The aim of speed training is to improve a player's ability to act quickly in situations where speed is essential. During speed training, players should perform maximally for a short period of time (<10 s). The periods between the exercise bouts should be long enough for the muscles to recover to near-resting conditions, so as to enable a player to perform maximally in a subsequent exercise bout. In soccer, speed is not merely dependent on physical factors; it also involves rapid decision making, which must then be translated into quick movements. Therefore, speed training should mainly be performed with a ball. Speed drills can be designed to promote a player's ability to perceive and predict situations as well as to decide on the opponents' responses in advance.

Speed endurance training can be separated into *production* and *tolerance (maintenance) training*. The purpose of *production training* is to improve the ability to perform maximally for a relatively short period of time, whereas the aim of *tolerance training* is to increase the ability to sustain exercise at a high intensity. The exercise intensity in *production training* should be almost maximal, to elicit major adaptations in the enzymes associated with anaerobic metabolism. The exercise bouts should be relatively short (15–40 s) and the rest periods in between should be comparatively long (1.5–4 min), in order to maintain a very high intensity during the exercise periods throughout the training session. In speed endurance *tolerance training*, the exercise bouts last 20–90 s, separated by relatively short recovery periods (1–3 times the exercise duration).

**Table 2.2** Principles of anaerobic training.

|  |  | Duration | | Intensity | Number of repetitions |
|---|---|---|---|---|---|
|  |  | Exercise | Rest |  |  |
| Speed training |  | 2–10 | >10 times the exercise duration | Maximal | 2–10 |
| Speed endurance training | Production | 15–40 | >5 times the exercise duration | Almost maximal | 2–10 |
|  | Tolerance (maintenance) | 20–90 | 1–3 times the exercise duration | High/very high | 2–10 |

The adaptations caused by speed endurance training are mostly localized to the exercising muscles. Thus, it is important that a player performs movements in a manner similar to match-play. Figure 2.3 illustrates a small-sided game within the tolerance category of speed endurance training. It also shows heart rate and blood lactate values for a player, illustrating that the game fulfils the criteria for speed endurance training. Speed endurance training is both physically and mentally demanding for players. Therefore, it is recommended that this type of training is used only by top-class players.

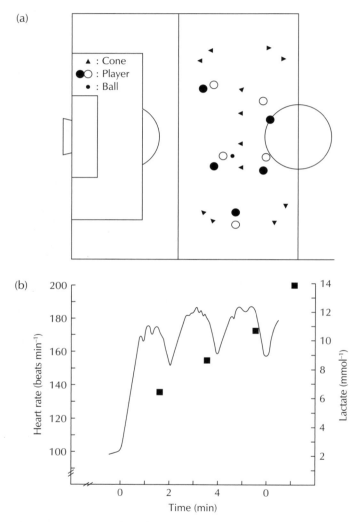

Notes:

Area of field: One-third of a soccer field

Number of players: Ten

Organization: A team consists of five players. The teams perform man-to-man marking. Six small 'goals' (pairs of cones) are placed at various positions on the field. Description: Ordinary soccer play. The players must try to play the ball through the goals to a team-mate.

Rule: The players are not allowed to run through the goals. Intervals: Exercise periods of 1 min and rest periods of 1 min. Scoring: A point is scored when passing the ball through one of the goals to a team-mate.

Comments: The players should be motivated to exercise continuously at a high intensity. If one player cannot cope with the marking of an opponent, the intensity of the other players can be affected. It is therefore important to have players of equal ability marking each other. In order to avoid delays, extra balls should be placed around the field. The exercise demands can be controlled by changing the number or the width of the goals.

**Figure 2.3** A speed endurance training small-sided game.

J. Bangsbo and F.M. Iaia

## Effects of anaerobic training

A period of speed training has been shown to increase the activity of the muscle enzymes creatine kinase (CK) (Mohr *et al.*, 2007; Thorstensson, Sjodin, and Karlsson, 1975) and myokinase (Dawson *et al.*, 1998; Thorstensson *et al.*, 1975). These adaptations lead to a quicker breakdown of high-energy phosphates, such as adenosine triphosphate (ATP) and creatinephosphate (CP) stored in the muscle, resulting in an improved capacity to generate power rapidly during short maximal bouts. Speed training does not appear to influence the concentration of ATP and CP (Dawson *et al.*, 1998; Linossier, Denis, Dormois, Geyssant, and Lacour, 1993; Thorstensson *et al.*, 1975). During speed endurance training, creatine kinase and glycolytic pathways are highly stimulated, as shown by an increased activity of some anaerobic enzymes such as phosphofructokinase (PFK), lactate dehydrogenase (LDH) and glycogen phosphorylase (Phos) (Ross and Leveritt, 2001). This increase in enzyme activity may improve the ability to sustain very intense work and to perform maximal runs repeatedly via a higher rate of anaerobic energy turnover.

A period of speed endurance training also elevates a number of muscle membrane transport proteins involved in pH regulation, such as the $Na^+/H^+$ exchanger isoform 1 (NHE1) as well as monocarboxylate transporters (MCT1 and MCT4) (Iaia *et al.*, 2008; Mohr *et al.*, 2007), and in some cases enhances muscle-buffering capacity (Edge, Bishop, and Goodman, 2006; Sharp, Costill, Fink, and King, 1986). These changes reduce the inhibitory effects of $H^+$ within the muscle cell and can be part of the explanation of an improved performance during repeated intense exercise observed after a period of speed endurance training. Anaerobic training increases also the expression of $Na^+,K^+$ pumps (Iaia *et al.*, 2008; McKenna *et al.*, 1993; Mohr *et al.*, 2007) which, by reducing the contraction-induced net loss of $K^+$ from the working muscles, may contribute to preserving the cell excitability and maintaining force development. Speed endurance tolerance training enhances the number of capillaries (Jensen *et al.*, 2004), having a positive effect on performance during intense exercise as described above. Thus, a player improves the ability to sustain very intense exercise for longer durations and perform more frequent high-intensity efforts during the game.

Speed endurance production training has been shown to be very effective in improving both the short- and long-term performance of runners (Iaia and Bangsbo, 2010). It also seems to be the case for soccer players. In a recent study, the effects of a 2-wk intensified training period were examined in trained soccer players (Thomassen, Christensen, Gunnarsson, Nybo, and Bangsbo, 2010). After the last match of the season 7 elite soccer players performed, during a 2-wk period, 10 training sessions mainly consisting of aerobic high-intensity training (8 x 2-min exercise bouts separated by 1 min of rest) and speed endurance training (10–12 x 30-s sprints separated by 3 min of rest). After the 2 weeks, performance in 10 repeated 20-m sprints was enhanced (Figure 2.4). In addition, the protein expression of the $Na^+/K^+$ pump $\alpha 2$ isoform was 15% higher after the intervention period. Furthermore, running economy was improved and the amount of pyruvate dehydrogenase was 17% higher. Apparently, intensified training of already well-trained soccer players can cause significant muscular adaptations and improve performance.

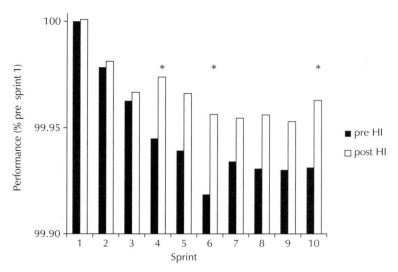

**Figure 2.4** Repeated sprint performance for elite soccer players before (pre) and after (post) a 2-week intensified training period (HI).

*Note*: * Significant difference between pre and post HI (P<0.05).

## SPECIFIC MUSCLE TRAINING

Specific muscle training involves training of muscles in isolated movements. The aim of this type of training is to increase performance of a muscle to a higher level than can be attained just by playing soccer. Specific muscle training can be divided into *muscle strength*, *muscle speed endurance* and *flexibility* training (Figure 2.1). The effect of this form of training is specific to the muscle groups that are engaged and the adaptation within the muscle is mainly limited to the kind of training performed. A brief description of muscle strength training is given below (see also Bangsbo, 1994a).

### Strength training

Many activities in soccer, such as jumping, kicking, tackling and turning, are forceful and explosive. The power output during these activities is related to the strength of the muscles involved in the movements. Thus, it is beneficial for a player to have a high level of muscular strength, which can be obtained by strength training.

The overall aim of muscle strength training is to develop the player's muscular make-up. The specific aims of muscle strength training are outlined below.

- To increase muscle power output during explosive activities such as jumping and accelerating.
- To prevent injuries.
- To regain strength after an injury.

J. Bangsbo and F.M. Iaia

## Components of strength training

Strength training can be divided into *functional strength training* and *basic strength training* (see Figure 2.1). In functional strength training, movements related to the sport are used. The training can consist of activities in which typical movements are performed under conditions more stressful than normal. During basic strength training, muscle groups are trained in isolated movements. For this training, different types of conventional strength training machines and free weights can be used, but body weight may also be used as resistance. Strength training should be carried out in a manner that resembles activities and movements specific to the sport. Strength training can be divided into isometric, concentric and eccentric work (see Figure 2.1). Several principles can be used in concentric strength training. Table 2.3 illustrates a principle that is based on determinations of five-repetition maximum (5-RM) and that allows for muscle groups to be trained at both slow and fast speeds. The exercises should be performed with a maximum effort. After each repetition the player should rest a few seconds to allow for a higher force production in the subsequent muscle contraction. The number of repetitions in a set should not exceed 15. During each training session, 3 to 5 sets should be performed with each muscle group, and rest periods between sets should be longer that 3 min. During this time, the athletes can exercise with other muscle groups.

## Effects of strength training

A period of strength training can result in hypertrophy of the muscle. When performed with heavy weights, all muscle fibres will be larger. Training with explosive movements and performed with high intensity will primarily lead to larger fast twitch (FT) fibres. Thus, the FT muscle fibres will take up relatively more of the total muscle cross-sectional area after the training period and the muscles will be able to produce more power. There is no evidence that the number of muscle fibres increases with training. However, fibres may be transformed in the direction of FT fibres (Andersen, Klitgaard, Bangsbo, and Saltin, 1994). A study involving elite sprinters who underwent 3 months of heavy explosive resistance training and intensive short-interval training showed a significant increase in the relative number of FT fibres and a decrease in the number of slow twitch (ST) fibres in a response to training (Andersen, Klitgaard, and Saltin, 1994). The increased number of FT fibres was a result of a marked increase in the amount of FTa fibres, while the number of FTx fibres decreased. Apparently, the training

Table 2.3 Types of strength training.

| Type of anaerobic training | Work load | Number of repetitions | Rest between repetitions | Number of sets |
|---|---|---|---|---|
| Concentric | | | | |
| Low speed | 5 RM | 5 | 2–5 | 2–4 |
| High speed | 50% of 5 RM | 15 | 1–3 | 2–4 |
| Isometric | 85–100% of max maintained for 5–15 s | 5–10 | 5–15 | 2–4 |

RM: repetition maximum

caused the ST and FTx fibres to be converted into FTa fibres, which was associated with improvements in strength and sprint performance (Andersen *et al.*, 1994).

There is also a neuromotor effect of strength training, and part of the increase in muscle strength can be attributed to changes in the nervous system. Improvements in muscular strength during isolated movements seem closely related to training speeds. However, significant increases in force development at very high speeds (10–18 rad/s) have also been observed in slow-speed high resistance training (Aagaard, Simonsen, Trolle, Bangsbo, and Klausen, 1994). One essential function of the muscles is to protect and stabilize joints of the skeletal system. Consequently, strength training helps to prevent new injuries as well as the re-occurrence of old injuries. A prolonged period of inactivity, for example during recovery from an injury, will considerably weaken the muscle. Thus, before a player returns to training after an injury, a period of strength training is needed. The length of time required to regain strength depends on the duration of the inactivity period, but often months are needed. For a group of soccer players observed 2 years after a knee operation, it was found that the maximal power of the quadriceps muscle of the injured leg was only 75% of the strength in the other leg (Ekstrand, 1982).

## PLANNING OF FITNESS TRAINING

The time course of adaptations in the various biological tissues should be taken into account when planning fitness training. A change in heart size is rather slow to manifest and there is a need for training over a long period of time (years) to get marked improvements in the pump capacity of the heart. Blood volume changes more quickly than the heart size, but this adaptation is optimal after a dimensional development of the cardiovascular system has first occurred. The content of oxidative enzymes and the degree of capillarization in skeletal muscle change more rapidly, but months of regular training are needed to obtain considerable increases in muscle capillaries and oxidative enzymes. On the other hand, a reduction in these parameters can occur with a time constant of weeks. The changes in glycolytic enzymes are rapid and they can be markedly elevated within a month of appropriate training (Bangsbo, Michalsik, and Petersen, 1993; Houston, Bentzen, and Larsen, 1979).

When planning fitness training in soccer, the year should be separated into off-season and in-season periods. The latter may be further divided into pre-season and competitive season. Table 2.4 shows how the different types of fitness training can be structured through the three periods of the year. The higher the number given, the more important is the form of training. The scheme is based on a 2-month off-season and a 10-month season of which the last 8 weeks before the season are spent in the club. The scheme is only a guideline, since there are differences in the duration of the season and off-season from country to country, and some countries have a mid-season break. It should also be emphasized that there may be deviation in the priority of the various aspects of fitness training, due to specific tactics and strategy employed by a team.

During the off-season, the players should regularly perform sessions with Aerobic$_{MO}$ training, since the oxidative enzyme capacity is rapidly lost with inactivity and it takes months to restore the enzyme levels. The training will reduce the decrease in fitness level, which always occurs on cessation of normal training and competition. A gradual transition between the off-season and pre-season also keeps the risk of injuries low and leaves time for other types of soccer

**Table 2.4** Planning of fitness training.

| | Off-season | | Pre-season | | | Competitive season | | | | | | | |
|---|---|---|---|---|---|---|---|---|---|---|---|---|---|
| **Aerobic training** | | | | | | | | | | | | | |
| Moderate-intensity | 3344 | 4445 | 5555 | 4433 | 4343 | 4343 | 4343 | 4343 | 4343 | 4343 | 4343 | 4343 | 434xx |
| High-intensity | 2223 | 3234 | 4445 | 4555 | 5545 | 5545 | 5545 | 5545 | 5545 | 5545 | 5545 | 5545 | 544xx |
| **Anaerobic training** | | | | | | | | | | | | | |
| Speed endurance | 1111 | 1111 | 2234 | 4555 | 4353 | 4353 | 4353 | 4353 | 4353 | 4353 | 4353 | 4353 | 345xx |
| Speed | 1111 | 1111 | 2234 | 4555 | 5555 | 5555 | 5555 | 5555 | 5555 | 5555 | 5555 | 5555 | 555xx |
| **Muscle strength training** | | | | | | | | | | | | | |
| Basic | 3334 | 5555 | 5543 | 2323 | 2323 | 2323 | 2323 | 2323 | 2323 | 2323 | 2323 | 2323 | 222xx |
| Functional | 2222 | 3333 | 3344 | 4343 | 4343 | 4343 | 4343 | 4343 | 4343 | 4343 | 4343 | 4343 | 432xx |
| Muscle speed training | 1111 | 1112 | 3333 | 3333 | 3333 | 3333 | 3333 | 3333 | 3333 | 3333 | 3333 | 3333 | 333xx |
| Flexibility training | 3232 | 3434 | 4444 | 4444 | 4444 | 4444 | 4444 | 4444 | 4444 | 4444 | 4444 | 4444 | 444xx |

Note:
Each single number represents a week. For practical purposes each month is given 4 weeks. The values represent the following priorities, 1, very low priority; 2, low priority; 3, moderate priority; 4, high priority; 5, very high priority.

training, such as tactical and technical training. In the first part of the off-season, it is reasonable to emphasize basic strength training, since the adaptations from this type of training can be maintained with minimal effort during the season. As the start of the season approaches, the amount of basic strength training is reduced and more time is allocated to functional strength training and playing soccer. During the last 6 weeks or so of the off-season, the players frequently perform sessions of Aerobic$_{HI}$ training, speed training and, for elite players, speed endurance training. Such training should be supplemented by regular matches at a high competitive level. During the season, Aerobic$_{HI}$ training is given a high priority (see Table 2.4). Speed training and, for top-class players, speed endurance training should be performed regularly. The total amount of training may be significantly reduced in periods. Then, by including intense training session, performance may even be improved (Bangsbo, Gunnarsson, Wendell, Nybo, and Thomassen, 2009; Iaia et al., 2008). Endurance capacity may be maintained by frequent prolonged training sessions with only short rest periods. The extent of strength training during the season should be determined by the total training time available.

## SUMMARY

With appropriate training, the physical performance of a player during a match can be increased and the risk of injury reduced. In order to design an efficient training programme, it is important to be aware of the requirements of the game and the different components of fitness training in soccer. Aerobic training increases the ability to exercise at an overall higher intensity during a match and minimizes a decrease in technical performance induced by fatigue towards the end of a game. Anaerobic training elevates a player's potential to perform maximal runs repeatedly and to sustain intense work during a game. Muscle strength training, combined with technical training, improves a player's power output during explosive activities in a match. Fitness training should mainly be performed as small-sided games or drills with the ball. The principle of specificity of training ensures that the specific muscles used in soccer are trained and that players develop their technical skills under conditions similar to those encountered during competition.

## REFERENCES

Aagaard, P., Simonsen, E. B., Trolle, M., Bangsbo, J., and Klausen, K. (1994). Moment and power generation during maximal knee extensions performed at low and high speeds. *European Journal of Applied Physiology and Occupational Physiology*, 69, 376–381.

Andersen, J. L., Klitgaard, H., and Saltin, B. (1994). Myosin heavy chain isoforms in single fibres from m. vastus lateralis of sprinters: influence of training. *Acta Physiologica Scandinavica*, 151, 135–142.

Andersen, J. L., Klitgaard, H., Bangsbo, J., and Saltin, B. (1994). Myosin heavy chain isoforms in single fibres from m. vastus lateralis of soccer players: effects of strength-training. *Acta Physiologica Scandinavica*, 150, 21–26.

Bailey, S. J., Wilkerson, D. P., Dimenna, F. J., and Jones, A. M. (2009). Influence of repeated sprint training on pulmonary O2 uptake and muscle deoxygenation kinetics in humans. *Journal of Applied Physiology*, 106, 1875–1887.

**J. Bangsbo and F.M. Iaia**

Bangsbo, J. (1994a). *Fitness Training in Soccer: A Scientific Approach*. Bagsvaerd, Denmark: HO+Storm.

Bangsbo J. (1994b). The physiology of soccer – with special reference to intense intermittent exercise. *Acta Physiologica Scandinavica*, 151, Suppl. 619.

Bangsbo, J. (1994c). Energy demands in competitive soccer. *Journal of Sports Science*, 12, S5–12.

Bangsbo, J. (2008). *Aerobic and Anaerobic Training in Soccer: With Special Emphasis on Training of Youth Players. Fitness Training in Soccer I*. Bagsvaerd, Denmark: HO+Storm.

Bangsbo, J. and Mizuno, M. (1988). Morphological and metabolic alterations in soccer players with detraining and retraining and their relation to performance. In T. Reilly, A. Lees, K. Davids and W.J. Murphy (eds), *Science and Soccer* (pp.114–124). London: E. & F.N. Spon.

Bangsbo, J., Iaia, F. M., and Krustrup, P. (2007). Metabolic response and fatigue in soccer. *International Journal of Sports Physiology and Performance* 2, 111–127.

Bangsbo, J., Iaia, F. M., and Krustrup, P. (2008). The Yo-Yo intermittent recovery test : a useful tool for evaluation of physical performance in intermittent sports. *Sports Medicine*, 38, 37–51.

Bangsbo, J., Michalsik, L., and Petersen, A. (1993). Accumulated O2 deficit during intense exercise and muscle characteristics of elite athletes. *International Journal of Sports Medicine*, 14, 207–213.

Bangsbo, J., Mohr, M., and Krustrup, P. (2006). Physical and metabolic demands of training and match-play in the elite football player. *Journal of Sports Science*, 24, 665–674.

Bangsbo, J., Norregaard, L., and Thorso, F. (1991). Activity profile of competition soccer. *Canadian Journal of Sport Science*, 16, 110–116.

Bangsbo, J., Gunnarsson, T. P., Wendell, J., Nybo, L., and Thomassen, M. (2009). Reduced volume and increased training intensity elevate muscle Na+-K+ pump α2-subunit expression as well as short- and long-term work capacity in humans. *Journal of Applied Physiology*, 107, 1771–1780.

Bassett, D. R., Jr, and Howley, E. T. (2000). Limiting factors for maximum oxygen uptake and determinants of endurance performance. *Medicine and Science in Sports and Exercise* 32, 70–84.

Bloomfield, J., Polman, R., and O'Donoghue, P. (2007). Physical demands of different positions in FA Premier League soccer. *Journal of Sports Science and Medicine*, 6, 63–70.

Bradley, P. S., Sheldon, W., Wooster, B., Olsen, P., Boanas, P., and Krustrup, P. (2009). High-intensity running in English FA Premier League soccer matches. *Journal of Sports Science*, 27, 159–168.

Buchheit, M., Mendez-Villanueva, A., Simpson, B. M., and Bourdon, P. C. (2010). Repeated-sprint sequences during youth soccer matches. *International Journal of Sports Medicine*, 31, 709–716.

Chamari, K., Hachana, Y., Kaouech, F., Jeddi, R., Moussa-Chamari, I., and Wisloff, U. (2005). Endurance training and testing with the ball in young elite soccer players. *British Journal of Sports Medicine*, 39, 24–28.

Dawson, B., Fitzsimons, M., Green, S., Goodman, C., Carey, M., and Cole, K. (1998). Changes in performance, muscle metabolites, enzymes and fibre types after short sprint training. *Eur.J.Appl.Physiol Occup.Physiol*, 78, 163–169.

Di Salvo, V., Gregson, W., Atkinson, G., Tordoff, P., and Drust, B. (2009). Analysis of high intensity activity in Premier League soccer. *International Journal of Sports Medicine*, 30, 205–212.

Di Salvo, V., Baron, R., Tschan, H., Calderon Montero, F. J., Bachl, N., and Pigozzi, F. (2007). Performance characteristics according to playing position in elite soccer. *International Journal of Sports Medicine*, 28, 222–227.

Edge, J., Bishop, D., and Goodman, C. (2006). Effects of chronic NaHCO3 ingestion during interval training on changes to muscle buffer capacity, metabolism, and short-term endurance performance. *Journal of Applied Physiology*, 101, 918–925.

Ekblom, B. (1968). Effect of physical training on oxygen transport system in man. *Acta Physiol Scand.Suppl,* 328, 1–45.

Ekblom, B. (1986). Applied physiology of soccer. *Sports Medicine*, 3, 50–60.

Ekstrand, J. (1982). 'Soccer injuries and their prevention' (doctoral dissertation). Linkoping Medical University, Sweden.

Ferrari, B. D., Impellizzeri, F. M., Rampinini, E., Castagna, C., Bishop, D., and Wisloff, U. (2008). Sprint vs. interval training in football. *International Journal of Sports Medicine*, 29, 668–674.

Henriksson, J. and Hickner, R. C. (1996). Skeletal muscle adaptation to endurance training. In D. A. D. MacLeod, R. J. Maughan, C. Williams, C. R. Madeley, J. C. M. Sharp, and R. W. Nutton (eds), *Intermittent High Intensity Exercise* (pp. 5–26). London: E. & F.N. Spon.

Hill-Haas, S. V., Dawson, B. T., Coutts, A. J., and Rowsell, G. J. (2009). Physiological responses and time-motion characteristics of various small-sided soccer games in youth players. *Journal of Sports Science*, 27, 1–8.

Houston, M. E., Bentzen, H., and Larsen, H. (1979). Interrelationships between skeletal muscle adaptations and performance as studied by detraining and retraining. *Acta Physiol Scand.,* 105, 163–170.

Iaia, F. M. and Bangsbo, J. (2010). Speed endurance training is a powerful stimulus for physiological adaptations and performance improvements of athletes. *Scandinavian Journal of Medicine and Science in Sports*, 20 Suppl 2, 11–23.

Iaia, F. M., Perez-Gomez, J., Thomassen, M., Nordsborg, N. B., Hellsten, Y., and Bangsbo, J. (2011). Relationship between performance at different exercise intensities and skeletal muscle characteristics. *Journal of Applied Physiology*, doi:10.1152/japplphysiol.00420.2010.

Iaia, F. M., Thomassen, M., Kolding, H., Gunnarsson, T., Wendell, J., Rostgaard, T. *et al.* (2008). Reduced volume but increased training intensity elevates muscle Na+-K+ pump α1-subunit and NHE1 expression as well as short-term work capacity in humans. *American Journal of Physiology – Regulatory, Integrative and Comparative Physiology*, 294, R966–R974.

Impellizzeri, F. M., Marcora, S. M., Castagna, C., Reilly, T., Sassi, A., Iaia, F. M. *et al.* (2006). Physiological and performance effects of generic versus specific aerobic training in soccer players. *International Journal of Sports Medicine*, 27, 483–492.

Jensen, J. M., Bredsgaard-Randers, M., Krustrup, P., and Bangsbo, J. (2009). Intermittent high-intensty drills improve in-seasonal performance of elite soccer players. In T. Reilly and F. Korkusuz (eds), *Science and Soccer VI* (pp. 296–301). London: Routledge.

Jensen, L., Bangsbo, J., and Hellsten, Y. (2004). Effect of high intensity training on capillarization and presence of angiogenic factors in human skeletal muscle. *Journal of Physiology*, 557, 571–582.

Kanstrup, I. L. and Ekblom, B. (1984). Blood volume and hemoglobin concentration as determinants of maximal aerobic power. *Medicine and Science in Sports and Exercise*, 16, 256–262.

40

Kelly, D. M. and Drust, B. (2009). The effect of pitch dimensions on heart rate responses and technical demands of small-sided soccer games in elite players. *Journal of Science, Medicine and Sport*, 12, 475–479.

Krustrup, P., Hellsten, Y., and Bangsbo, J. (2004). Intense interval training enhances human skeletal muscle oxygen uptake in the initial phase of dynamic exercise at high but not at low intensities. *Journal of Physiology*, 559, 335–345.

Krustrup, P., Aagaard, P., Nybo, L., Petersen, J., Mohr, M., and Bangsbo, J. (2010). Recreational football as a health promoting activity: a topical review. *Scandinavian Journal of Medicine and Science in Sports*, 20 Suppl 1, 1–13.

Krustrup, P., Mohr, M., Steensberg, A., Bencke, J., Kjaer, M., and Bangsbo, J. (2006). Muscle and blood metabolites during a soccer game: implications for sprint performance. *Medicine and Science in Sports and Exercise*, 38, 1165–1174.

Laughlin, M. H. and Armstrong, R. B. (1983). Rat muscle blood flows as a function of time during prolonged slow treadmill exercise. *American Journal of Physiology*, 244, H814–H824.

Linossier, M. T., Denis, C., Dormois, D., Geyssant, A., and Lacour, J. R. (1993). Ergometric and metabolic adaptation to a 5-s sprint training programme. *European Journal of Applied Physiology and Occupational Physiology*, 67, 408–414.

McKenna, M. J., Schmidt, T. A., Hargreaves, M., Cameron, L., Skinner, S. L., and Kjeldsen, K. (1993). Sprint training increases human skeletal muscle Na(+)-K(+)-ATPase concentration and improves K+ regulation. *Journal of Applied Physiology*, 75, 173–180.

Mohr, M., Krustrup, P., and Bangsbo, J. (2003). Match performance of high-standard soccer players with special reference to development of fatigue. *Journal of Sports Science*, 21, 519–528.

Mohr, M., Krustrup, P., and Bangsbo, J. (2005). Fatigue in soccer: a brief review. *Journal of Sports Science*, 23, 593–599.

Mohr, M., Krustrup, P., Nielsen, J. J., Nybo, L., Rasmussen, M. K., Juel, C. *et al.* (2007). Effect of two different intense training regimens on skeletal muscle ion transport proteins and fatigue development. *American Journal of Physiology – Regulatory, Integrative and Comparative Physiology*, 292, R1594–R1602.

Rampinini, E., Coutts, A. J., Castagna, C., Sassi, R., and Impellizzeri, F. M. (2007a). Variation in top level soccer match performance. *International Journal of Sports Medicine*, 28, 1018–1024.

Rampinini, E., Impellizzeri, F. M., Castagna, C., Abt, G., Chamari, K., Sassi, A. *et al.* (2007b). Factors influencing physiological responses to small-sided soccer games. *Journal of Sports Science*, 25, 659–666.

Rampinini, E., Impellizzeri, F. M., Castagna, C., Azzalin, A., Ferrari, B. D., and Wisloff, U. (2008). Effect of match-related fatigue on short-passing ability in young soccer players. *Medicine and Science in Sports and Exercise*, 40, 934–942.

Rampinini, E., Impellizzeri, F. M., Castagna, C., Coutts, A. J., and Wisloff, U. (2009). Technical performance during soccer matches of the Italian Serie A league: effect of fatigue and competitive level. *Journal of Science, Medicine and Sport*, 12, 227–233.

Ross, A. and Leveritt, M. (2001). Long-term metabolic and skeletal muscle adaptations to short-sprint training: implications for sprint training and tapering. *Sports Medicine*, 31, 1063–1082.

Rostgaard, T., Iaia, F. M., Simonsen, D. S., and Bangsbo, J. (2008). A test to evaluate the physical impact on technical performance in soccer. *The Journal of Strength and Conditioning Research*, 22, 283–292.

Sharp, R. L., Costill, D. L., Fink, W. J., and King, D. S. (1986). Effects of eight weeks of bicycle ergometer sprint training on human muscle buffer capacity. *International Journal of Sports Medicine*, 7, 13–17.

Talanian, J. L., Galloway, S. D., Heigenhauser, G. J., Bonen, A., and Spriet, L. L. (2007). Two weeks of high-intensity aerobic interval training increases the capacity for fat oxidation during exercise in women. *Journal of Applied Physiology*, 102, 1439–1447.

Thomassen, M., Christensen, P. M., Gunnarsson, T. P., Nybo, L., and Bangsbo, J. (2010). Effect of 2-wk intensified training and inactivity on muscle Na+-K+ pump expression, phospholemman (FXYD1) phosphorylation, and performance in soccer players. *Journal of Applied Physiology*, 108, 898–905.

Thorstensson, A., Sjodin, B., and Karlsson, J. (1975). Enzyme activities and muscle strength after 'sprint training' in man. *Acta Physiologica Scandinavica*, 94, 313–318.

Williams, A., Williams, A. M., and Horn, R. (2003) Physical and technical demands of different playing positions. *Insight: FA Coaches Association Journal*, 2, 24–28.

# CHAPTER 3

## FITNESS TESTING

B. Drust and W. Gregson

### INTRODUCTION

Performance in soccer is a consequence of a number of inter-dependent factors that include the technical and tactical abilities of the player, their psychological make-up and their physiological capabilities. The physiological demands of soccer require players to be competent in several aspects of fitness. Important attributes include high levels of aerobic fitness, the ability to sprint (in repeated bouts as well as one-off efforts), anaerobic power, good force-generating capabilities (muscle strength) and flexibility (Svensson and Drust, 2005).

A player's physiological capabilities can be modified as a consequence of the type and amount (frequency, duration, intensity) of activity that they complete at specific times of the season (Stolen et al., 2005). At specific stages of the year, it is therefore important to obtain objective information about a player's physical status in order to provide potentially useful data on his/her prospective performance(s) and to clarify the objectives of both short- and long-term training programmes. Such objective information may be obtained by implementing tests that attempt to evaluate physical performance capacity in relevant areas of fitness. The aims of this chapter are to present a rationale for testing soccer players and to describe and evaluate several laboratory and field tests used by trainers and sports scientists within soccer. It is not the intention of this chapter to provide information on all of the tests that are used within the sport by scientists and practitioners. The content here reflects some of the more commonly used assessments within the scientific literature and those procedures for which there is something of an evidence base for their appropriateness as assessment tools.

### PURPOSE OF PHYSIOLOGICAL TESTING

Physiological performance in soccer is no different to most sports, in that it is the result of a blend of several factors that include genetic endowment, training and the health status of the individual athlete (MacDougall and Wenger, 1991). The sports scientist, the strength and conditioner and the coach can, through physiological testing, analyse these factors and use the data to inform a number of important elements of the performance plan for a given team. The use of physiological testing programmes in soccer is common, as the complex multi-factorial nature of the game makes it very difficult to use the performance within competitive matches to evaluate each player's physiological capabilities.

The tactical requirements placed on players will vary markedly between matches, though it is unlikely that an individual's physiological capacities are taxed fully in any game, despite these varied requirements. This idea is supported by the large variability that is associated with a range of performance variables commonly used as indicators of a player's match activity. For example, the coefficient of variation (CV) for high-speed running and sprinting was around 16% and 31%, respectively, in the large sample of players analysed by Gregson et al. (2010) using a commercially available computer-automated system. These data would indicate that such variables are difficult to implement as a model of performance unless a large sample of games are available for a given individual. This requirement may be impractical for all but the best-resourced professional teams in the elite leagues around the world who can record, monitor and evaluate large numbers of players simultaneously across prolonged time periods.

Such complications necessitate alternative performance assessment strategies such as the implementation of physiological assessment programmes. Physiological testing programmes attempt to decompose the physical demands placed on players during games into discrete physiological capabilities and then devise appropriate assessment protocols to evaluate each specific parameter in isolation. The underlying assumption of such approaches is that analysing the function of a number of relevant components can give us some idea of the capabilities in a discrete element of physiological function and the potential to perform in a soccer-specific context. Such tests clearly need to be specific to the sport, as unsuitable protocols (e.g., mode of exercise) will limit the relevance of the data for the competitive situation. The two main general areas that physiological testing may inform are: (a) the development of individual physical profiles for each player in the squad; and (b) the provision of a framework for the evaluation of strategies used to improve the physical performance of players (e.g., training programmes).

## Developing individual physical profiles for players

Incorporating suitable physiological assessments can identify both strengths and weaknesses in individuals in relation to other players within the squad or across teams. If individuals have weaknesses in any particular fitness component relative to their sport, these components can be remedied by employing appropriate training programmes (MacDougall and Wenger, 1991). Training prescription should be based on the strengths/weaknesses of the individual player and the specific requirements of the player's playing position. Position-specific training programmes result in improvements in the most relevant fitness measures, thereby ensuring that players are better able to fulfil their tactical responsibilities during the game (Di Salvo and Pigozzi, 1998). These improvements may not, however, overcome individual deficiencies in genetic potential for the physiological characteristics required for the position. This may mean that the player may need to be employed in a more tactically suitable role for his/her capabilities if it is deemed important for the overall performance of the team.

**B. Drust and W. Gregson**

## Study the effectiveness of a training programme

Objective data are required with respect to changes in performance over time, in order to study the effectiveness of a training programme and/or the readiness of the individual to return to normal training and match-play following rehabilitation (Balsom, 1994). Results from a fitness test provide valuable feedback to the coach both on the usefulness of the intervention programme and on the responses of each individual athlete (MacDougall and Wenger, 1991). Such outcomes are dependent on the validity and reliability of the test (Boddington et al., 2001).

Atkinson and Nevill (1998) outline suitable definitions for the concepts of both validity and reliability. They suggest that validity is generally seen as the ability of a measurement to reflect the parameter which it was designed to measure. Validity can be difficult to assess, as a consequence of the number of different approaches that can be adopted to investigate the links between a test and its relevance to the performance of an athlete. Reliability relates to the consistency of an individual's performance on a test. As such, reliability can be evaluated by adopting a systematic approach aimed at quantifying the measurement error (both systematic bias and random error) associated with two or more trials of an identical assessment. Atkinson and Nevill (1998) state that reliability should be assessed before validity, since any measurement tool will not be valid if it does not produce consistent values in repeated measurements. As a consequence of this latter observation, sport scientists and practitioners should ensure that all tests follow suitable data collection and analysis procedures in an attempt to determine and limit the acceptable amount of error that is suitable for the test(s). As the changes in performance that may be meaningful for any given player could be very small (e.g., 1–5%), it is imperative that the error in any tests is reduced as much as possible.

Pre- and post-programme assessments should be specific to the aims of the intervention. For example, if a specific sprint-training programme is performed, the fitness test used should tax the appropriate energy system (e.g., anaerobic in nature). Anaerobic performance can also be differentiated into specific components according to the energy system that predominates (e.g., high-energy phosphates or glycolytic pathway) in the actual activity. The specificity of the test should include an assessment of this relevant energy system. It is also recommended to wait until the residual fatigue associated with the training programme has subsided, in order to prevent data from tests being affected by individuals not fully adapting to the training stimulus. Individuals should therefore be allowed the maximal time possible to allow for the remodelling associated with the training stimulus before assessment (Hoffman, 2002). Such specific time points are, however, generally poorly characterised in the majority of tests that have been used in soccer.

## FIELD TESTS

Fitness tests performed in the field have a greater degree of specificity, though they may provide less accurate measurements, as compared to laboratory tests (MacDougall and Wenger, 1991). Sport scientists and other relevant staff can therefore use field tests to evaluate specific aspects of soccer performance. For example, the Hoff test (Chamari et al., 2005) represents a good example of a soccer-specific test of aerobic performance. Such tests may therefore be more valid, as they could provide a better indication of the ability to perform in a soccer match than do laboratory-based evaluations. However, it is important to remember that no field test will determine performance during soccer match-play, as it is difficult to isolate the importance of individual physical parameters when the overall demands of the sport are so complex.

Field-based tests have the benefit of requiring minimal equipment and the potential to be carried out anywhere relatively easily. It is recommended that any testing should be performed under standardised conditions to ensure reliability. These considerations will include standardisation of the surface and, where possible, similar environmental conditions (e.g., wind speed or temperature). While equipment considerations are not essential for effective field testing, careful consideration of the approaches used is important, especially during tests which involve the recording of the time to complete a set distance (Balsom, 1994). For example, if stop-watches are used in recording sprint times, there can be an element of human error, which may affect accuracy. Such problems can be avoided by the use of electronic timing gates. Performance assessment with field tests may be most effective when carried out at regular intervals throughout the season to monitor changes in soccer-specific performance rather than on one-off occasions in an attempt to characterise specific fitness characteristics. Such approaches may, however, provide inadequate information when players start to underperform and more detailed laboratory assessments may need to be completed.

Outlined in the next section are some examples of field tests used to evaluate important components of fitness for soccer players. The assessment of muscle strength in the field is difficult, albeit some useful information can be collected using resistance equipment (both free weights and machines).

## Common field tests used in the assessment of soccer-specific fitness

### Multistage fitness test

The 20-m shuttle run has been used extensively to test soccer players (e.g., Strudwick et al., 2002; Davis et al., 1992; Tumilty, 2000; Castagna et al., 2010). The multistage fitness test (20-m shuttle run) was designed by Leger et al. (1988) to estimate $\dot{V}O_{2max}$ and has been validated by Ramsbottom et al. (1988). The test is based on repeated shuttle runs between two lines 20 m apart. The running speed is incremental and dictated by audio signals from a tape recorder. The aim of the test is for players to complete as many shuttles as possible. The 20-m shuttle run has the advantage of evaluating more than one individual at a time, can be performed with relative ease by anyone and needs minimal equipment. Performance on the test only provides an estimated $\dot{V}O_{2max}$, as opposed to laboratory tests, where a precise measurement of oxygen consumption is recorded, as expired air is not collected. It is also possible to report the test result as the number of shuttles completed during the test, though this approach is less frequently used despite its providing a more direct indicator of a player's performance.

A number of studies were completed in the years following the development of the shuttle run test that attempted to support its effective use as a field-based assessment for soccer. Ramsbottom et al. (1988) found a significant positive correlation between $\dot{V}O_{2max}$ established by direct measurements on the treadmill and performance on the 20-m shuttle test. However, other investigations have demonstrated a lack of consistency in correlations of test performance to $\dot{V}O_{2max}$ (St Clair-Gibson *et al.*, 1998). Castagna *et al.* (2010) noted a relationship between the performance on the 20-m shuttle run test and both other field-based assessments of endurance fitness (e.g., Yo-Yo test) and match performance in young soccer players. This finding may indicate that the test has a better relationship with other field-based assessments of aerobic fitness than with laboratory-based measures. It may also indicate that the test result may help to select players to perform in games, though such suggestions are probably limited by a range of assumptions associated with correlations and causality. The 20-m shuttle run does not seem to be sensitive to training interventions or to differentiate between playing standards. Odetoyinbo and Ramsbottom (1997) found that there was no significant improvement in 20-m shuttle run performance following eight weeks of high-intensity training in soccer players. There was also no significant difference in the 20-m shuttle run performance of English academy scholars (who play full time) and recreational soccer players (Edwards *et al.*, 2003).

The available published reports would seem to suggest that while the 20-m shuttle may relate to performance on other field tests, it may not be suitable for either the estimation of $\dot{V}O_{2max}$ in soccer players or to study the effects of a training intervention, especially in high-level performers in certain sports. This fact may be partly a consequence of a failure to demonstrate a maximal effort for a number of individuals completing the test. It may also be due to problems associated with predicting $\dot{V}O_{2max}$ from the number of levels and shuttle runs completed. In addition to the problems of estimating $\dot{V}O_{2max}$, the continuous activity pattern of the 20-m shuttle run does not fully represent the intermittent activity profile of soccer or soccer-specific endurance per se. This issue is important, as the pattern of exercise can play an important role in determining the physiological responses to exercise. This limitation suggests that data from the 20-m shuttle run may not be useful in predicting soccer-specific endurance.

The Yo-Yo tests

The concept of shuttle running was used by Bangsbo (1993) to devise a more soccer-specific assessment. The Yo-Yo test (Figure 3.1) includes two levels and can be used to assess an individual's endurance capacity (Yo-Yo IR1) or the ability to perform repeated intense bouts of exercise (Yo-Yo IR2) (Bangsbo *et al.*, 2008). The difference between the multistage fitness test and the Yo-Yo tests is the intermittent exercise pattern used in the Yo-Yo tests. In both of the Yo-Yo tests, a recovery period is incorporated after each pair of 20-m shuttle runs. This activity profile clearly provides a defined intermittent pattern with both an exercise and a recovery period. The difference between the Yo-Yo IR1 and the Yo-Yo IR2 primarily relates to the initial starting speed and the increases in speed that are used within the test. The Yo-Yo IR1 test starts at a lower running speed and incorporates relatively slow increases in intensity, whereas the Yo-Yo IR2 is initiated at a faster speed and includes more rapid speed changes. This difference results in the average test time being longer in the Yo-Yo IR1 (around 10–20 min) than the Yo-Yo IR2 (5–15 min). Performance in the Yo-Yo tests is indicated in a similar way to that in the multistage fitness test, with the level and number of shuttles completed being recorded. These values are then translated into a total distance covered. Both Yo-Yo tests can be performed with limited equipment and conducted in most applied settings, though again, standardised testing conditions (including surface) are important for reliability.

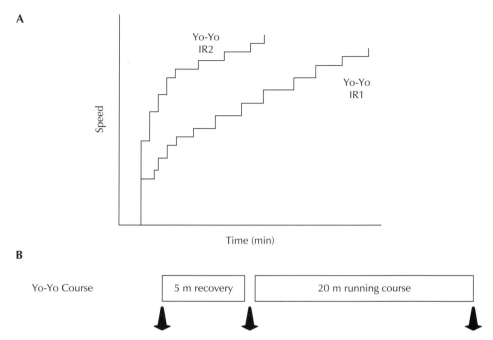

A

Yo-Yo
IR2

Yo-Yo
IR1

Speed

Time (min)

B

Yo-Yo Course | 5 m recovery | 20 m running course

**Figure 3.1** The Yo-Yo test. (A) Diagrammatic representation of the protocols for both the Yo-Yo IR1 and Yo-Yo IR2 tests; (B) illustration of the test course.

The Yo-Yo tests are amongst the most extensively studied of all fitness assessments in soccer, especially in relation to both the validity and reliability of the evaluation. Bangsbo *et al.* (2008) provide a detailed insight into the various approaches used in their research outputs to demonstrate the validity of the Yo-Yo IR1 and Yo-Yo IR2. These approaches include examining the difference between athletic groups and levels of soccer players as well as evaluating the ability of the tests to identify seasonal changes in fitness. The test scores can also be related to match-specific indicators of performance such as the high-intensity distance covered within a match. Other approaches have included examining, in detail, the physiological and metabolic responses to the Yo-Yo IR2 (Krustrup *et al.*, 2003) in an attempt to identify the energetic pathways that support the activity. A number of researchers have also attempted to quantify the reliability of both tests (see Bangsbo *et al.*, 2008 for details), with the data reporting smaller coefficients of variation for the Yo-Yo IR1 (between 5 and 9%) than the Yo-Yo IR2 (7–13%). On the whole, these assessments have supported the idea that the Yo-Yo tests are simple, relatively reliable, effective and valid ways (more so than other field-based evaluations) to evaluate important components of soccer-specific fitness. While the weight of this evidence is compelling, it would be inappropriate to accept this information without question, as such studies are not (in the majority of cases) exempt from methodological limitations that might influence the certainty with which the data can be interpreted.

**B. Drust and W. Gregson**

Sprint tests

The ability to sprint is important for crucial match actions such as reaching passes that lead to goal-scoring opportunities or making last-ditch goal-saving tackles. The ability of players to complete one-off sprint bouts has been a commonly assessed fitness parameter. While it is clear that the protocols for such assessments should relate to the sprinting activities observed in games, it is more common for sprint performance to be assessed over longer distances (e.g., 30–40 m). These sprint lengths are probably used because they are more likely to provide better information on the maximal sprint speeds of players than shorter test distances. Such strategies are also able to provide information on the acceleration of players if split times are recorded for specific components of the total sprint distance (e.g., 5 or 10 m). As there is no general consensus as to the specific nature of the protocols that can be used for sprint assessments, it is usually left to individual researchers to decide on their own approach to player evaluation, making it difficult to compare between different populations of players and establish normative values.

During a soccer match, players should be able to recover rapidly between sprints, as the exercise pattern in a match frequently requires multiple sprints with limited rest periods (Gregson et al., 2010). For example, failure to recover after a sprint when attacking may lead to an increased time in taking up a tactical defensive position, leaving the team vulnerable defensively. A number of different multiple-sprint tests have been developed to evaluate an individual's ability to repeatedly perform intense efforts. These protocols will frequently vary with respect to the number of sprints that a player completes, the length of these sprints and the recovery duration that is incorporated between each sprint. There is currently no gold-standard assessment of repeated sprint ability identified in the literature, making it difficult to evaluate the performance of specific players against a comprehensive normative reference data base. An excellent review of a range of approaches to the assessment of repeated sprint performance can be obtained from Spencer et al. (2005).

The key characteristics of a multiple-sprint test can be outlined using just one of the range of tests that are available (Bangsbo, 1994). This particular test consists of 7 x 35 m sprints separated by 25 s recovery. The test results include the fastest sprint time, mean sprint time (the average time taken to complete the seven sprints) and a fatigue index (calculated by subtracting the fastest time of the first two sprints from the slowest time for the last two sprints). The rationale behind the inclusion of a range of specific performance indicators in such a test is a consequence of the ability of each discrete variable to provide different information on a player's repeated sprint performance. The best sprint time and mean sprint time should both be low, as they each represent the player's ability to perform explosive actions on an individual basis and within a short period of time during match-play. The fatigue index is believed to be representative of a player's ability to recover between sprints. A high fatigue index may be due to physiological factors such as an inability to replenish phosphagen stores and remove blood lactate between sprints (Spencer et al., 2005). A low fatigue index is advantageous, as it indicates the ability to recover rapidly between high-intensity exercise bouts.

The approach to the analysis of the data from repeated sprint tests can also vary. It is clear from publications such as Pyne et al. (2008) that this data is sensitive to the method of analysis that is employed. This can be illustrated by the problems associated with specific variables such as fatigue indexes. These variables are a consequence of the underlying methodologies that are used to calculate such parameters (Oliver, 2009). Other variables (such as total sprint time, the cumulative time taken to complete all the sprints in the protocol) may therefore provide a better approximation of the physiological potential of the individual in this area. Such statistical manipulations of the data will not, however, compensate for individuals developing 'pacing' strategies throughout the test and therefore not exerting maximal efforts in each of the sprints. Additions to the methodological procedures associated with the test, such as ensuring that the initial sprints are within a pre-determined percentage of the fastest time, may help to alleviate such issues.

Such multiple sprint tests stimulate the anaerobic pathways (Spencer et al., 2005). For example, lactate values between 9 and 14 mmol.l$^{-1}$ were reported immediately after the seventh sprint in a group of elite players in Denmark (Bangsbo, 1994). Multiple-sprint tests are also sensitive enough to discriminate between different standards of players and to be used as an indicator of changes in physical performance (Reilly et al., 2000; Mujika et al., 2007). Such data would imply that these tests have the potential to be important components of soccer-specific test batteries, though the lack of convincing reliability assessments for a number of the test protocols does limit a conclusive view on their effectiveness.

*Tests for the determination of agility*

Agility tests are important to soccer, as they can supposedly discriminate elite soccer players from the general population better than any other field test for strength, power or flexibility (Raven et al., 1976). Elite players also perform significantly better on a 40-m agility test, as compared to sub-elite players in a talent identification study by Reilly et al. (2000). Such evidence may suggest that agility tests are not only a good indicator of performance in soccer but are also able to identify talented players by providing the clearest differentiation between elite, recreational and non-players. A close inspection of the more recent available literature does not, however, provide additional evidence to support such claims. The failure to build on these original research papers with anything more than additional testing protocols (e.g., Sheppard et al., 2006) has limited the development of our understanding of this specific fitness parameter. As a consequence, our understanding of its importance to the modern-day player is based on an ageing research base that may not reflect the performance of the contemporary player or requirements of the modern game.

Agility is the ability to change the direction of the body rapidly and is a result of a combination of strength, speed, balance and co-ordination (Draper and Lancaster, 1985). Agility tests incorporate rapid and frequent changes in direction (Figure 3.2). Since agility is a result of a number of neuro-physiological factors, it is difficult to determine exactly which variables contribute to a changed result on a test (Buttifant et al., 2002). Some agility tests have a strong correlation to velocity (e.g., Illinois Agility Run), while others have a good correlation with acceleration (the 505 test) (Draper and Lancaster, 1985). These different relationships may influence the choice of assessment if the correlations that are observed in such studies are meaningful physiologically. This may mean that the coach or sports scientist should choose a test which examines the physical components of agility they consider most important for their individual player or the specific aspect of soccer performance they are most interested in. If

# 50

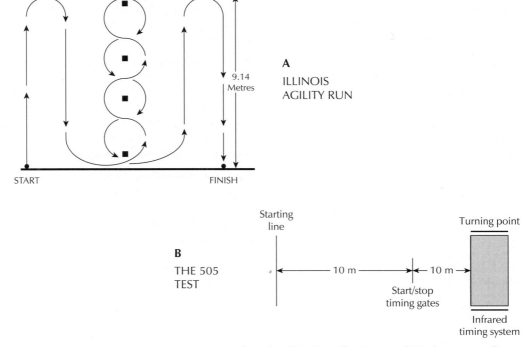

**Figure 3.2** Diagrammatic representation of (A) the Illinois Agility Run and (B) the 505 Agility Test.

*Source*: Highton *et al*. (2009).

a number of components are of interest, a number of different agility tests may need to be included so as to provide a comprehensive evaluation of an individual's agility. Future research may provide clearer guidelines on the specific requirements of tests in this area.

## LABORATORY TESTING

Laboratory tests are performed in a controlled environment to reduce the impact of extraneous variables. In contrast to field protocols, such testing procedures generally provide more accurate and reliable data in relation to isolated fitness components. The more detailed information arising from such assessments may also provide an insight into the physiological changes that arise in response to systematic training.

Due to some of the limitations of laboratory tests, such forms of assessment are often used by sport scientists to generate an idea of the general physical capabilities of the player at certain points in the season. For example, a laboratory-based assessment may be carried out at the beginning and end of pre-season to evaluate the status of the player on his return to the club after the off-season break and the subsequent effectiveness of the training that has been completed in pre-season. During the in-season period, there are probably fewer opportunities to conduct time-consuming laboratory tests across entire squads. However, more detailed laboratory assessments may be required at certain times where field-based testing has identified individual players who may be underperforming in certain areas.

Another major drawback of laboratory-based testing lies in the financial outlay needed to purchase the expensive equipment, as well as the need for specific space requirements. Furthermore, unlike the delivery of field testing, such forms of testing often require expertise that may lie outside the club's existing staff base. As a consequence, access to laboratory facilities may be difficult for clubs outside of the top level. Increasingly, many clubs draw upon the expertise and facilities available within universities or other specialist environments (e.g., hospitals, clinics), either on a consultancy basis or as part of a research programme.

The issues highlighted above have probably prevented significant developments in the approaches to laboratory testing within the sport of soccer. As a consequence, our understanding of the effectiveness of such strategies in the assessment of soccer players is probably limited in relevance, depth and currency. The data that is available comes predominantly from specific published research projects, as opposed to more 'real world' applied interventions. Such approaches may not provide the best framework with which to evaluate the usefulness of a testing philosophy that has at its core a focus on individual player performance changes. The content below therefore represents an overview of a selection of the available information on common laboratory tests that have been frequently used within the sport.

## Common laboratory tests used in the assessment of general fitness

### Tests for the determination of maximal aerobic power

Maximal aerobic power ($\dot{V}O_{2max}$) is the highest amount of oxygen that the body can utilise during exhaustive exercise while breathing air at sea level. Maximal oxygen uptake is one of the most commonly used indicators of aerobic metabolism and power, as it provides an indication on the functional limit of the oxygen transport system (Howley et al., 1995). During soccer match-play, the majority of energy provision is derived from the aerobic energy system (Stolen et al., 2005). The determination of a soccer player's maximal aerobic power is therefore important, as the oxygen transport system underpins the ability to play for 90 minutes, as well as the ability to recover between short bouts of high-intensity exercise (Stone and Kilding, 2009). When maximal aerobic power is evaluated in athletes, it is important that the test resembles the activity pattern of the specific sport. Therefore, $\dot{V}O_{2max}$ tests for soccer players should be performed on a treadmill, as opposed to a cycle ergometer, to increase the specificity of the active musculature to that used in the activity patterns observed in soccer.

The average values of $\dot{V}O_{2max}$ for top-level soccer players tend to be high, with results lying in the region of 55–70 ml kg$^{-1}$ min$^{-1}$. This range supports the belief that there is a large contribution from the aerobic energy system in playing the game (Hoff and Helgerud, 2004). Data reported in the literature for the $\dot{V}O_{2max}$ levels of elite soccer players suggest that players competing at a higher standard of competition may possess higher $\dot{V}O_{2max}$ values (Apor, 1988; Wisløff et al., 1998). Maximal oxygen uptake levels also vary with playing position,

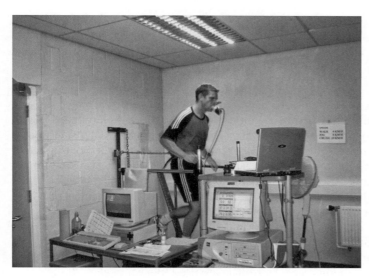

**Figure 3.3** Participant completing a $\dot{V}O_{2max}$ test on a treadmill.

with the highest and lowest values often reported in mid-fielders and central defenders, respectively, while full backs and strikers have values that are intermediate (Stolen *et al.*, 2005). The $\dot{V}O_{2max}$ of elite players is also sensitive to training regimens, with significant increases observed in the pre-season period, when there is emphasis on aerobic training (Helgerud *et al.*, 2011). Maximal oxygen uptake also seems to be related to the total amount of work done during match-play (Hoff *et al.*, 2002), with improvements in $\dot{V}O_{2max}$ corresponding to increases in the total distance covered during a match (Helgerud *et al.*, 2001).

Analysis of this information would suggest that $\dot{V}O_{2max}$ is a valid tool in the assessment of soccer players. However, $\dot{V}O_{2max}$ may not be a sensitive measure of performance in important aspects of soccer match-play (Bangsbo and Lindquist, 1992) or in the detection of training-related improvements in performance across the season (Casajus, 2001). The lack of a relationship between $\dot{V}O_{2max}$ and match-specific indicators of match performance may partly reflect methodological limitations which stem from the inherent variability of match performance (Gregson *et al.*, 2010). However, this deficiency may also be due to discrepancies in the activity patterns, as well as the underlying physiology associated with soccer-specific exercise relative to the $\dot{V}O_{2max}$ test. Limitations to $\dot{V}O_{2max}$ have been the subject of much debate, although the available evidence appears to suggest a predominantly central limitation (Hoppeler and Weibel, 2000). The intermittent nature of soccer-specific exercise often necessitates performance at exercise intensities in excess of those achieved during a $\dot{V}O_{2max}$ test (Stolen *et al.*, 2005). As a result, energy must be derived at the onset of exercise from substrates and oxygen supplies within the active musculature (Bangsbo *et al.*, 2002). Such evidence indicates that the oxidative potential of muscle is important for the performance of intense bouts of intermittent exercise in addition to $\dot{V}O_{2max}$. Maximal oxygen uptake may therefore be useful for describing players in relation to different populations and/or for evaluating changes in fitness when such alterations are expected to be large (e.g., pre-season).

It does not, however, seem to be a sensitive enough indicator of fitness for regular use within the competitive season, when changes in performance will be small and may reflect peripheral rather than central adaptations.

## Lactate threshold test

The concept of a 'lactate threshold' can be defined as the $\dot{V}O_2$ above which blood lactate exceeds resting concentrations during incremental exercise (Wasserman et al., 1973), and so marks the transition between moderate and heavy exercise. The determination of the lactate threshold is important, as this reference point indicates the onset of lactate accumulation in the blood. Such a transition may also mark the change between the predominance of aerobic and anaerobic metabolism (Jones and Doust, 2001). The lactate threshold and the 4 mmol.l$^{-1}$ reference points, also known as the onset of blood lactate accumulation (OBLA), are determined from responses during a graded treadmill test. The use of the 4 mmol.l$^{-1}$ OBLA reference point was introduced as a more objective means of analysing lactate data (Sjödin et al., 1982) as the lactate threshold inflection point requires a subjective interpretation of the threshold, unless complicated mathematical formulae are used (Beaver et al., 1985).

In endurance sports, the lactate threshold is a more useful indicator of aerobic endurance performance than is $\dot{V}O_{2max}$ (Allen et al., 1985), as the lactate threshold appears to be sensitive to changes in training, with the lactate threshold occurring at higher running speeds during a graded exercise test following a training intervention for both track athletes (Jones and Doust, 2001) and soccer players (Helgerud et al., 2001). The lactate threshold can also be used to provide information to athletes in respect to the intensity of training. By monitoring physiological variables such as heart rate during graded exercise tests, training intensities can be pre-selected according to the discrete aims of the training sessions. Such procedures may help to ensure the effectiveness of the isolated stimulus and any intervention.

The lactate threshold concept is infrequently applied to current testing programmes in the sport of soccer. Differences in the exercise pattern associated with soccer-specific intermittent exercise and steady-state exercise limit the application of the lactate threshold as an assessment tool. During intermittent exercise, the physiological response is dependent on the type of activity and/or the exercise protocol that is performed (Ballor and Volovsek, 1992). The manipulation of these variables can induce higher or lower levels of physiological stress than those associated with steady-state exercise, leading to occasions when blood lactate concentrations are above or below the lactate threshold. For example, a 2:1 exercise:rest ratio at an intensity of 110% $\dot{V}O_{2max}$ will produce higher (10.7 mmol.l$^{-1}$) blood lactate concentrations compared to a 1:2 exercise:rest ratio performed at the same intensity (2.7 mmol.l$^{-1}$) on a cycle ergometer (Ballor and Volovsek, 1992). The application of the lactate threshold will be further restricted during soccer-specific intermittent exercise, due to the additional physiological demands of game skills over and above the physiological cost of locomotion (Stolen et al., 2005). The relationship between the lactate threshold and other physiological variables (e.g., heart rate) is therefore altered under such conditions when compared to those associated with steady-state exercise. This dissociation between physiological parameters during intermittent exercise when compared to steady-state exercise will therefore affect the usefulness of tests such as the lactate threshold to predict and monitor optimal training intensity during soccer-specific intermittent exercise (Akubat and Abt, 2011).

**B. Drust and W. Gregson**

Careful considerations of methodology and the use of repeated assessments may help in the application of the lactate threshold in fitness assessment. However, its suitability for training-intensity prescription may not extend beyond steady-state exercise as a result of changes in the physiological response to exercise when the exercise pattern is intermittent, particularly soccer-specific intermittent exercise where additional energy demands are associated with unorthodox movements and game-related skills. This statement suggests that the lactate threshold is at best capable of providing a general descriptor of fitness rather than a specific indicator of physiological potential for match performance. As a result of these observations, the use of the lactate threshold may be limited to periods of assessment in which gross changes in aerobic fitness are expected (e.g., pre-season, following prolonged periods of injury), as opposed to regular use within the competitive season, when changes in performance will be small and likely associated with different pathways of adaptation.

*Tests for the determination of muscle strength*

Muscle strength is defined as the amount of force or tension a muscle or muscle group exerts against a resistance at a specified velocity during a maximal voluntary contraction (Bell and Wenger, 1992). In soccer, upper body strength is employed in throw-ins and helpful in preventing being knocked off the ball. Isometric strength is also important for stabilising the trunk, thereby providing a platform for more dynamic muscular activity of the lower body to take place. For the goalkeeper, almost all the body's muscle groups are important. In outfield players, however, strength in the lower limbs is of obvious concern: the quadriceps, hamstrings, gastrocnemius and soleus must generate high forces for jumping, kicking, tackling and changing direction as well as game-specific technical skills. These activities put great stress on the lower limbs, and developing strength in soccer players is of great importance in reducing the risk of injury (Askling et al., 2003).

Various tests of muscle strength have been employed in the assessment of soccer players. These range from performance tests using resistance equipment (both free weights and machines) and measurement of isometric strength to more contemporary measures obtained using specialist equipment. In the laboratory, isokinetic apparatus can be used in the assessment of the muscle strength of performers across most sports. Isokinetic dynamometry provides a controlled environment where the neuromuscular performance of the joint system can be stressed (Forbes et al., 2009). The muscular force against the motor-driven lever arm, or the torque, is measured with the angular velocity controlled when performing movements in the vertical plane such as knee flexion and extension. Force production during eccentric and concentric actions can also be assessed. The assessment of strength via isokinetic dynamometry will be the focus of this section, as this is the most popular approach used within soccer (Figure 3.4). Yet, a limited amount of contemporary research is available on the application of this form of strength assessment to the assessment of players, especially at the elite level.

One of the greatest advantages of isokinetic dynamometry is the accuracy in assessment provided by the constant pre-selected velocity of movement. It is also relatively sensitive in detecting changes in muscle strength during a rehabilitation programme (Kaufman et al., 1991). Isokinetic systems also permit muscle function tests to be completed across a variety of different angular velocities and joint angles. Such procedures improve its flexibility as an

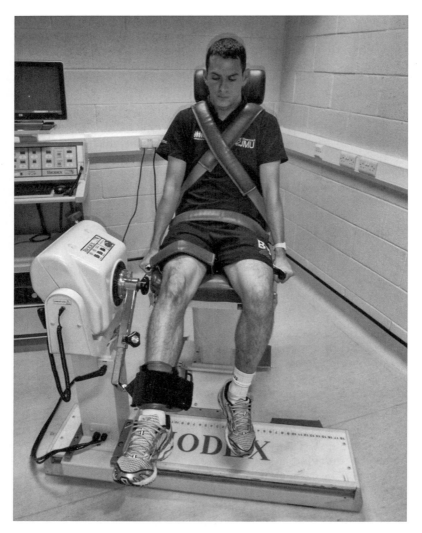

**Figure 3.4** Participant completing a muscle-strength assessment protocol on an isokinetic dynamometer.

assessment tool, but can make inter-individual comparisons difficult (Wisløff *et al.*, 1998). Appropriate filters are needed for the correction of gravity and inertial effects, to eliminate errors. Such standardised protocols are now commonplace in computerised systems such as the BioDex and Lido devices (Baltzopoulos and Gleeson, 2001).

There are some methodological limitations associated with isokinetic assessment. During the assessment, the relevant muscle group is isolated (e.g., quadriceps), and this restricts any assessment to the specific joint being examined. The isolation of muscle groups will reduce the validity of the measurements to functional performance, as the multi-joint movements

*B. Drust and W. Gregson*

involved in most sports will not be re-created. As a result, isokinetic dynamometry does not fully reflect performance in the specific movement patterns of the limbs in sports such as soccer (Cometti et al., 2001). Assessment involving free weights may be more accurate in determining the functional strength in a soccer context (Wisløff et al., 1998), as the individual has a greater freedom of movement, though such procedures may not be easy to control.

Isokinetic dynamometry can be used to assess the balance of strength between the hamstrings (H) and quadriceps (Q) muscle groups about the knee joint, calculated as either the conventional or functional H/Q ratio (Aagaard et al., 1995; 1998). The conventional H/Q ratio is calculated by dividing maximal knee flexion strength by maximal knee extension strength. However, this ratio is calculated at the same angular velocity and contraction mode (eccentric, concentric or isometric), which does not provide adequate information on agonist–antagonist muscle contraction. Therefore, the functional H/Q ratio or dynamic control ratio (DCR) was introduced as a descriptor of the agonist–antagonist balance of strength during knee flexion or extension (Aagaard et al., 1995). The functional H/Q ratio is calculated as maximal eccentric hamstring strength divided by maximal concentric quadriceps strength (during extension) or vice versa during flexion (Aagaard et al., 1998). The ideal functional H/Q ratio should be 1.0, which indicates that the hamstrings can resist as much force as the quadriceps can produce (Graham-Smith and Lees, 2002). The H/Q ratio may, however, have limited practical application in rehabilitation settings, as H/Q ratios can be identical for both injured and healthy individuals (Kannus, 1994). This may make it difficult to determine optimal H/Q ratios that can be used with injured individuals undergoing rehabilitation programmes.

Nevertheless, conventional and, especially, the functional H/Q ratio may be helpful for soccer players in identifying the functional muscle balance and stability at the knee joint (Zakas et al., 1995). Combining data on conventional H/Q ratios with those on functional H/Q ratios and values of absolute strength will result in a more thorough description of the muscular strength properties at the knee joint than that revealed by the conventional H/Q ratio alone (Aagaard et al., 1998). A high level of muscle strength relative to the functional H/Q ratio in order to stabilise the knee joint seems to be important to prevent injury (Orchard et al., 1997) with the H/Q ratio ranging between 41% and 81% in soccer players, depending on the angular velocity of movement (Rahnama et al., 2003). An ideal H/Q ratio of 60% has been suggested (Ekstrand and Gillquist, 1983). Also, it seems that H/Q ratio deficits may be more accurately determined at lower speeds, as compared to faster speeds (Orchard et al., 1997).

There is evidence to suggest that muscle strength can differentiate between age categories (Forbes et al., 2009), levels of play (Öberg et al., 1986) and playing positions (Öberg et al., 1984). Goalkeepers and defenders were reported to have a higher knee extension torque compared to mid-fielders and forwards, but differences for most players were attributed to body size (Öberg et al., 1984). These findings suggest that high levels of absolute isokinetic muscle strength in the lower limbs are important components of fitness for successful soccer play and that muscle strength increases with progressive standards of play. It seems that the H/Q ratio can also differentiate between different levels of play, as Cometti et al. (2001) reported that French elite players had a higher H/Q ratio, as compared to sub-elite players at different angular velocities from -2.09 rad.s$^{-1}$ to 5.23 rad.s$^{-1}$, except at 5.23 rad.s$^{-1}$. Similar findings have been reported for English players (Rahnama et al., 2003). A likely explanation for the higher H/Q ratios in elite players as compared to amateur players is an increased training load and specialised strength training programmes, which result in better strength balances between different muscle groups.

It is clear that the data from the assessment of muscle strength in soccer players using isokinetic dynamometers can be employed to assess muscle strength, compare positional differences in strength and evaluate the effect of resistance training. It is recommended that data from both conventional and functional H/Q ratios are combined to provide a thorough evaluation of knee joint stability and subsequent risk of injury in individuals. Test criteria may be improved by taking the angle of occurrence of peak torque into account. Due to the expensive and time-consuming nature of accommodating a whole squad for isokinetic assessment, tests should be performed at strategic intervals both pre-, in- and off-season. Such tests may be especially important when monitoring rehabilitation of muscle strength in injured players. Extensive familiarisation is required in order that a true indication of the performance capacity of the individual player may be established.

## Important considerations for fitness testing programmes

### Planning testing periods

One of the main aims of physiological testing is to monitor the effectiveness of training. It is therefore essential that tests are repeated at certain stages in the season. Unlike in many other sports, the short preparation period and long competitive season in soccer means that opportunities to undertake testing, particularly exhaustive testing, are restricted. This is particularly evident at the senior level in leading clubs, where the increased frequency of competition means that the majority of the available training time is spent recovering from matches and performing technical and tactical preparation as the next game approaches. The timing and type of testing across the season will to some extent be influenced by the level of competition and the competitive demands placed upon the squad.

Squad testing is often scheduled at key stages across the season where marked changes in physical performance are expected (e.g., pre-season phase). As such, both field and, where available, laboratory-based testing will often occur in order to provide the coaches and sport science team with detailed information on the players' fitness as the competitive phase approaches. Such testing sessions will frequently include a range of different test parameters that are important to the sport so that a comprehensive overview of the players' physical status is obtained. More detailed testing on an individual basis may also occur where under-performance is reported in players or where a player has recently returned from injury. The 'detail' of such testing sessions can be manipulated by either the inclusion of additional testing sessions or the implementation of more comprehensive assessment techniques. Both approaches attempt to provide additional information to either coach(es) or sport scientist(s) about the player(s) in question. These data facilitate the decision-making process regarding the physiological loads that the player may be able to handle in training or the reduction in the return to play time of players. Improvements in both these areas will ultimately improve the player availability data. Reserve and youth team players may also undergo such test batteries throughout the competitive phase (e.g., at 2–3 month intervals). With such populations the focus may be on their on-going development, in addition to reducing the risk of injury.

# 58

Extensive and exhaustive fitness testing is often difficult with all squads located within a professional club, particularly successful teams that have increased competitive demands. With the exception of individuals who may require special attention, only tests for fitness parameters that do not lead to high a degree of fatigue (e.g., strength and power assessments) are likely to be undertaken frequently. Modified test protocols that are sub-maximal in nature may be utilised to provide information on fitness parameters (e.g., aerobic) that have traditionally required the player to work to exhaustion (Bangsbo et al., 2008). Limited data are currently available on the comprehensive usefulness of such low-intensity surrogates in testing players, especially at the elite level. This may be an interesting area for future research.

## Organisation of testing

Testing sessions in soccer frequently involve conducting assessments on a large number of players. The use of field tests is therefore favoured. Whilst certain phases of the season (e.g., beginning and the end of pre-season) often afford the time to undertake more time-consuming laboratory tests, during the in-season phase, time is often at a premium and therefore the amount of information derived from testing needs to be maximised while ensuring that the required scientific rigour is applied. In most clubs, this approach usually involves the players rotating through a number of field tests. Completing a number of different testing stations in a single session allows data to be collected on a range of fitness parameters in a time- and space-efficient manner. If this approach is to be employed, it is vital for both the test order and timing between tests to be standardised. While there is no perfect combination of these variables, it is usually essential for any exhaustive tests (e.g., 20-m shuttle run test) to be arranged at the end of the session, to prevent fatigue affecting other performances.

## Quality assurance for fitness assessment

In order to facilitate test reliability, test administration, including the type of instruction given to the athlete, warm-up procedures, test order and the recovery time between successive tests should be standardised. This standardisation is essential for assessing any aspect of fitness in both field and laboratory evaluations. Similarly, the time of day when testing occurs, prior exercise (e.g., previous day training load) and nutritional and hydration status should be controlled where possible. This is often difficult in the elite environment, when the time with players is very limited. The test environment should be also standardised, with tests preferably performed indoors using a surface that best simulates turf (e.g., Fieldturf®). If this is not available, then wooden gym floors provide a suitable alternative because they will not change as a result of differences in environmental conditions, as outdoor turf fields will.

## Providing feedback

The final stage in the assessment process requires the test results to be communicated back to coaches and players. This step is crucial and often one that is poorly handled by the scientist. Feedback on test results should occur at the earliest possible convenience, with data presented in a format that can be easily understood by the coach and player. This frequently requires the omission of overly scientific terminology and excessively long reports. Including data from

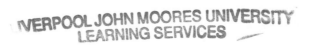

previous testing sessions, to allow trends in the player's performance across time, is a useful addition. This is a fundamentally important aspect of the testing process, as it can both educate and motivate individuals. Appropriate interventions should then be implemented in order to address any issues highlighted from the test data.

## SUMMARY

The physiological demands and the dynamic nature of soccer require players to be adept in various fitness components. Laboratory tests provide a means for coaches and sport scientists to establish the general fitness of players. Through the use of specialised equipment in the laboratory, accurate test results can be obtained on isolated fitness components. It is therefore recommended that players are tested in the laboratory, for example, at the beginning and end of pre-season, to evaluate the effectiveness of training. During the season, there are probably fewer opportunities to conduct time-consuming laboratory tests. Results from field tests provide information on specific performance changes related to the sport. Field tests therefore provide more sport-specific measures than do laboratory tests. The use of field tests restricts the interpretation of physiological mechanisms, since very limited physiological data can be measured in the field. Field tests require basic equipment, can be performed with relative ease and are relatively cost-effective. Field tests should therefore be conducted more extensively throughout the season, as opposed to laboratory tests, as testing can be carried out easily on the training ground. It is important to consider that even though data from laboratory and field tests are useful in providing information on general physical profile and soccer-specific fitness, test results can never be used to predict the overall performance during match-play, due to the complex nature of the demands of the game.

## REFERENCES

Aagaard, P., Simonsen, E.B., Magnusson, S.P., Larsson, B., and Dyhre-Poulsen, P. (1998). A new concept for isokinetic hamstring: quadriceps muscle strength ratio. *American Journal of Sports Medicine* 26, 231–237.

Aagaard, P., Simonsen, E.B., Trolle, M., Bangsbo, J., and Klausen, K. (1995). Isokinetic hamstring/quadriceps strength ratio: influence from joint angular velocity, gravity correction and contraction mode. *Acta Physiologica Scandinavica* 154, 421–427.

Akubat, I. and Abt, G. (2011). Intermittent exercise alters the heart rate–blood lactate relationship used for calculating the training impulse (TRIMP) in team sport players. *Journal of Science and Medicine in Sport* 14(3), 249–253.

Allen, W.K., Seals, D.R., Hurley, B.F., Ehsani, A.A., and Hagberg, J.M. (1985). Lactate threshold and distance-running performance in young and older endurance athletes. *Journal of Applied Physiology* 58, 1281–1284.

Apor, P. (1988). Successful formulae for fitness training. In T. Reilly, A. Lees, K. Davids and W.J. Murphy (eds), *Science and Football* (pp. 95–107). London: E. and F.N. Spon.

Askling, C., Karlsson, J., and Thorstensson, A. (2003). Hamstring injury occurrence in elite soccer players after preseason strength training with eccentric overload. *Scandinavian Journal of Medicine and Science in Sports* 13, 244–250.

**B. Drust and W. Gregson**

Atkinson, G., and Nevill, A.M. (1998). Statistical methods for assessing measurement error (reliability) in variables relevant to sports medicine. *Sports Medicine* 26, 217–238.

Ballor, D.L., and Volovsek, A.J. (1992). Effect of exercise to rest ratio on plasma lactate concentration at work rates above and below maximum oxygen uptake. *European Journal of Applied Physiology and Occupational Physiology* 65, 365–369.

Balsom, P.D. (1994). Evaluation of physical performance. In B. Ekblom (ed.), *Football (soccer)* (pp. 102–123). London: Blackwell.

Baltzopoulos, V. and Gleeson, N. (2001). Skeletal muscle function. In. R. Eston and T. Reilly (eds), *Kinanthropometry and Exercise Physiology Laboratory Manual. Vol. 2: Exercise Physiology* (pp. 1–35). London: Routledge.

Bangsbo, J. (1993). *Yo-Yo Testene*. Brondby: Danmarks Idraetsforbund.

Bangsbo, J. (1994). *The Physiology of Soccer with Special Reference to High-intensity Intermittent Exercise*. Copenhagen: H + O Storm.

Bangsbo, J., and Lindquist, F. (1992). Comparison of various exercise tests with endurance performance during soccer in professional players. *International Journal of Sports Medicine* 13, 125–132.

Bangsbo, J., Iaia, F.M., and Krustrup, P. (2008). The Yo-Yo intermittent recovery test: a useful tool for evaluation of physical performance in intermittent sports. *Sports Medicine* 38, 37–51.

Bangsbo, J., Gibala, M.J., Krustrup, P., Gonzalez-Alonso, J., and Saltin, B. (2002). Enhanced pyruvate dehydrogenase activity does not affect muscle $O_2$ uptake at the onset of intense exercise. *American Journal of Physiology* 282, R273–R280.

Beaver, W.L., Wasserman, K., and Whipp, B.J. (1985). Improved detection of lactate threshold during exercise using a log-log transformation. *Journal of Applied Physiology* 59, 1936–1940.

Bell, G.J., and Wenger, H.A. (1992). Physiological adaptations to velocity-controlled resistance training. *Sports Medicine* 13, 234–244.

Boddington, M.K., Lambert, M.I., St Clair Gibson, A. and Noakes, T.D. (2001). Reliability of a 5-m multiple shuttle test. *Journal of Sports Science* 19, 223–228.

Buttifant, D., Graham, K., and Cross, K. (2002). Agility and speed in soccer players are two different performance parameters. In W. Spinks, T. Reilly and A. Murphy (eds), *Science and Football IV* (pp. 329–333). London: Routledge.

Casajus, J.A. (2001). Seasonal variation in fitness variables in professional soccer players. *Journal of Sports Medicine and Physical Fitness* 41, 463–469.

Castagna, C., Manzi, V., Impellizzeri, F., Weston, M., and Barbero Alvarez, J.C. (2010). Relationship between endurance field tests and match performance in young soccer players. *Journal of Strength and Conditioning Research* 24, 3227–3233.

Chamari, K., Hachana, Y., Kaouech, F., Jeddi, R., Moussa-Chamari, I. and Wisloff, U. (2005). Endurance training and testing with the ball in young elite soccer players. *British Journal of Sports Medicine* 39, 24–28.

Cometti, G., Maffiuletti, N.A., Pousson, M., Chatard, J.C., and Maffulli, N. (2001). Isokinetic strength and anaerobic power of elite, subelite and amateur French soccer players. *International Journal of Sports Medicine* 22, 45–51.

Davis, J.A., Brewer, J., and Atkin, D. (1992). Pre-season physiological characteristics of English first and second division soccer players. *Journal of Sports Science* 10, 541–547.

Di Salvo, V., and Pigozzi, F. (1998). Physical training of football players based on their positional rules in the team. *Journal of Sports Medicine and Physical Fitness* 38, 294–297.

Draper, J.A. and Lancaster, M.G. (1985). The 505 test: a test for agility in the horizontal plane. *Australian Journal of Science and Medicine in Sport* 17, 15–18.

Edwards, A.M., MacFayden, A.M., and Clark, N. (2003). Test performance indicators from a single soccer-specific test differentiate between highly trained and recreationally active soccer players. *Journal of Sports Science and Medicine* 2, 23–29.

Ekstrand, J., and Gillquist, J. (1983). The avoidability of soccer injuries. *International Journal of Sports Medicine* 4, 124–128.

Forbes, H., Bullers, A., Lovell, A., McNaughton, L., Polman, R.C., and Siegler, J.C. (2009). Relative torque profiles of elite young male youth footballers: effects of age and pubertal development. *International Journal of Sports Medicine* 30, 592–597.

Graham-Smith, P. and Lees, A. (2002). Risk assessment of hamstring injury in Rugby Union place kicking. In W. Spinks, T. Reilly, and A Murphy (eds), *Science and Football IV* (pp.182–189). London: Routledge.

Gregson, W., Drust, B., Atkinson, G., and Salvo, V.D. (2010). Match-to-match variability of high-speed activities in premier league soccer. *International Journal of Sports Medicine* 31, 237–242.

Helgerud, J., Engen, L.C., Wisloff, U., and Hoff, J. (2001). Aerobic endurance training improves soccer performance. *Medicine and Science in Sports and Exercise* 33, 1925–1931.

Helgerud, J., Rodas, G., Kemi, O.J., and Hoff, J. (2011). Strength and endurance in elite football players. *International Journal of Sports Medicine.* EPub ahead of print.

Highton, J.M., Twist, C., and Eston, R.G. (2009). The effects of exercise-induced muscle damage on agility and sprint running performance. *Journal of Exercise Science and Fitness* 7, 24–30.

Hoff, J., and Helgerud, J. (2004). Endurance and strength training for soccer players: physiological considerations. *Sports Medicine* 34, 165–180.

Hoff, J., Wisloff, U., Engen, L.C., Kemi, O.J., and Helgerud, J. (2002). Soccer specific aerobic endurance training. *British Journal of Sports Medicine* 36, 218–221.

Hoffman, J. (2002). *Physiological Aspects of Sports Training and Performance.* Champaign, IL: Human Kinetics.

Hoppeler, H., and Weibel, E.R. (2000). Structural and functional limits for oxygen supply to muscle. *Acta Physiol Scand* 168, 445–456.

Howley, E.T., Bassett, D.R. Jr, and Welch, H.G. (1995). Criteria for maximal oxygen uptake: review and commentary. *Medicine and Science in Sports and Exercise* 27, 1292–1301.

Jones, A.M., and Doust, J. (2001). Limitations to sub-maximal exercise performance. In R. Eston and T. Reilly (eds), *Kinanthropometry and Exercise Physiology Laboratory Manual. Vol 2: Exercise Physiology* (pp. 235–262). London: Routledge.

Kannus, P. (1994). Isokinetic evaluation of muscular performance. *International Journal of Sports Medicine* 15, S11-S18.

Kaufman, K.R., An, K.N., Litchy, W.J., Morrey, B.F., and Chao, E.Y. (1991). Dynamic joint forces during knee isokinetic exercise. *American Journal of Sports Medicine* 19, 305–316.

Krustrup, P., Mohr, M., Amstrup, T., Rysgaard, T., Johansen, J., Steensberg, A., Pedersen, P.K. and Bangsbo, J. (2003). The Yo-Yo intermittent recovery test: physiological response, reliability and validity. *Medicine and Science in Sport and Exercise* 35 (4), 697–705.

**B. Drust and W. Gregson**

Leger, L.A., Mercier, D., Gadoury, C., and Lambert, J. (1988). The multistage 20 metre shuttle run test for aerobic fitness. *Journal of Sports Science* 6, 93–101.

MacDougall, J.D., and Wenger, H.A. (1991). The purpose of physiological testing. In J.D. MacDougall, H.A. Wenger and H.J. Green (eds), *Physiological Testing of the High-performance Athlete* (2nd edn, pp.1–5). Champaign, IL: Human Kinetics.

Mujika, I., Santisteban, J., Angulo, P., and Padilla, S. (2007). Individualised aerobic-power training in an underperforming youth elite association football player. *International Journal of Sports Physiology and Performance* 2, 332–335.

Öberg, B., Ekstrand, J., Moller, M., and Gillquist, J. (1984). Muscle strength and flexibility in different positions of soccer players. *International Journal of Sports Medicine* 5, 213–216.

Öberg, B., Moller, M., Gillquist, J., and Ekstrand, J. (1986). Isokinetic torque levels for knee extensors and knee flexors in soccer players. *International Journal of Sports Medicine* 7, 50–53.

Odetoyinbo, K., and Ramsbottom, R. (1997) 'Aerobic' and 'anaerobic' field testing of soccer players. In T. Reilly, J. Bangsbo and M. Hughes (eds), *Science and Football III* (pp. 21–26). London: E. and F.N. Spon.

Oliver, J.L. (2009). Is fatigue index a worthwhile measure of repeated sprint ability? *Journal of Science and Medicine in Sport* 12, 20–23.

Orchard, J., Marsden, J., Lord, S., and Garlick, D. (1997). Preseason hamstring muscle weakness associated with hamstring muscle injury in Australian footballers. *American Journal of Sports Medicine* 25, 81–85.

Pyne, D.B., Saunders, P.U., Montgomery, P.G., Hewitt, A.J. and Sheehan, K. (2008). Relationships between repeated sprint testing, speed and endurance. *Journal of Strength and Conditioning Research* 22, 1633–1637.

Rahnama, N., Reilly, T., Lees, A., and Graham-Smith, P. (2003). A comparison of musculoskeletal function in elite and sub-elite English soccer players. In T. Reilly and M. Marfell-Jones (eds), *Kinanthropometry VIII: Proceedings of the Eighth International Conference of the International Society for the Advancement of Kinanthropometry* (pp. 151–164). London: Taylor and Francis.

Ramsbottom, R., Brewer, J., and Williams, C. (1988). A progressive shuttle test run to estimate oxygen uptake. *British Journal of Sports Medicine* 22, 141–144.

Raven, P., Gettman, L., Pollock, M., and Cooper, K. (1976). A physiological evaluation of professional soccer players. *British Journal of Sports Medicine* 109, 209–216.

Reilly, T., Williams, A.M., Nevill, A., and Franks, A. (2000). A multidisciplinary approach to talent identification in soccer. *Journal of Sports Science* 18, 695–702.

Sheppard, J.M., Young, W.B., Doyle, T.L., Sheppard, T.A., and Newton, R.U. (2006). An evaluation of a new test of reactive agility and its relationship to sprint speed and change of direction speed. *Journal of Science and Medicine in Sport* 9, 342–349.

Sjödin, B., Jacobs, I., and Svedenhag, J. (1982). Changes in onset of blood lactate accumulation (OBLA) and muscle enzymes after training at OBLA. *European Journal of Applied Physiology and Occupational Physiology* 49, 45–57.

Spencer, M., Bishop, D., Dawson, B., and Goodman, C. (2005). Physiological and metabolic responses of repeated-sprint activities specific to field-based team sports. *Sports Medicine* 35, 1025–1044.

St Clair-Gibson, A., Broomhead, S., Lambert, M.I. and Hawley, J.A. (1998). Prediction of maximal oxygen uptake from a 20-m shuttle run as measured directly in runners and squash players. *Journal of Sports Science* 16, 331–335.

Stolen, T., Chamari, K., Castagna, C., and Wisloff, U. (2005). Physiology of soccer: an update. *Sports Medicine* 35, 501–536.

Stone, N.M., and Kilding, A.E. (2009). Aerobic conditioning for team sports ahtletes. *Sports Medicine* 39, 615–642.

Strudwick, A., Reilly, T., and Doran, D. (2002). Anthropometric and fitness characteristics of elite players in two football codes. *Journal of Sports Medicine and Physical Fitness* 42, 239–242.

Svensson, M., and Drust, B. (2005). Testing soccer players. *Journal of Sports Science* 23, 601–618.

Tumilty, D. (2000). Protocols for the physiological assessment of male and female soccer players. In C.J. Gore (ed.), *Physiological Tests for Elite Athletes* (pp. 356–362). Champaign, IL: Human Kinetics.

Wasserman, K., Whipp, B.J., Koyl, S.N., and Beaver, W.L. (1973). Anaerobic threshold and respiratory gas exchange during exercise. *Journal of Applied Physiology* 35, 236–243.

Wislöff, U., Helgerud, J., and Hoff, J. (1998). Strength and endurance of elite soccer players. *Medicine and Science in Sports and Exercise* 30, 462–467.

Zakas, A., Mandroukas, K., Vamvakoudis, E., Christoulas, K., and Aggelopoulou, N. (1995). Peak torque of quadriceps and hamstring muscles in basketball and soccer players of different divisions. *Journal of Sports Medicine and Physical Fitness* 35, 199–205.

# CHAPTER 4

## RECOVERY FROM TRAINING AND MATCHES

I. Mujika, S. Halson, C. Argus and P. Krustrup

### INTRODUCTION

Professionalism in soccer has provided the foundation for elite athletes to focus purely on training and competition. Optimal recovery from training and performance provides numerous benefits during repetitive high-level training and competition, and the rate and quality of recovery in professional athletes may be as important as the training itself. Therefore, investigating different recovery interventions and their effect on fatigue, muscle injury, recovery and performance is important. A number of recovery strategies are considered important for the elite athlete. While the amount of research into recovery has increased substantially in recent years, there is little scientific information specifically focused on this topic in soccer. Therefore, evidence from other team sports will be presented when considering potential implications for elite soccer players.

### DEMANDS OF MATCH PLAY

Like most team sports (e.g., basketball, hockey, rugby, team handball), soccer can be described as moderate-to-long duration exercise including repeated bouts of high-intensity activity interspersed with periods of low-to-moderate intensity active recovery or passive rest. From a physiological perspective, soccer is characterised by the moderate-to-long distances covered by players during match play (e.g., 8 to 12 km), as well as the variable activity pattern with 800–1500 speed changes, including 125–500 high-intensity runs and 20–40 maximal sprints per match (Bangsbo, 1994; Bradley et al., 2009; Di Salvo et al., 2007; Reilly and Thomas, 1976). In addition, hundreds of specific intense actions with a high concentric and eccentric muscle force are performed in each match, including tackles, jumps, turns, shots, and dribbles (Bloomfield et al., 2007; Mohr et al., 2003). The ability of players to perform repeated sprints with short-duration recovery in between is an important determinant of performance in intermittent team sports (Krustrup et al., 2003; Rampinini et al., 2007; Spencer et al., 2005). This activity pattern determines to a great extent the physiological requirements of match-play and the recovery needs after matches. Physiological measurements conducted during match-play have shown that aerobic loading is high throughout games and that a high anaerobic energy turnover occurs during the intense running bouts and the specific intense actions. Average heart rate is ~85% and 20–35% of the total time is spent with heart rate values >90% of individual maximal heart rate (Bangsbo, 1994; Ekblom, 1986; Krustrup et al., 2005, 2011).

At the same time, average blood lactate values are 3–8 mM with individual values of 10–14 mM (Krustrup et al., 2006, 2010; Mohr et al., 2010).

Researchers have also investigated the muscle metabolite changes that occur during real and simulated soccer games, recording individual muscle lactate and creatine phosphate values >35 and <10 mmol/kg dw, respectively, confirming periodically high rates of glycolysis as well as creatine phosphate degradation (Krustrup et al., 2006; Bendiksen et al., 2012). The studies also revealed increases in muscle IMP and plasma ammonia towards the end of games, suggesting an activation of adenosine monophosphate deaminase (Krustrup et al., 2006). In accordance with the findings of a high aerobic energy turnover and periods with a high rate of glycolysis, a significant muscle glycogen depletion has been shown to occur over the course of a match (Bangsbo et al., 2006; Gunnarsson et al., 2011; Saltin, 1973). Furthermore, histochemical muscle analyses have shown that about half of the individual slow-twitch and fast-twitch muscle fibres are empty or almost empty of glycogen after a soccer match (Gunnarsson et al., 2011; Krustrup et al., 2006, 2011), and reduced fuel stores may well have implications for the ability to perform repeated intense exercise towards the end of, and in the recovery period after, soccer matches (Figure 4.1).

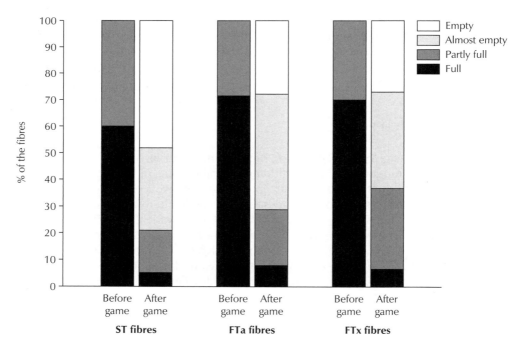

**Figure 4.1** Fibre type-specific glycogen depletion after a soccer match (n=30).

*Source*: Krustrup et al. (2006, 2011); Gunnarsson et al. (2011).

I. Mujika, S. Halson , C. Argus and P. Krustrup

## PERFORMANCE DECREMENTS DURING AND AFTER MATCH PLAY

Major performance decrements are observed towards the end of soccer matches at elite and sub-elite level. Activity profile analyses show that the amount of high-intensity running and sprinting is reduced by 25–50% in the last 15-min period of a game (Bradley *et al.*, 2009; Krustrup *et al.*, 2005, 2010; Mohr *et al.*, 2003, 2010). Various test procedures performed before and after competitive and friendly games have revealed that repeated sprint and jump performance is reduced by 2–8% (Andersson *et al.*, 2008; Krustrup *et al.*, 2006, 2010; Mohr *et al.*, 2004, 2010) and that Yo-Yo intermittent endurance performance is reduced by 50–60% after soccer matches (Krustrup *et al.*, 2010). Some researchers have shown performance decrements in single muscle actions such as isometric and dynamic knee-extensions (Andersson *et al.*, 2008; Krustrup *et al.*, 2011; Thorlund *et al.*, 2009) and single jump performance (Andersson *et al.*, 2008), although single jump performance is not always affected (Krustrup *et al.*, 2010; Mohr *et al.*, 2010). While some of the game-induced performance decrements are temporary (Mohr *et al.*, 2003), others have a slow recovery. For example, knee-extensor force/torque was still lowered 24 and 27 h after soccer matches (Andersson *et al.*, 2008; Krustrup *et al.*, 2011), and in the study by Andersson *et al.* (2008) counter-movement jump performance was not fully recovered 69 h after a match.

## MUSCLE RECOVERY AFTER MATCH PLAY

It has been known for several decades that muscle glycogen resynthesis is impaired after soccer matches and training, and this may be one of the reasons why players train less than athletes in endurance sports (Saltin, 1973; Jacobs *et al.*, 1982). The glycogen resynthesis rate after a soccer match is only one-third to one-half of the resynthesis rate observed after long-term endurance exercise such as cycling, and muscle glycogen levels are not fully recovered until 48 h or even 72 h after matches (Bangsbo *et al.*, 2006; Gunnarsson *et al.*, 2011; Jacobs *et al.*, 1982; Krustrup *et al.*, 2011). A recent study has shown that although none of the individual muscle fibres was empty of glycogen after 48 h of recovery, the average glycogen content was still significantly lowered in the fast-twitch fibre pool (Gunnarsson *et al.*, 2011). Potential reasons for failure to refuel effectively after competition include interference with glycogen storage, due to the presence of muscle damage arising from eccentric activities (Zehnder *et al.*, 2004) or contact injuries, a non-optimal diet (Bangsbo *et al.*, 2006; Burke, 2010; Jacobs *et al.*, 1982) and excessive intake of alcohol (Burke, 2007).

Inevitably, blood markers of muscle damage, such as creatine kinase (CK) are elevated for as long as 48–72 h and quadriceps muscle soreness is reported for as long as 72 h after matches (Andersson *et al.*, 2008; Krustrup *et al.*, 2011), whereas the match-induced reduction in muscle sarcoplasmatic reticulum function was no longer present 24 h after a soccer match (Krustrup *et al.*, 2011) (Figure 4.2). A recent study using a simulated soccer protocol including 90 min of soccer-like activities with no body contact but multiple running activities, unorthodox running modes and soccer-specific intense actions such as shots, headers and turns, observed similar slow rates of glycogen resynthesis as are observed after high-level competitive soccer games (Bendiksen *et al.*, 2012), suggesting that body contact and contact injuries are not the cause of delayed glycogen resynthesis. Additional studies are warranted

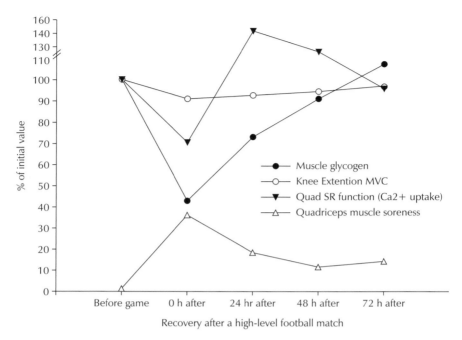

**Figure 4.2** Recovery of muscle glycogen, maximal voluntary contraction (MVC) performance, sarcoplasmic reticulum (SR) function and muscle soreness during the first 72 hours after a competitive soccer game.

*Source*: Adapted from Krustrup *et al*. (2011).

to elucidate the underlying mechanisms and the time-course for muscle recovery after soccer match-play and training.

## NUTRITION

A mismatch between the carbohydrate needs of training and competition and dietary intake can be a cause of poor performance in soccer. The current guidelines for carbohydrate intakes amended to suit a range of needs for team sport players are summarised in Table 4.1.

There are several published reports from both field and laboratory viewpoints which have examined the value of fuelling up in preparation for soccer match-play. In one investigation, professional soccer players completed an intermittent high-intensity protocol of field and treadmill running lasting ~90 min, after a 48-h intake of high-carbohydrate (~8 g/kg/d) or moderate carbohydrate (~4.5 g/kg/d) diets. The high-carbohydrate diet increased intermittent running to fatigue at the end of the protocol by ~1 km, although the performance enhancement was more marked in some participants than others (Bangsbo *et al*., 1992). Similarly, movement analysis of a four-a-side indoor soccer game lasting 90 min was undertaken following 48 h of high (~8 g/kg/d) or moderate (~3 g/kg/d) carbohydrate intake. The high-carbohydrate diet increased muscle glycogen by 38% and allowed soccer players to complete ~33% more high-intensity work during the game (Balsom *et al*., 1999).

# 68

**Table 4.1** Fuel requirements for training and match-play adapted for team players.

| | Situation | Carbohydrate targets per kg of the player's body mass |
|---|---|---|
| | *Daily needs for fuel and recovery\** | |
| Minimal | Light training programme (low-intensity or skill-based exercise) | 3–5 g per kg each day |
| Moderate | Moderate exercise programme (i.e., ~1 h per day) | 5–7 g per kg each day |
| High | Endurance program (i.e., 1–3 h per day of moderate- to high-intensity exercise) | 6–10 g per kg each day |
| Very High | Extreme exercise (i.e., >4–5 h per day of moderate- to high-intensity exercise) | 10–12 g per kg each day |

*Note*: \* Players with high body mass or players undertaking a weight-loss programme may be better suited to reduce their fuel intake to the needs of the previous category.

| | *Special situations requiring fuel* | |
|---|---|---|
| Maximal daily refuelling | Post-event recovery or aggressive fuelling ('carbohydrate loading') before the game | 7–12 g per kg for each 24 h |
| Speedy refuelling | Less than 8 h recovery between 2 demanding workouts | 1–1.2 g per kg immediately after first session. Repeated each hour until the normal meal schedule is resumed |
| Pre-game fuelling | Before the game | 1–4 g per kg eaten 1–4 h before exercise |
| During game | Short games or small fuel demands. Moderate game demands (e.g., games 60–90 min). Large game fuel demands (e.g., games >2 h for mobile players). May also include players who start match poorly fuelled | Small amounts of carbohydrate – including simply tasting carbohydrate. 30–60 g/h. Perhaps up to 80–90 g/h |

*Source*: Mujika and Burke (2010).

Abt *et al*. (1998) examined the effect of a high-carbohydrate diet on the dribbling and shooting skills of soccer players using a simulated game protocol. The findings indicated that a high-carbohydrate diet did not increase the ability of players to shoot or dribble. Several explanations are possible: either muscle glycogen depletion may not impair the ability of the player to execute game skills; alternative fatigue mechanisms such as dehydration or increased lactate production may be causative factors in the reduction in skill performance; or the treadmill protocol employed failed to induce a degree of glycogen depletion or fatigue large enough to cause a significant fall in performance.

Rapid refuelling after the completion of the game will be important in situations where there is only a short interval between matches or where the player needs to undertake a significant training load between matches (see Table 4.1). There are few published reports focusing on actual glycogen restoration following real or simulated competition in soccer, most of which show failure to replenish glycogen stores within 24 h (Bangsbo et al., 2006; Bendiksen et al., 2012; Gunnarsson et al., 2011; Jacobs et al., 1982; Krustrup et al., 2011), with the exception of the study by Zehnder et al. (2001). In the study by Gunnarsson et al. (2011), 10 high-level players were provided a diet high in glycogen (~10 g/kg/d) as well as protein (~3 g/kg/d whey protein) during the first 48 h after a competitive match, and in the study by Krustrup et al. (2011) 7 high-level players were given a carbohydrate-rich diet (~9 g/kg/d) and creatine supplementation (0.2–0.25 g/kg/d) during the first 5 days after a competitive match. However, the glycogen resynthesis for those players was below 6 and 3.5 mmol/kg dw/h during the first and second 24-h period and not higher than what has been observed for players with normal diets. Lack of fuelling does not seem to be the primary cause of the delayed muscle resynthesis after matches. Nonetheless, current sports nutrition guidelines for everyday eating recommend that team sport athletes consume adequate carbohydrate to meet the fuel requirements of their training programme, thus allowing training sessions to be undertaken with high carbohydrate availability (Burke, 2010).

However, some researchers have found that when exercise is undertaken with low muscle glycogen content, the transcription of a number of genes involved in training adaptations is enhanced (Barr and McGee, 2008). This information explains the recently described 'train low, compete high' paradigm: training with low glycogen/carbohydrate availability to enhance the training response, but competing with high fuel availability to promote performance. There are a number of potential ways to reduce carbohydrate availability for the training environment, including doing two training sessions in close succession without opportunity for refuelling (Hansen et al., 2005; Yeo et al., 2008), or training in a fasted state with only water intake (Cox et al., 2010). As reviewed by Burke (2010), it should be pointed out that these do not always promote a low carbohydrate diet per se, nor restrict carbohydrate availability for all training sessions, and some researchers have reported a reduction in self-chosen training intensity (Yeo et al., 2008; Hulston et al., 2010).

One study has applied the 'train low' theory to a team sport model. Morton and colleagues (2009) followed the progress of 3 groups of recreationally active men who undertook 4 weekly sessions of a set programme of high-intensity running with either high carbohydrate availability (1 session per day), train low (twice a week training with two training sessions in succession), or train low + glucose (as before, but with glucose intake before and during the second session). All groups recorded a similar improvement in $\dot{V}O_{2max}$ (~10%) and distance run during a Yo-Yo Intermittent Recovery Test 2 protocol (~18%), although the group that trained with low availability of exogenous and endogenous carbohydrate sources showed greater metabolic advantages such as increased activity of oxidative enzymes. Clearly, more work is needed on this topic.

I. Mujika, S. Halson , C. Argus and P. Krustrup

## HYDROTHERAPY

Although hydrotherapy is incorporated widely into post-exercise recovery regimes, information regarding these interventions is largely anecdotal. The human body responds to water immersion with changes in cardiac response, peripheral resistance, skin, core and muscle temperature alterations and changes in blood flow (Wilcock et al., 2006). Hydrotherapy may thus have an effect on inflammation, body temperature, immune function, muscle soreness and perception of fatigue.

Two published reports have examined recovery in soccer players. Tessitore et al. (2007) examined the effects of four different recovery interventions (passive, aerobic exercise, water-based aerobic exercise and electrostimulation) on jump and sprint performance as well as perceptions of recovery in elite junior soccer players. The time between exercise sessions was 5 h, with recovery interventions lasting 20 min. There were no effects of any of the recovery strategies on subsequent performance; however aerobic exercise and electrostimulation were more effective than passive rest and water-based aerobic exercise in reducing perceptions of muscle pain. It is important to note that perceived muscle pain was low in all trials (between 1 and 2 out of a possible 10), therefore levels of muscle damage may have been minimal, allowing recovery to occur in the 5-h timeframe. Similarly, Rowsell et al. (2009) conducted a study in high-performance junior soccer players, with 4 matches played over 4 days and recovery completed after each match. No effect of cold water immersion was observed when compared to thermoneutral water immersion on indicators of soccer performance. However, the perception of fatigue and muscle soreness was lower in the cold water immersion group.

In other team sports, researchers have reported that contrast water therapy has no beneficial effect on performance during repeated sprinting (Hamlin, 2007). Twenty rugby players performed 2 repeated sprint tests separated by 1 h; between trials they completed either contrast water therapy or active recovery. While substantial decreases in blood lactate concentration and heart rate were observed following contrast water therapy, compared to the first exercise bout, performance in the second exercise bout was decreased regardless of the intervention (Hamlin, 2007).

When examining the effect of various recovery strategies (passive, active, cold water immersion, contrast water immersion), King and Duffield (2009) reported no significant effects of strategies on performance during a simulated netball circuit (vertical jump, 20-m sprint, 10-m sprint and total circuit time). However, effect sizes showed trends for a smaller decline in sprint performance and vertical jumps with both cold water immersion and contrast water immersion. The timeframe between testing sessions was 24 h, suggesting that complete recovery may have occurred prior to repeat testing. It is possible that the water immersion protocols were not substantial enough to have an effect, with immersion to the iliac crest only and showers used for the hot water exposure in the contrast water therapy. This finding may suggest that muscle temperature is a key factor when considering the timing of recovery strategies.

The effectiveness of three recovery strategies (carbohydrate and stretching, cold water immersion and full leg compression garments) was examined pre and post a 3-day tournament-style basketball competition in state-level players (Montgomery et al., 2008). Recovery was performed each day and the athletes played one full 48-min game per day. Sprint, vertical jump and agility performance decreased across the 3-day tournament, indicating accumulated fatigue. Cold water immersion was substantially better than other strategies in maintaining 20-m acceleration. Cold water immersion and compression showed similar benefits in maintaining line-drill performance when compared to carbohydrate and stretching. It should be noted that in well-controlled laboratory studies, positive effects of various forms of hydrotherapy have been demonstrated. Limited studies in team sports, combined with differences in methodology, have resulted in differences between the above studies and previous laboratory research.

## SLEEP

The need for athletes to achieve an appropriate quality and/or quantity of sleep may have significant implications on performance and recovery, and reduce the risk of developing overreaching or overtraining. However, the fundamental question of *why* humans require sleep is largely unanswered. As the duration and timing of sleep are tightly regulated, it is assumed that sleep provides a number of important psychological and physiological benefits. It is probable that sleep has multiple functions across a diverse range of physical and cognitive aspects and that these functions are strongly interrelated.

While the exact function of sleep may not be clear, the effects of sleep deprivation on exercise performance are somewhat clearer. Researchers have demonstrated changes in exercise performance following partial sleep deprivation (Reilly and Deykin, 1983; Sinnerton and Reilly, 1992). It appears that sustained exercise may be more affected than single maximal efforts, and thus longer submaximal exercise tasks may be affected following sleep deprivation (Reilly and Edwards, 2007). With respect to recovery, the suggested recuperative and restorative effects of sleep may have necessary beneficial effects on athletic recovery. In particular, impairments in the immune and endocrine system (Reilly and Edwards, 2007) that result from sleep deprivation may impair the recovery process, and hence adaptation to training. Appropriate sleep quality and quantity is anecdotally reported to be the single best recovery strategy available to elite athletes.

In a recent study, athletes and coaches ranked sleep as the most prominent problem when they were asked about the causes of fatigue/tiredness (Fallon, 2007). Sleep characteristics ranked first when athletes were asked about the aspects of the clinical history that they thought were important. Thus, although there is almost no scientific evidence to support the role of sleep in enhancing recovery, elite athletes and coaches often identify sleep as a vital component of the recovery process.

## ACTIVE RECOVERY

An active recovery consists of low-intensity aerobic exercise that can be performed using different modes such as cycling, jogging, aqua jogging or swimming. Additionally, some athletes perform low-intensity resistance training as another form of active recovery. The superiority of an active recovery over a passive recovery has been regularly reported and attributed to enhanced blood flow and clearance of lactic acid and other metabolic byproducts. However, the removal of lactate may not be a valid indicator of enhanced recovery and performance (Bond et al., 1991). Other possible benefits attributed to an active recovery include facilitation

I. Mujika, S. Halson , C. Argus and P. Krustrup

of a smoother decline in body temperature (as body temperature continues to rise if exercise is stopped abruptly), reductions in post-exercise muscle soreness and suppressing nervous system activity, potentially promoting sleep (Carter et al., 2002; Reilly and Brooks, 1986; Smith and Reilly, 2004).

Research examining the effects of active recovery following soccer training or competition has produced inconsistent findings. Tessitore et al. (2008) reported that the implementation of an active recovery protocol (16 min walking, jogging and running, plus 4 min stretching) immediately following an indoor soccer game (futsal) was no more beneficial in improving anaerobic performance and muscle pain than a passive recovery. Similarly, Andersson et al. (2008) reported that a combined active recovery of sub-maximal cycling and low-intensity resistance training performed 22 h and 46 h following a soccer match did not enhance recovery, as compared to passive recovery. Tessitore et al. (2007) reported that an active recovery was ineffective in improving recovery following a 2-h soccer training session. In contrast, Reilly and Rigby (2002) investigated the effects of active and passive recoveries following a soccer match. Immediately following recovery, there was a 50% greater decrement in the fatigue index of a repeated 30-m sprint test in the passive condition when compared to an active recovery. Additionally, at 24 h post match, 30-m sprint time was 5% slower in the passive condition. Furthermore, active recovery significantly reduced the decline in horizontal and vertical jump performance, as compared to passive recovery at all time points.

The effectiveness of an active cycle recovery (7 min at 80–100 rpm, ~150 W) on levels of creatine kinase (CK), a marker of muscle damage, has been assessed following a rugby union match (Gill et al., 2006). Eighty-four h post match, CK had returned to 88% of post match values, whilst at the same time point following passive recovery CK had only returned to 39%, indicating a faster recovery when an active recovery was performed. The active recovery was not significantly different to contrast water therapy or compression recovery strategies, which had returned to 85% and 84% of post match values, respectively. No performance measures were assessed (Gill et al., 2006).

There are mixed findings on the effects of an active recovery between training sessions or following competition in team sport athletes. However, as no detrimental effects on performance have been reported following an active recovery (when compared to a passive recovery) between training sessions, along with a small amount of literature reporting enhanced performance (and possible sleep benefits), we would recommend an active recovery following training and competition.

## MASSAGE

Massage has been suggested to aid in recovery through increased peripheral blood flow, reduced inflammation, faster healing, reduced muscle pain and increased joint flexibility and range of motion. However, the use of massage as a recovery intervention has been shown to have limited performance benefits.

Hilbert et al. (2003) reported that a 20-min massage 2 h following a muscle-damaging protocol had no effect on recovery of peak torque. However, soreness was lower following massage relative to the control group at 48 h post exercise. Farr et al. (2002) assessed the effects of massage following downhill walking and reported improved perceptions of soreness, albeit it did not prevent the decline in isometric strength and vertical jump height. Zainuddin *et al.* (2005) reported that following eccentric exercise, massage significantly improved perceived soreness and reduced CK levels. However, no significant effects on recovery of muscle strength and range of motion were observed.

In less damaging exercise protocols, more consistent with typical sporting competition, Hemmings *et al.* (2000) observed that a reduction in average boxing punch force was not prevented by a 20-min massage, despite greater perceptions of recovery between bouts. Additionally, Dawson *et al.* (2004) reported that 30 min of massage immediately following a half marathon had no effect on peak torque, muscle soreness and swelling. In contrast, Brooks *et al.* (2005) indicated that forearm and hand massage following fatiguing isometric exercise significantly improved grip-strength, as compared to a passive control. Mancinelli *et al.* (2006) observed that receiving massage following 2 days of pre-season training, and immediately prior to post-testing, significantly improved vertical jump displacement, reduced soreness and prevented a decrease in shuttle run time. However, findings from this study would be impossible to replicate, as the training performed was not reported. Lane and Wenger (2004) reported that massage reduced the decline in total work completed between 2 cycle bouts. Although not significantly different, active recovery and cold water immersion improved recovery of performance more than the massage treatment.

It appears that the use of massage for enhancing recovery of performance may be limited. However, as massage may have potential benefits in injury prevention and management and also in psychological aspects of recovery (such as perceptions of soreness and perceived recovery), it may still be beneficial for soccer players.

## COMPRESSION

Compression clothing has been adapted from the medical setting, where it is used to treat various lymphatic and circulatory conditions. Athletes commonly wear elastic compression clothing during long-haul travel and/or following strenuous exercise. Compression garments are thought to improve venous return through application of graduated compression to the limbs from proximal to distal (Bochmann *et al.*, 2005). The external pressure created may reduce the intramuscular space available for swelling and promote stable alignment of muscle fibres, attenuating the inflammatory response and reducing muscle soreness (Bochmann *et al.*, 2005; Davies *et al.*, 2009; Kraemer *et al.*, 2001).

There is limited research in the area of compression for exercise recovery. In a fatiguing protocol consisting of 10 sets of 10 drop jumps, full leg compression worn for 12 h following exercise significantly improved recovery of countermovement jump-squat performance, isokinetic strength and muscle soreness. No differences were observed in CK levels (Jakeman *et al.*, 2010). Kraemer *et al.* (2010) reported that wearing full body compression for 24 h following a typical resistance training session resulted in significant improvements in perceived fatigue and muscle soreness, reduced swelling and CK levels and improved bench throw power. No differences were observed in lower body power, as compared to the control (Figure 4.3). Duffield *et al.* (2010) investigated the use of lower body compression worn during and following high-intensity sprint and plyometric exercise. Wearing compression resulted in a

74

smaller performance decline in a repeated jump task, along with reduced muscle soreness and CK levels. However, no differences were observed for repeat sprint performance, as compared to the control group. These authors examined the effects of wearing compression both during and after an 80-min high-intensity exercise circuit in rugby union players. It was reported that compression garments did not improve or hamper subsequent performance (speed and power), although participants reported reduced levels of perceived muscle soreness (Duffield et al., 2008). Montgomery et al. (2008) reported that wearing lower body compression following 3 basketball matches over 3 days did not enhance recovery of performance measures, as compared to a control group.

Research on the effects of compression on recovery from exercise has produced inconsistent findings, but no detrimental effects have been reported. Compression is likely to be beneficial for improving psychological and perceptual aspects of recovery and it may enhance recovery of both performance and physiological measures.

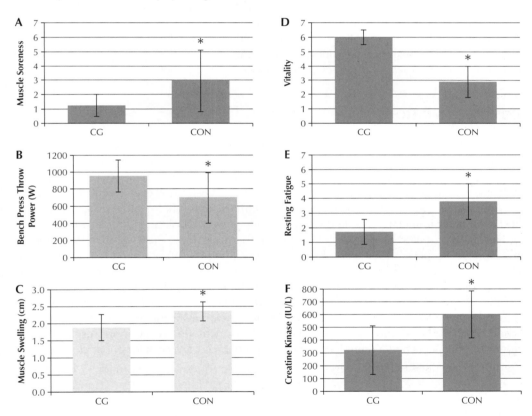

**Figure 4.3** Mean ± SD of various parameters (A–F) for trained men assessing the effectiveness of a compression garment (CG), compared to a control condition (CON) 24 h following a typical heavy resistance training workout.

*Source*: Kraemer *et al.* (2010).
*Note*: * p < 0.05 from corresponding CG condition

## STRETCHING

Stretching following training is one of the most commonly used recovery strategies. Stretching can improve flexibility and range of motion, whilst appropriate (dynamic) stretching performed prior to exercise can improve performance (Amiri-Khorasani et al., 2010). Anecdotal evidence suggests that stretching post training or competition enhances muscle relaxation, reduces muscle stiffness and soreness and helps to prevent injury in subsequent training bouts. However, the scientific evidence in support of stretching during recovery is unclear (Andersen, 2005; Thacker et al., 2004).

Kinugasa and Kilding (2009) assessed the effects of 7 min of static stretching following a soccer game. Stretching was not as effective as contrast water therapy or a combined recovery (contrast water therapy and active recovery) for improving players' perceived recovery. Similarly, Montgomery et al. (2008) reported that a combined recovery strategy (stretching plus carbohydrate ingestion) performed immediately after 3 basketball games over 3 days was not as effective as cold water immersion for restoring physical performance (20-m sprint, basketball-specific running drill, sit and reach). Although stretching is commonly used as a recovery strategy, researchers have indicated that stretching following exercise may not provide any benefit for improving subsequent performance (Barnett, 2006).

## COMBINED METHODS

A combined-method approach may be more beneficial for improving recovery than when recovery methods are performed in isolation. A combined recovery of active cycling and massage was significantly better at maintaining repeated cycle performance than active cycling or massage individually (Monedero and Donne, 2000). Al Nawaiseh et al. (2007) reported that a combined recovery of nutrition (antioxidant vitamins), anti-inflammatory drugs (ibuprofen) and cold water immersion resulted in significantly greater absolute and relative mean cycle power than a passive recovery. Combined methods have been shown to improve psychological aspects of recovery. Kinugasa and Kilding (2009) observed that a combined recovery of active cycling and cold water immersion was more effective at improving perceptions of recovery following a soccer match than when each strategy was performed in isolation. Similarly, Jakeman et al. (2010) reported that a combination of compression and massage significantly improved perceptions of soreness following intense plyometric exercise, when compared to compression or a passive recovery alone. While more research is still required, it appears that a combined-method approach is beneficial for enhancing recovery following training or competition.

## SUMMARY

Optimal recovery from training and matches may provide numerous benefits during repetitive high-level training and competition. Soccer is characterised by a high-intensity intermittent activity pattern over a fairly long duration, with high aerobic loading and a high anaerobic energy turnover inducing glycogen depletion, creatine phosphate degradation and adenine

I. Mujika, S. Halson , C. Argus and P. Krustrup

nucleotide deamination. Fatigue and performance decrements are observed towards the end of soccer matches. Glycogen resynthesis is impaired after soccer matches and training, and a mismatch between the carbohydrate needs of training and competition and dietary intake can be a cause of poor performance in soccer. There is limited evidence that training with low glycogen availability may induce greater metabolic adaptations, but current sports nutrition guidelines recommend that soccer players consume a high-carbohydrate diet to meet the fuel requirements of their training programme. Appropriate sleep quality and quantity is the single best recovery strategy available to soccer players. Other recovery strategies such as hydrotherapy, low-intensity active recovery, massage, compression garments, stretching or various combinations of these methods may have merit as recovery-enhancing strategies, but research has produced inconsistent findings and more investigation is needed before authoritative recommendations can be made.

## REFERENCES

Abt, G., Zhou, S. and Weatherby, R. (1998). The effect of a high-carbohydrate diet on the skill performance of midfield soccer players after intermittent treadmill exercise. *Journal of Science and Medicine in Sport*, 1, 203–212.

Al Nawaiseh, A.M., Bishop, P.A., Pritchett, R.C. and Porter, S. (2007). Enhancing short-term recovery after high intensity anaerobic exercise. *Medicine and Science in Sports and Exercise*, 39, S307.

Amiri-Khorasani, M., Sahebozamani, M., Tabrizi, K.G. and Yusof, A.B. (2010). Acute effect of different stretching methods on Illinois agility test in soccer players. *Journal of Strength and Conditioning Research*, 24, 2698–2704.

Andersen, J.C. (2005). Stretching before and after exercise: effect on muscle soreness and injury risk. *Journal of Athletic Training*, 40, 218–220.

Andersson, H., Raastad, T., Nilsson, J., Paulsen, G.R., Garthe, I. and Kadi, F. (2008). Neuromuscular fatigue and recovery in elite female soccer: effects of active recovery. *Medicine and Science in Sports and Exercise*, 40, 372–380.

Balsom, P.D., Wood, K., Olsson, P. and Ekblom, B. (1999). Carbohydrate intake and multiple sprint sports: with special reference to football (soccer). *International Journal of Sports Medicine*, 20, 48–52.

Bangsbo, J. (1994). The physiology of soccer: with special reference to intense intermittent exercise. *Acta Physiologica Scandinavica*, 619, 1–155.

Bangsbo, J., Mohr, M. and Krustrup, P. (2006). Physical and metabolic demands of training and match-play in the elite football player. *Journal of Sports Sciences*, 24, 665–674.

Bangsbo, J., Norregaard, L. and Thorsoe, F. (1992). The effect of carbohydrate diet on intermittent exercise performance. *International Journal of Sports Medicine*, 13, 152–157.

Barnett, A. (2006). Using recovery modalities between training sessions in elite athletes: does it help? *Sports Medicine*, 36, 781–796.

Barr, K. and McGee, S. (2008). Optimising training adaptations by manipulating glycogen. *European Journal of Sport Science*, 8, 97–106.

Bendiksen, M., Bischoff, R., Randers, M.B., Mohr, M., Rollo, I., Suetta, C., Bangsbo, J. and Krustrup, P. (2012). The Copenhagen Soccer Test: physiological response and fatigue development. *Medicine and Science in Sports and Exercise*, 44, 1595–1603.

Bloomfield, J., Polman, R. and O'Donoghue, P.G. (2007). Reliability of the Bloomfield Movement Classification. *International Journal of Performance Analysis in Sport*, 7, 20–27.

Bochmann, R.P., Seibel, W., Haase, E., Hietschold, V., Rödel, H. and Deussen, A. (2005). External compression increases forearm perfusion. *Journal of Applied Physiology*, 99, 2337–2344.

Bond, V., Adams, R.G., Tearney, R.J., Gresham, K. and Ruff, W. (1991). Effects of active and passive recovery on lactate removal and subsequent isokinetic muscle function. *Journal of Sports Medicine and Physical Fitness*, 31, 357–361.

Bradley, P.S., Sheldon, W., Wooster, B., Olsen, P., Boanas, P. and Krustrup, P. (2009). High-intensity running in English FA Premier League soccer matches. *Journal of Sports Sciences*, 27, 159–168.

Brooks, C.P., Woodruff, L.D., Wright, L.L. and Donatelli, R. (2005). The immediate effects of manual massage on power-grip performance after maximal exercise in healthy adults. *Journal of Alternative and Complementary Medicine*, 11, 1093–1101.

Burke, L. (2007) Field-based team sports. In L. Burke, *Practical Sports Nutrition* (pp. 185–219). Champaign, IL: Human Kinetics.

Burke, L.M. (2010). Fuelling strategies to optimise performance: training high or training low? *Scandinavian Journal of Medicine and Science in Sports*, 20 (Suppl. 2), 48–58.

Carter, R. 3rd, Wilson, T.E., Watenpaugh, D.E., Smith, M.L. and Crandall, C.G. (2002). Effects of mode of exercise recovery on thermoregulatory and cardiovascular responses. *Journal of Applied Physiology*, 93, 1918–1924.

Cox, G.R., Clark, S.A., Cox, A.J., Halson, S.L., Hargreaves, M., Hawley, J.A., Jeacocke, N., Snow, R.J., Yeo, W.K. and Burke, L.M. (2010). Daily training with high carbohydrate availability increases exogenous carbohydrate oxidation during endurance cycling. *Journal of Applied Physiology*, 109, 126–134.

Davies, V., Thompson, K.G. and Cooper, S.M. (2009). The effects of compression garments on recovery. *Journal of Strength and Conditioning Research*, 23, 1786–1794.

Dawson, B., Dawson, K. and Tiidus, P.M. (2004). Evaluating the influence of massage on leg strength, swelling, and pain following a half marathon. *Journal of Science and Medicine in Sport*, 3, 37–43.

Di Salvo, V., Baron, R., Tschan, H., Calderon Montero, F.J., Bachl, N. and Pigozzi, F. (2007). Performance characteristics according to playing position in elite soccer. *International Journal of Sports Medicine*, 28, 222–227.

Duffield, R., Cannon, J. and King, M. (2010). The effects of compression garments on recovery of muscle performance following high-intensity sprint and plyometric exercise. *Journal of Science and Medicine in Sport*, 13, 136–140.

Duffield, R., Edge, J., Merrells, R., Hawke, E., Barnes, M., Simcock, D. and Gill, N. (2008). The effects of compression garments on intermittent exercise performance and recovery on consecutive days. *International Journal of Sports Physiology and Performance*, 3, 454–468.

Ekblom, B. (1986). Applied physiology of soccer. *Sports Medicine*, 3, 50–60.

Fallon, K.E. (2007). Blood tests in tired elite athletes: expectations of athletes, coaches and sport science/sports medicine staff. *British Journal of Sports Medicine*, 41, 41–44.

Farr, T., Nottle, C., Nosaka, K. and Sacco, P. (2002). The effects of therapeutic massage on delayed onset muscle soreness and muscle function following downhill walking. *Journal of Science and Medicine in Sport*, 5, 297–306.

78

Gill, N.D., Beaven, C.M. and Cook, C. (2006). Effectiveness of post-match recovery strategies in Rugby players. *British Journal of Sports Medicine*, 40, 260–263.

Gunnarsson, T.P., Bendiksen, M., Bischoff, R., Christensen, P.M., Lesivig, B., Madsen, K., Stephens, F., Greenhaff, P., Krustrup, P. and Bangsbo, J. (2011). Effect of whey protein and carbohydrate enriched diet on glycogen resynthesis during the first 48 h after a soccer game. *Scandinavian Journal of Medicine and Science in Sports*, doi: 10.1111/j.1600-0838.2011.01418.x.

Hamlin, M.J. (2007). The effect of contrast temperature water therapy on repeated sprint performance. *Journal of Science in Medicine and Sport*, 10, 398–402.

Hansen, A.K., Fischer, C.P., Plomgaard, P., Andersen, J.L., Saltin, B. and Pedersen, B.K. (2005). Skeletal muscle adaptation: training twice every second day vs. training once daily. *Journal of Applied Physiology*, 98, 93–99.

Hemmings, B., Smith, M., Graydon, J. and Dyson, R. (2000). Effects of massage on physiological restoration, perceived recovery, and repeated sports performance. *British Journal of Sports Medicine*, 34, 109–114.

Hilbert, J.E., Sforzo, G.A. and Swensen, T. (2003). The effects of massage on delayed onset muscle soreness. *British Journal of Sports Medicine*, 37, 72–75.

Hulston, C.J., Venables, M.C., Mann, C.H., Martin, C., Philp, A., Baar, K. and Jeukendrup, A.E. (2010). Training with low muscle glycogen enhances fat metabolism in well-trained cyclists. *Medicine and Science in Sports and Exercise*, 42, 2046–2055.

Jacobs, I., Westlin, N., Karlsson, J., Rasmusson, M. and Houghton, B. (1982). Muscle glycogen and diet in elite soccer players. *European Journal of Applied Physiology*, 48, 297–302.

Jakeman, J.R., Byrne, C. and Eston, R.G. (2010). Efficacy of lower limb compression and combined treatment of manual massage and lower limb compression on symptoms of exercise-induced muscle damage in women. *Journal of Strength and Conditioning Research*, 24, 3157–3165.

King, M. and Duffield, R. (2009). The effects of recovery interventions on consecutive days of intermittent sprint exercise. *Journal of Strength and Conditioning Research*, 23, 1795–1802.

Kinugasa, T. and Kilding, A.E. (2009). A comparison of post-match recovery strategies in youth soccer players. *Journal of Strength and Conditioning Research*, 23, 1402–1407.

Kraemer, W.J., Bush, J.A., Wickham, R.B., Denegar, C.R., Gómez, A.L., Gotshalk, L.A., Duncan, N.D., Volek, J.S., Putukian, M. and Sebastianelli, W.J. (2001). Influence of compression therapy on symptoms following soft tissue injury from maximal eccentric exercise. *Journal of Orthopaedic & Sports Physical Therapy*, 31, 282–290.

Kraemer, W.J., Flanagan, S.D., Comstock, B.A., Fragala, M.S., Earp, J.E., Dunn-Lewis, C., Ho, J.Y., Thomas, G.A., Solomon-Hill, G., Penwell, Z.R., Powell, M.D., Wolf, M.R., Volek, J.S., Denegar, C.R. and Maresh, C.M. (2010). Effects of a whole body compression garment on markers of recovery after a heavy resistance workout in men and women. *Journal of Strength and Conditioning Research*, 24, 804–814.

Krustrup, P., Mohr, M., Ellingsgaard, H. and Bangsbo, J. (2005). Physical demands during an elite female soccer game: importance of training status. *Medicine and Science in Sports and Exercise*, 37, 1242–1248.

Krustrup, P., Zebis, M., Jensen, J.M. and Mohr, M. (2010). Game-induced fatigue patterns in elite female soccer. *Journal of Strength and Conditioning Research*, 24, 437–441.

Krustrup, P., Mohr, M., Steensberg, A., Bencke, J., Kjaer, M. and Bangsbo, J. (2006). Muscle and blood metabolites during a soccer game: implications for sprint performance. *Medicine and Science in Sports and Exercise*, 38, 1165–1174.

Krustrup, P., Mohr, M., Amstrup, T., Rysgaard, T., Johansen, J., Steensberg, A., Pedersen, P.K. and Bangsbo, J. (2003). The Yo-Yo intermittent recovery test: physiological response, reliability, and validity. *Medicine and Science in Sports and Exercise*, 35, 697–705.

Krustrup, P., Ortenblad, N., Nielsen, J., Nybo, L., Gunnarsson, T.P., Iaia, F.M., Madsen, K., Stephens, F., Greenhaff, P. and Bangsbo, J. (2011). Maximal voluntary contraction force, SR function and glycogen resynthesis during the first 72 h after a high-level competitive soccer game. *European Journal of Applied Physiology*, 111: 2987–2995.

Lane, K.N. and Wenger, H.A. (2004). Effect of selected recovery conditions on performance of repeated bouts of intermittent cycling separated by 24 hours. *Journal of Strength and Conditioning Research*, 18, 855–860.

Mancinelli, C.A., Davis, D.S., Aboulhosn, L., Brady, M., Eisenhofer, J. and Foutty, S. (2006). The effects of massage on delayed onset muscle soreness and physical performance in female collegiate athletes. *Physical Therapy in Sport*, 7, 5–13.

Mohr, M., Krustrup, P. and Bangsbo, J. (2003). Match performance of high-standard soccer players with special reference to development of fatigue. *Journal of Sports Sciences*, 21, 519–528.

Mohr, M., Krustrup, P., Nybo, L., Nielsen, J.J. and Bangsbo, J. (2004). Muscle temperature and sprint performance during soccer matches – beneficial effect of re-warm-up at half-time. *Scandinavian Journal of Medicine and Science in Sports*, 14, 156–162.

Mohr, M., Mujika, I., Santisteban, J., Randers, M.B., Bischoff, R., Solano, R., Hewitt, A., Zubillaga, A., Peltola, E. and Krustrup, P. (2010). Examination of fatigue development in elite soccer in a hot environment: a multi-experimental approach. *Scandinavian Journal of Medicine and Science in Sports*, 20 (suppl. 3), 125–132.

Monedero, J. and Donne, B. (2000). Effect of recovery interventions on lactate removal and subsequent performance. *International Journal of Sports Medicine*, 21, 593–597.

Montgomery, P.G., Pyne, D.B., Hopkins, W.G., Dorman, J.C., Cook, K. and Minahan, C.L. (2008). The effect of recovery strategies on physical performance and cumulative fatigue in competitive basketball. *Journal of Sports Sciences*, 26, 1135–1145.

Morton, J.P., Croft, L., Bartlett, J.D., Maclaren, D.P., Reilly, T., Evans, L., McArdle, A. and Drust, B. (2009). Reduced carbohydrate availability does not modulate training-induced heat shock protein adaptations but does upregulate oxidative enzyme activity in human skeletal muscle. *Journal of Applied Physiology*, 106, 1513–1521.

Mujika, I. and Burke, L.M. (2010). Nutrition in team sports. *Annals of Nutrition and Metabolism* 57 (suppl.), 26–35.

Rampinini, E., Bishop, D., Marcora, S.M., Ferrari Bravo, D., Sassi, R. and Impellizzeri, F.M. (2007). Validity of simple field tests as indicators of match-related physical performance in top-level professional soccer players. *International Journal of Sports Medicine*, 28, 228–235.

Reilly, T. and Brooks, G.A. (1986). Exercise and the circadian variation in body temperature measures. *International Journal of Sports Medicine*, 7, 358–362.

Reilly, T. and Deykin, T. (1983). Effects of partial sleep loss on subjective states, psychomotor and physical performance tests. *Journal of Human Movement Studies*, 9, 157–170.

Reilly, T. and Edwards, B. (2007). Altered sleep–wake cycles and physical performance in athletes. *Physiology and Behaviour*, 90, 274–284.

# 80

Reilly, T. and Rigby, M. (2002). Effect of an active warm-down following competitive soccer. In W. Spinks (ed.), *Science and Football IV* (pp. 226–229). London: Routledge.

Reilly, T. and Thomas, V. (1976). A motion analysis of work-rate in different positional roles in professional football match-play. *Journal of Human Movement Studies*, 2, 87–97.

Rowsell, G.J., Coutts, A.J., Reaburn, P. and Hill-Haas, S. (2009). Effects of cold-water immersion on physical performance between successive matches in high-performance junior male soccer players. *Journal of Sports Sciences*, 27, 565–573.

Saltin, B. (1973). Metabolic fundamentals in exercise. *Medicine and Science in Sports*, 5, 137–146.

Sinnerton, S. and Reilly, T. (1992). Effects of sleep loss and time of day in swimmers. In D. Maclaren, T. Reilly and A. Lees (eds), *Biomechanics and Medicine in Swimming: Swimming Science IV* (pp. 399–405). London: E. and F.N. Spon.

Smith, R.S. and Reilly, T. (2004). Sleep deprivation and the athlete. In C. Kushida (ed.), *Sleep Deprivation* (pp. 313–334). New York: Marcel Dekker.

Spencer, M., Bishop, D., Dawson, B. and Goodman, C. (2005). Physiological and metabolic responses of repeated-sprint activities: Specific to field-based team sports. *Sports Medicine*, 35, 1025–1044.

Tessitore, A., Meeusen, R., Cortis, C. and Capranica, L. (2007). Effects of different recovery interventions on anaerobic performances following preseason soccer training. *Journal of Strength and Conditioning Research*, 21, 745–750.

Tessitore, A., Meeusen, R., Pagano, R., Benvenuti, C., Tiberi, M. and Capranica, L. (2008). Effectiveness of active versus passive recovery strategies after futsal games. *Journal of Strength and Conditioning Research*, 22, 1402–1412.

Thacker, S.B., Gilchrist, J., Stroup, D.F. and Kimsey, C.D. Jr (2004). The impact of stretching on sports injury risk: a systematic review of the literature. *Medicine and Science in Sports and Exercise*, 36, 371–378.

Thorlund, J.B., Aagaard, P. and Madsen, K. (2009). Rapid muscle force capacity changes after soccer match play. *International Journal of Sports Medicine*, 30, 273–278.

Wilcock, I.M., Cronin, J.B. and Hing, W.A. (2006). Physiological response to water immersion: a method for sport recovery? *Sports Medicine*, 36, 747–765.

Yeo, W.K., Paton, C.D., Garnham, A.P., Burke, L.M., Carey, A.L. and Hawley, J.A. (2008). Skeletal muscle adaptation and performance responses to once a day versus twice every second day endurance training regimens. *Journal of Applied Physiology*, 105, 1462–1470.

Zainuddin, Z., Newton, M., Sacco, P. and Nosaka, K. (2005). Effects of massage on delayed-onset muscle soreness, swelling, and recovery of muscle function. *Journal of Athletic Training*, 40, 174–180.

Zehnder, M., Rico-Sanz, J., Kuhne, G. and Boutellier, U. (2001). Resynthesis of muscle glycogen after soccer specific performance examined by 13C-magnetic resonance spectroscopy in elite players. *European Journal of Applied Physiology*, 84, 443–447.

Zehnder, M., Muelli, M., Buchli, R., Kuehne, G. and Boutellier, U. (2004). Further glycogen decrease during early recovery after eccentric exercise despite a high carbohydrate intake. *European Journal of Nutrition*, 43, 148–159.

# CHAPTER 5

## ENVIRONMENTAL STRESS

W. Gregson and B. Drust

### INTRODUCTION

Soccer is played worldwide and in highly varied environmental conditions which are rarely conducive to optimal performance. In some instances, the climatic conditions are too hostile or unsuitable for playing and there is an enforced break in the competitive programme, particularly in northern climates during winter and tropical countries during the rainy season. In the former, it becomes impossible to maintain playing pitches and the weather is too cold to play in comfort. At the other extreme is the stress imposed by a hot environment and the difficulty of coping with high heat and humidity. The hottest part of the day is usually avoided and matches are scheduled for evening kick-offs, albeit this is not always feasible in highly competitive international tournaments and teams are obliged to compete in conditions to which they are unaccustomed. This factor was illustrated by the final match of the 2008 Beijing Olympic Games, were air temperatures on the field reached 42°C.

Altitude is another environmental variable that can increase the physiological demands placed upon teams. This factor has applied to those teams who have competed at the World Cup in Mexico in 1970 and 1986, and to a lesser extent in South Africa in 2010. It applies also to teams playing friendly or international qualifying matches at moderate altitude. Additionally, training camps for top teams are sometimes located at altitude and this constitutes a particular novel challenge to sea-level dwellers.

The human body has mechanisms that allow it to acclimatise to some extent to environmental challenges. In the course of history it has evolved to match the environmental changes associated with the solar day. Consequently, many physiological functions wax and wane in harmony with cyclical changes in the environment every 24 h. The sleep–wake cycle is dovetailed with alternation of darkness and light and the majority of the body's activities are controlled by biological clocks. These are disturbed when the body is forced to exercise at a time it is unused to, for example, after crossing multiple time zones to compete overseas. It is also disturbed if the normal sleep pattern is altered.

In this chapter, the major environmental variables that impinge on soccer performance are considered. These include heat, cold, hypoxia and circadian rhythms. The biological background is provided, prior to describing the consequences of environmental conditions for the soccer player.

## TEMPERATURE

### Physiology of thermoregulation

Human core body temperature is normally maintained within a narrow range around a mean of 37°C. Core temperature is measured usually as a rectal, tympanic or oesophageal temperature. Intestinal temperature, measured via a disposal ingestible temperature sensor, provides a valid and reliable non-invasive measure of internal temperature (Gant et al., 2006). This latter method is particularly useful in the field or for assessing core body temperature over extended periods of time. The temperature in the periphery of the body is more variable than the core and responds to changes in environmental temperatures; however, mean skin temperature is normally around 4°C below core temperature, providing a gradient for dissipating heat from the internal environment. The size of gradient between skin and environment is one of the factors that influence the amount of heat that is lost or gained by the body.

The human body gains or loses heat according to prevailing conditions and can modify heat exchange with the environment in various ways to achieve equilibrium (Figure 5.1). The heat balance equation is expressed as:

$$M - S = E \pm C \pm R \pm K$$

Where M = metabolic rate, S = heat storage, E = evaporation, C = convection, R = radiation and K = conduction

Thermal equilibrium is attained by a balance between heat loss and gain mechanisms (Figure 5.1). Heat is produced as a by-product of metabolic processes, basal metabolic rate being around 1 kcal kg$^{-1}$h$^{-1}$. One kilocalorie (4.186 kJ) is the energy required to raise 1 kg water through 1°C. During soccer, energy expenditure might increase this by a factor of 15, with only 20–25% of the energy expended reflected in external power output. The rest is dissipated as heat within the active tissues and, as a result, body heat storage increases. In order to avoid overheating, the body is equipped with mechanisms for losing heat. It also has in-built responses to safeguard the body's thermal status under conditions where heat may be lost too rapidly to the environment, for example, in very cold conditions.

Heat generated in the muscle may be transferred through adjacent tissue to the skin surface by means of conduction. The transfer of heat through this physical mechanism also occurs from the skin surface to materials (e.g., clothing), surfaces or to the air that is in direct contact with the skin surface. The material of the clothing and subcutaneous adipose tissue constitutes barriers against heat loss by conduction. Films of stationary air or water in immediate contact with clothing, along with the air trapped in the clothing itself, provide barriers between the body and the environment. In contrast to conduction, the transfer of heat by movement of gas or fluid is referred to as convective heat exchange. Alongside conduction, heat produced in the working muscle can be transferred to the skin surface via convection in the arterial blood. The movement of air over the skin surface also represents an important means of cooling the body when competing in hot conditions, since this movement dispels the layer of warm air adjacent to the skin. The greater the air movement, the faster the rate of heat removal

83

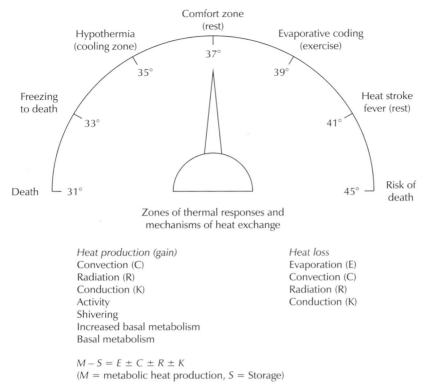

Zones of thermal responses and
mechanisms of heat exchange

*Heat production (gain)*
Convection (C)
Radiation (R)
Conduction (K)
Activity
Shivering
Increased basal metabolism
Basal metabolism

*Heat loss*
Evaporation (E)
Convection (C)
Radiation (R)
Conduction (K)

$M - S = E \pm C \pm R \pm K$
(M = metabolic heat production, S = Storage)

**Figure 5.1** Heat loss and heat gain mechanisms.

by convection. When the air temperature remains lower than skin temperature, conduction and convection constantly remove heat from the body; however, their combined contribution to total heat loss in air at rest is relatively small (~10–20%) and is further reduced during exercise.

Heat is also lost by the process of evaporation, the rate being determined by the vapour pressure gradient across the film of stationary air surrounding the skin and by the thickness of the stationary film. Evaporation is the primary avenue for heat loss during exercise (~80%) and becomes more important with increasing environmental temperatures. Some evaporation arises without our awareness; it is referred to as insensible water loss and occurs with breathing, as water from moist mucous membranes in the upper respiratory tract is vaporised. The result is a gradual dehydration, as can happen in dry air, especially at altitude or on board aircraft. Evaporative loss from the lungs is in fact dependent on the minute ventilation, the barometric pressure and dryness of the air. There is also insensible water loss through the skin. Insensible water loss is relatively stable; consequently, as body temperature rises there is an increase in secretion of sweat onto the skin surface for the purpose of losing heat by the process of evaporation. As sweat arrives on the skin, it is converted from a liquid to a vapour by heat from the skin, consequently sweat evaporation becomes increasingly important as body temperature rises.

**W. Gregson and B. Drust**

Body temperature is controlled by specialised nerve cells within the hypothalamus. The neurones in the anterior portion constitute the heat-loss centre, since they trigger initiation of heat-loss responses. The hypothalamus is sensitive to the temperature of the blood that bathes these cells controlling thermoregulatory responses. In addition to this direct information, the cells receive signals from warm and cold receptors located in the skin. In this way, heat-loss and heat-gain centres receive information about both the body's internal thermal state and environmental conditions (Figure 5.2).

### Exercise in the heat

An increase in body temperature markedly influences exercise performance, with the effects highly dependent upon the type of exercise performed (Racinais and Oksa, 2010). Heat stress reduces the capacity to perform prolonged, intermittent, high-intensity running (Morris et al., 2000). The factors responsible for this earlier onset of fatigue have yet to be fully elucidated;

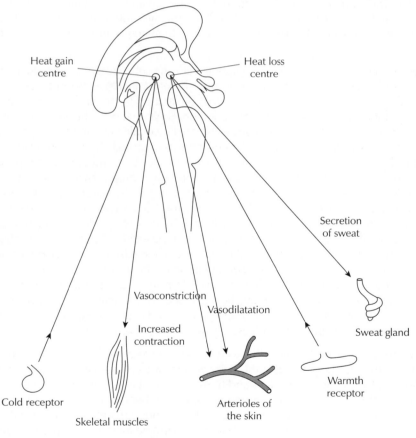

**Figure 5.2** Control of human thermoregulation.

however, the attainment of a high core body temperature which serves to reduce the central nervous system's drive to the active musculature is thought to be involved (Nybo and Nielsen, 2001). These detrimental effects contrast with improvements in the capacity to perform single or short-term periods of maximal exercise in heat stress where increases in muscle temperature enhance the contractile properties of the muscle and, subsequently, performance (Davies and Young, 1983).

Post-match rectal temperatures in excess of 39°C are frequently observed (Edwards and Clark, 2006), with individual values in excess of 40°C reported in the literature (Ekblom, 1986). Continuous observations of body temperature during match-play suggest that core body temperature may peak (> 40°C) at certain time points within the game (e.g., half-time period) rather than at the end of the game (Özgünen et al., 2010). These high internal temperatures are likely to negatively impact on the player's physical performance during match-play. Any improvements in the ability to undertake high-intensity bouts due to increases in temperature of the working muscles are likely to be overridden by high levels of core body temperature as the match progresses (Drust et al., 2005a). The inherent difficulties in quantifying performance (Gregson et al., 2010) mean that few attempts have been made to study the influence of heat stress on match-play. There are, however, indications from motion analysis of players that heat stress may reduce total distance (Özgünen et al., 2010) and the high-intensity (Ekblom, 1986; Mohr et al., 2010) distance covered by players, as compared to matches undertaken in cooler conditions.

During demanding exercise such as soccer, the metabolic rate and subsequent heat production are markedly increased. Delivery of heat to the skin must therefore increase proportionally to re-establish thermal balance. This requirement for heat dissipation is increased in the heat, where a rise in thermal strain occurs as a result of the additional heat gain from the environment. As a result, competitive soccer in the heat may stress the cardiovascular system to its capacity. Under such conditions, the primary cardiovascular challenge is to provide both adequate skin blood flow for the dissipation of heat and sufficient blood flow to the muscles to support exercise. In an attempt to sustain the high levels of skin blood flow, a progressive redistribution of the central blood volume to the skin occurs. These central circulatory changes are characterised by a decline in stroke volume and a compensatory increase in heart rate in order to maintain blood pressure and cardiac output (Montain and Coyle, 1992). If heat loss increases sufficiently to balance heat production, core temperature can be essentially maintained. This level of thermal strain is largely proportional to the intensity of exercise and independent of environmental conditions under non heat stress conditions. In the heat, concomitant increases in skin temperature reduce the thermal gradient for heat transfer between the skin and the external environment. Consequently, evaporative heat loss becomes critical for the dissipation of heat and changes in circulatory functioning are more pronounced as the ambient temperature (Nadel et al., 1979) and exercise intensity increase (Shaffrath and Adams, 1984).

Without replenishment of the body water lost as a consequence of sweating, progressive dehydration occurs, which further increases the level of cardiovascular strain. In attempting to maintain cardiovascular functioning under conditions of thermal strain and dehydration, a decrease in skin blood flow may arise, consequently the rate of heat loss declines and core temperature continues to rise (Gonzalez-Alonso et al., 1997). Thus, athletes exercising in the heat with severe levels of dehydration are less able to cope with the increasing hyperthermia developed during exercise, due to reductions in the ability to dissipate heat (Gonzalez-Alonso

86

*et al.*, 1997). Heat is lost only when sweat is vaporised on the surface of the body; no heat is being exchanged if sweat drips off or is wiped away. When heat is combined with humidity, the possibilities of losing heat by evaporation are reduced, since the air is already highly saturated with water vapour. Consequently, hot, humid conditions are detrimental to performance and increase the risk of heat injury.

Limited information is available with respect to sweat loss in soccer players during competitive match-play, due to difficulties in obtaining measurements. Soccer players may lose on average around 3L or more of fluid during 90-min of play, which varies with the climatic conditions and between individuals. Some players may sweat little and will be at risk when competing in the heat, due to hyperthermia. Those who sweat profusely may be dehydrated near the end of the game. For example, mean sweat losses of 3.1L have been reported while playing matches in the heat (~34°C; Kurdak *et al.*, 2010). However, depending on individual variation, exercise type and particularly intensity, sweat rates may exceed 3 L/h (Rehrer, 2001). Such losses would seriously impair performance if fluid ingestion did not occur to alleviate the hypohydration incurred.

It is important that players are adequately hydrated prior to playing and training in the heat. Water is lost through sweat at a faster rate than it can be restored by means of drinking and subsequent absorption through the small intestine. Thirst is not a very sensitive indicator of the level of dehydration. Consequently, players should be encouraged to drink regularly, about 200 ml every 15–20 min when training in the heat. The primary need is for water, since sweat is hypotonic. Although drinking plain water does confer advantages, the use of properly formulated sports drink is likely to have more advantages (Maughan *et al.*, 2010).

The thermal strain on the individual player is a function of the relative exercise intensity (% $\dot{V}O_{2max}$) rather than the absolute work-load. Therefore, the higher the maximal aerobic power and cardiac output, the lower the thermal strain on the player. A well-trained individual has a highly developed cardiovascular system to cope with the dual roles of thermoregulation and exercise. The highly trained individual will acclimatise more quickly than one who is unfit. Training improves exercise tolerance in the heat, but does not eliminate the necessity of heat acclimatisation. Strategies that can reduce body temperature before exercise may facilitate performance by alleviating the degree of thermoregulatory strain experienced during match-play. These include reducing the intensity of the pre-match warm-up (Gregson *et al.*, 2005) and the application of external cooling modalities, including cold water immersion (Minett *et al.*, 2011), cooling vests (Price *et al.*, 2009) and the ingestion of cold fluids (Ross *et al.*, 2011). In soccer, the half-time break presents opportunities for the application of external cooling modalities, though the limited time available may only permit the use of time-efficient strategies such as hand and forearm immersion (Barr *et al.*, 2010).

## Heat acclimatisation

Acclimatisation refers to reactions to the natural climate. The term *acclimation* is used to refer to physiological changes which occur in response to experimentally induced changes in one particular factor (Nielsen, 1994). Repeated heat exposure promotes a number of physiological adaptations which reduce physiological strain, improves exercise performance and reduces the risk of heat injury during subsequent heat exposures.

The classic signs of heat acclimatisation include a lower heart rate, lower core body temperature and increased sweat rates during exercise-heat stress. The increased evaporative heat loss serves to counteract the reduced dry heat exchange and is characterised by an earlier onset of sweating (sweat produced at a lower rise in body temperature) and a more dilute solution from the sweat glands. The heat-acclimatised individual sweats more than an unacclimatised counterpart at a given exercise intensity. There is also an earlier increase in blood flow to the skin after a period of acclimatisation, so that heat transfer from core to skin is maintained, although the acclimatised player depends more on evaporative sweat loss than on distribution of blood flow.

Exercise in the heat represents the most effective strategy for inducing heat acclimatisation, although resting in the heat can promote some degree of acclimatisation. Optimal heat acclimation in dry heat is associated with a daily exposure of 100-min, with little further benefit gained from extending this period (Lind and Bass, 1963). In trained individuals, similar degrees of acclimation may be obtained by completing shorter periods of moderate-intensity exercise (Houmard et al., 1990). Heat acclimatisation occurs relatively quickly, with a good degree of adaptation developed within 7 days and generally complete within 10–14 days of the initial exposure. Further adaptations will enhance the athlete's capability to perform well in heat-stress conditions (Nielsen, 1994). Ideally, therefore, the athlete or team should be exposed to the climate of the host country for at least several weeks before the event. An alternative strategy is to have an acclimatisation period of 2 weeks or so well before the event with subsequent shorter exposures as training is tapered before competition. If these are not practical, players should attempt some degree of heat acclimatisation before leaving for the host country. This may be achieved by pre-acclimatisation, which may include:

1   exposure to hot and humid environments, the player seeking out the hottest time of day to train at home;

2   exercise in an environmental chamber for periodic bouts of heat exposure exercise rather than rest – about 3 h per week exercising in an environmental chamber should provide a good degree of acclimatisation (Reilly et al., 1997);

3   the heat load imposed under cool environmental conditions may be increased by wearing heavy training suits or windbreakers during training so as to induce a degree of adaptation to thermal strain.

On first exposure to a hot climate, players should be encouraged to drink copiously to maintain pale straw-coloured rather than dark urine (de Looy et al., 1988). They should drink much more fluid than they need, since thirst is often a very poor indicator of real need. When they arrive in the hot country they should be discouraged strongly from sunbathing, as this itself does not help acclimatisation except by the development of a suntan, which will eventually protect the skin from damage via solar radiation. This is a long-term process and is not beneficial in the short term, but negative effects of sunburn can cause severe discomfort and a decline in performance. Players should therefore be protected with an adequate sunscreen if they are likely to be exposed to the sun.

Initially, training should be undertaken in the cooler parts of the day so that an adequate work-load can be achieved and fluid must be taken regularly. If sleeping is difficult, arrangements should be made to sleep in an air-conditioned environment. However, to facilitate acclimatisation, the rest of the day should be partly spent exposed to the ambient temperature other than in air-conditioned rooms. Although sweating will increase as a result of acclimatisation, there should be no need to take salt tablets, provided adequate amounts of salt are taken with normal food. In the period of acclimatisation, players should regularly monitor body weight and try to compensate for weight loss with adequate fluid intake. Alcohol is inappropriate for rehydration purposes, since it acts as a diuretic and increases urine output. Although there is no ideal measure of hydration status, the most suitable methods include specific gravity, osmolality and conductivity (Shirreffs and Maughan,1998).

## Heat injury

Hyperthermia (overheating) and loss of body water (hypohydration) lead to abnormalities that are referred to as heat injuries. Progressively they may be manifest as three fairly distinct clinical syndromes known as muscle cramps, heat exhaustion and heat stroke. These syndromes overlap and frequently occur in combinations. They are observed more frequently in individual events such as distance running and cycling than in soccer, but can occur in matches or training sessions in the heat.

Heat cramps are the least serious of the three heat disorders and are associated with loss of body fluid, particularly in games where players compete in intense heat (Reilly, 2000). Although the body loses electrolytes in sweat, such losses cannot adequately account for the occurrence of cramps. These occurrences seem to coincide with low energy stores as well as reduced body water levels. Generally, the muscles employed in exercise are affected, but most vulnerable are the leg (upper or lower) and abdominal muscles. The cramp can usually be treated by moving the individual to a cooler location and administering fluids. Stretching the involved muscle and sometimes massage may also be effective.

Heat exhaustion is often characterised by core temperatures of 39–40°C, though poorly conditioned individuals or those unacclimatised to the heat may exhibit internal temperatures below 39°C. Associated with this are symptoms such as extreme fatigue, dizziness and breathlessness, hypotension and a weak, rapid pulse. These symptoms reflect the inability of the cardiovascular system to meet the dual demand for increased blood to both the working muscle and skin for heat dissipation. This effect typically arises when blood volume decreases as a consequence of excessive fluid loss. Victims of heat exhaustion are typically moved to a cooler location with their feet elevated and fluids provided. Where individuals are unconscious, medically supervised intravenous infusion of saline solution often occurs.

Heat stroke is a life-threatening heat disorder that requires immediate medical attention. It is characterised by core temperatures of 40°C or higher. Hypohydration due to loss of body water in sweat and associated with a high core body temperature can be driven so far as to threaten life. Heat stroke is characterised by cessation of sweating, total confusion or loss of consciousness. In such cases treatment is urgently needed to reduce body temperature. There may also be circulatory instability and loss of vasomotor tone as the regulation of blood pressure begins to fall.

## Competing in the cold

In many places, soccer is a winter sport and is often played in near-freezing conditions. Core temperature and muscle temperature may fall and exercise performance will be increasingly affected. Muscle power output is reduced by 5% for every 1°C fall in muscle temperature below normal levels (Bergh and Ekblom, 1979). A fall in core temperature to hypothermic levels is life threatening and the body's heat-gain mechanisms are designed to arrest the decline.

Among the responses to cold initiated by the posterior hypothalamus is a generalised vasoconstriction of the skin circulation, mediated by the sympathetic nervous system. Blood is displaced centrally away from the peripheral circulation and this increases the temperature gradient between the core and shell. The reduction in skin temperature in turn decreases the gradient between skin and environment, which protects against a massive loss of heat from the body. Superficial veins are also affected in that blood returning from the limbs is diverted to the vena comitantes that lie adjacent to the main arteries. The arterial blood is cooled by the venous return almost immediately it enters the limb by means of counter-current heat exchange.

One of the consequences of the fall in limb temperature is that motor performance is adversely affected. In addition to the drop in muscular strength and power output as the temperature in the muscle falls, there is impairment of conduction velocity of nerve impulses to the muscles. The sensitivity of muscle spindles declines and there is a loss of manual dexterity. For these reasons, it is important to preserve limb temperature in soccer players during competition. The goalkeeper in particular must maintain manual dexterity for handling the ball.

Shivering is a response of the body's autonomic nervous system to the fall in core temperature. It constitutes involuntary activity of skeletal muscle in order to generate metabolic heat. Shivering tends to be intermittent and may persist during exercise if the intensity is insufficient to maintain core temperature. It may be evident during stoppages in play, especially when cold conditions are compounded by sleet. The early symptoms of hypothermia include shivering, fatigue, loss of strength and coordination and an inability to sustain work-rate. Once fatigue develops, shivering may decrease and the condition worsens. Later symptoms include collapse, stupor and loss of consciousness. This risk applies more to recreational rather than professional soccer, as some players may not be able to sustain work-rate to keep them warm in extreme cold. In such events, the referee would be expected to abandon play before conditions became critical.

Cold is less of a problem than heat, in that the body can be protected against exposure to ambient environmental conditions. The important climate is the microclimate next to the skin and this can be maintained by appropriate choice of clothing. Behaviourally, players may respond to cold conditions by maintaining a high work-rate. Alternatively, they can be spared exposure to the cold by conducting training sessions in indoor facilities, where these are available.

Clothing of natural fibre (cotton or wool) is preferable to synthetic material in cold and cold-wet conditions. The clothing should allow sweat produced during exercise in these conditions to flow through the garment. The best material will allow sweat to flow out through the cells

90

of the garment while preventing water droplets from penetrating the clothing from the outside. If the fabric becomes saturated with water or sweat, it loses its insulating properties and in cold-wet conditions the body temperature may quickly drop.

Players training in the cold should ensure that the trunk area of the body is well insulated. The use of warm undergarments beneath a full tracksuit may be needed. Dressing in layers is well advised; outer layers can be discarded as body temperature rises and if ambient temperature gets warmer. When layers of clothing are worn, the outer layer should be capable of resisting both wind and rain. The inner layer should provide insulation and wick moisture from the skin to promote heat loss by evaporation. Polypropylene and cotton thermal underlay has good insulation and wicking properties and so is suitable for wearing next to the skin.

Immediately prior to competing in the cold, players should endeavour to stay as warm as possible. A thorough warm-up regimen (performed indoors if possible) is recommended. It is thought that cold conditions increase the risk of muscle injury in sports involving intense anaerobic efforts; warm-up exercise may afford some protection in this respect. Competitors may need to wear more clothing than they normally do during matches.

Aerobic fitness does not necessarily offer protection against the cold. Nevertheless, it will enable games players to keep more active when not directly involved in play and not increase the level of fatigue. Outfield players with a high level of aerobic fitness will be able to maintain activity at a satisfactory level to achieve heat balance. On the other hand, the individual with poor endurance may be at risk of hypothermia if the pace of activity falls dramatically. Shivering during activity signals the onset of danger.

## ALTITUDE

### Altitude

A large number of international tournaments have been held in countries that are above sea level. These include both international youth and World Cup tournaments (e.g., 1970, 1986 and 2010). The height above sea level can be classified as low altitude (1250 m), moderate altitude (1250–3000 m), high altitude (3000–6000 m) or severe altitude (6000 m+). The highest recorded official international game was held in La Paz in Bolivia (3600 m).

The main physiological challenge caused by exercise at altitude is hypoxia, or a relative lack of oxygen. The air is less dense as ambient pressure decreases and, as there are fewer oxygen molecules in a given volume of air, less oxygen is inspired. The decrease in oxygen tension in the lungs results in a lowered oxygen delivery by the red blood cells to the active tissues. With time, the body does demonstrate some adaptive responses which can compensate for the relative lack of oxygen in the air, though these responses may not be fully observed until weeks or months at altitude. The sea-level visitor to altitude is never as completely adapted as the individual born and bred there. This factor may lead to changes in a player's ability to perform the required activities during match-play, and hence reduce performance. In this section the major physiological challenges facing soccer players upon immediate exposure to altitude and the potential impact of such changes on performance are outlined. Approaches to preparing players for tournaments at altitude are also covered.

### The acute physiological challenge of altitude

The reduction in the partial pressure of oxygen ($PO_2$) in the inspired air at altitude is the source of the unique stress placed on soccer players during competition and training. Reductions in the ambient pressure and, consequently, tension in the alveolar in the lungs lead to a fall in gradient across the pulmonary capillaries for transferring oxygen into the blood. This effect will result in a desaturation of the red blood cells and an impairment of oxygen transport once the ambient pressure drops to a point corresponding to an altitude of around 1200 m. This effect occurs because the sigmoid shape of the oxygen disassociation curve of haemoglobin (Hb) protects the oxygen-carrying capacity of the blood for the first 1000 m or so increase above sea level. Above this altitude, the curve starts to decline steeply, affecting the oxygen transport in increasing levels.

The immediate physiological adjustment to altitude exposure is an increase in ventilation (both depth and frequency of breathing) to boost the $PO_2$ in the pulmonary alveoli. This factor helps in part to offset the fall in oxygen saturation that follows the reduction in alveolar $PO_2$. The hyperventilation that occurs leads to a rise in blood pH as a consequence of the increased loss of carbon dioxide ($CO_2$). As $CO_2$ in solution is a weak acid, the blood becomes more alkaline than normal and there is an excess of bicarbonate ions (Henderson-Hasselbach equation). The kidneys respond by excreting bicarbonate over the course of several days, which helps to restore blood pH towards normal. The temporary decrease in the body's alkaline reserve means that the blood has a poorer capability for buffering additional acids that may be released. For example, lactic acid diffusing from active muscles into the blood during exercise at altitude will not be neutralised as easily by buffering, meaning that high-intensity exercise may be harder to maintain than at sea-level.

### Altitude and performance

The impact of altitude on the outcome of soccer matches has been investigated by McSharry (2007). The approach in these investigations was to analyse 104 years of home and away games played in South America (a continent in which games are played across a range of altitudes (sea level to 3600 m), in an attempt to model the effect of altitude on the probability of winning. Such analysis, while providing useful information on the relative probabilities of teams from different altitudes winning against opponents from the same or different altitudes, does not provide any real information on the influence of hypoxia on each of the specific components that determine soccer performance, more specifically the psychological, technical, tactical and physiological demands.

Soccer players face relatively unique physiological challenges when competing at altitude. The physical performance of an invasive team sport such as soccer requires players to complete intermittent exercise patterns. The activities completed range from those that are performed at a low-sub-maximal intensity and stress predominantly the aerobic energy systems (e.g., walking, jogging) to those completed maximally using anaerobic metabolism (e.g., sprinting). There seems to be little literature currently available that has specifically attempted to evaluate the impact of altitude on intermittent exercise patterns, especially those that are associated with soccer. Levine *et al.* (2008) recommended that soccer players would have to adjust their

W. Gregson and B. Drust

pacing strategies at altitude in response to the observed declines in maximal aerobic power ($\dot{V}O_{2max}$) to prevent excessive fatigue during games. The $\dot{V}O_{2max}$ is reduced by about 15% at an altitude of 2.3 km and it is estimated that $\dot{V}O_{2max}$ declines by about 1–2% for every 100 m above 1.5 km, though these values can vary considerably between individuals. After 3–4 weeks at altitude, a portion of this impairment is recovered but the $\dot{V}O_{2max}$ remains below sea-level values. For example, the 15% initial drop in $VO_2$ at an altitude of 2.3 km is reversed to a reduction by 9% of the sea-level value within 4 weeks. These average values mask a wide variation across individuals. The fall in maximal aerobic power as a consequence of the reduction in ambient air pressure means that a fixed exercise challenge imposes a greater physiological stress on the athlete. Consequently, higher heart rate, ventilation and blood lactate values are observed, as compared with the same work-rate at sea-level and the increase corresponds to the decline in $\dot{V}O_{2max}$. This effect will mean that players will need longer periods than normal to clear the lactate that is produced and accumulated in the bloodstream. Alongside the increased relative physiological stress is a rise in the perceived exertion. This perceptual change in the player's response to the activity profile makes him/her less likely to complete voluntary runs to either create space or execute on the ball actions, and require longer recovery periods before they can repeat high-intensity efforts.

These observations would seem to indicate that some concessions in game tactics are needed to compensate for reductions in performance, particularly for individuals who are more vulnerable to altitude deterioration. Such concessions include more suitable timing of attacking movements and a willingness to concede possession to the opposition for longer periods than normal, in an attempt to offset the need for longer recovery periods. The evidence used to develop the recommendations presented by Levine et al. (2008) is, however, predominantly based on research studies that have examined the impact of increasing altitude on maximal and sub-maximal exercise performance completed as distinct bouts of activity. This approach is clearly limited, as the physiological and metabolic responses associated with intermittent exercise are not the same as those observed with exercise bouts performed at similar intensities completed as isolated exercise sessions. This observation does not invalidate these recommendations, but merely illustrates the need for more sport-specific research to be completed and published before we can fully evaluate the impact of altitude on team sport performance.

In contrast, the reduction in air density at altitude means that performance may be improved in events where air resistance may be a limiting factor. In soccer, this factor may predominantly apply to high-intensity activities such as sprinting. The nature of the sprinting activity in soccer match-play is very different from those athletic events that have benefitted from reduced air resistance at the Olympics (e.g., track events at all distances up to 800 m and field events such as the long jump). These differences may mean that any potential advantage associated with reduced air resistance is offset by the increased metabolic challenge in hypoxic conditions and its negative effects on performance, especially when sprints are repeated.

Altitude can also present difficulties to soccer players when completing important elements of technical performance. The decreasing air density associated with increasing altitude results in changes in the aerodynamics of ball flight. These alterations include a reduction in the lateral deflection or 'curve' of the ball and an increased flight, as the ball will travel more easily through the thinner air (Levine et al., 2008). This effect can cause difficulty for all outfield positions when shooting, chasing the ball, controlling long passes and clearing the ball using long kicks out of defence. The goalkeeper in soccer may also be more easily deceived by shots at goal, owing to the faster flight of the ball and its altered trajectory. These changes in ball flight may become especially important when a team prepare for competition at one altitude but have to contest a competitive game at a very different height without a suitable time period to re-adjust to the new flight characteristics. Such problems faced teams in World Cups staged in Mexico (1986) and South Africa (2010).

## Preparing players for competitions at altitude

Players who are required to compete at altitude should prepare appropriately for the additional physiological stresses that accompany both training and match-play. Suitable strategies include the completion of a period of acclimatisation either at the specific venue of competition or a suitable alternative (though this may lead to other problems, such as travel fatigue or jet lag prior to competition if travel is inappropriately timed). One of the most important considerations for the choice of acclimatisation venue would seem to be the suitability of the level of altitude for this initial exposure, as this seems to be a fundamental factor in determining the physiological changes that accompany any exposure to a hypoxic environment. Another key consideration is the time period that should be allowed prior to competition and following arrival, as this must be balanced to enable suitable physiological adaptations to be made, but not long enough to lead to a loss of fitness through de-training.

The physiological rationale for acclimatisation periods comes from the immediate changes that the body makes upon exposure to altitude, in an attempt to offset the reductions in the oxygen-carrying capacity of the blood. Adaptations to altitude may occur at any of the steps in the oxygen cascade between the lungs and the muscle cells. One of the major physiological adaptations to hypoxia is an increase in the number of red blood cells. Within a few days of reaching an altitude location, a rise in haemoglobin concentration is apparent, though this initial increase is a result of haemoconcentration from reductions in plasma volume. This fall in blood volume arises from increased water loss due to hyperventilation and decreased water intake due to loss of appetite. Nevertheless, there is a gradual increase in haemoglobin which is mediated by stimulation of the bone marrow to release slightly immature red blood cells (reticulocytes) and promote the early stages of erythropoiesis (Bergland, 1992). Both ventilatory and circulatory adaptations complement increases in the oxygen-carrying capacity of the blood. Such adjustments include a reduction in the heart rate response to sub-maximal exercise from that initially observed at altitude and a decrease in cardiac output. A number of morphological changes are observed in the muscle, such as reductions in muscle mass and increases in tissue myoglobin and capillary density to facilitate oxygen transport, and there are increases in mitochondrial density and efficiency enzyme activities to promote aerobic metabolism. Additionally, substrate utilisation is enhanced by mobilisation of free fatty acids and increased use of blood glucose, thereby saving muscle glycogen (Brooks et al., 1991).

Prolonged stays at altitude may be disadvantageous to performance, as the physiological changes associated with hypoxia can negatively affect training loads that can be completed by the players. The available research suggests that around 14 days should be allowed for acclimatisation for altitudes around 1500–2000 m. This should be extended by around 7 days

94

for higher venues (2000–2500 m). It is not advisable to train hard for the first 2–3 days following arrival since such sessions will increase the likelihood of illness and injury (based on Gore *et al.*, 2008). During this time, it may be beneficial to focus training sessions on technical/tactical issues, as this type of work is frequently less physiologically stressful than fitness-orientated work. Following this initial period, the intensity of training sessions can be gradually increased across the next 7–10 days until the intensity matches that usually completed. These increases in intensity may reflect a return to normal recovery periods between high-intensity efforts, as well as increases in the intensity or volume of the exercise bouts. Careful attention should be given to adequate nutrition and fluid replacement during these initial stages of acclimatisation, to prevent glycogen depletion (as carbohydrate will be the dominant fuel for exercise during the first exposures to altitude) and to offset any excessive losses in plasma volume. The need for iron supplementation should also be considered to support the changes in red blood cells.

The demands of the modern game may make such prolonged stays at altitude unrealistic for anything other than the most important international tournaments. In such situations, alternative approaches may be employed in an attempt to acclimatise players to hypoxic conditions. These simulated options are usually created with nitrogen-enriched mixtures of air, as it is more difficult to reduce the atmospheric pressure. Such equipment is frequently found in the training centres of high-level professional soccer teams for use with both fit players during normal training and injured players in rehabilitation. Such approaches include the frequent exposure of players to simulated altitude in environmental chambers or using specially designed equipment that lower the inspired-oxygen tension. A wide range of potential exposure strategies to such equipment have been identified in the literature, including intermittent hypoxic resting exposure, intermittent hypoxic training and live high train low strategies (see Gore *et al.*, 2008). A comprehensive review of these approaches is beyond the scope of this chapter, though Millet and colleagues (2010) outline the effectiveness of a range of such strategies in supporting the preparation for competition at altitude.

## Circadian variation

A large number of physiological functions in the body exhibit cyclical changes in relation to time. These rhythms are characterised by the length of their cycle, which can range from a fraction of a second to a number of days. One of the most commonly studied biological rhythms is the circadian rhythm. A circadian rhythm is one which recurs around the solar day, exhibiting a length of around 24 hours. A good example of a circadian rhythm is core temperature. Figure 5.3 illustrates the pattern of the daily variation in core temperature and includes an illustration of both the peak value (acrophase) that occurs around 17:00 to 18:00 and the minimum noted around 6:00. Such rhythms are influenced by both endogenous (internal control mechanisms that are a consequence of a 'body clock' located in the brain) and exogenous factors (external factors such as light, ambient temperature, timing of meals, social activity), indicating that these rhythms have both internal and environmental influences in their control.

Researchers have suggested that many measures of human performance follow closely the curve in body temperature (Drust *et al.* 2005b). These measures include components of motor

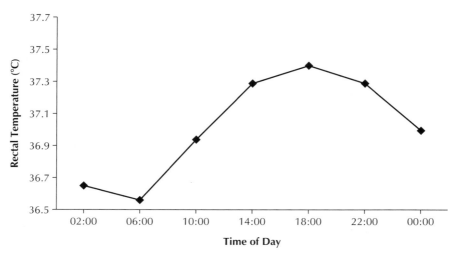

**Figure 5.3** Circadian rhythm in rectal temperature.

performance that are important in soccer play such as strength, reaction time, jumping and endurance (Drust *et al.*, 2005b). These daily variations have the potential to influence important physiological determinants of performance, albeit this factor has not been investigated in any detail within the available scientific literature. Another major biological rhythm that is of major importance to soccer performance is the sleep–wake cycle. The sleep–wake cycle results in sharp contrasts in arousal, with peak values occurring around mid-day, at the time that the concentrations of adrenaline are at their highest. These changes in arousal may influence factors such as the decision-making abilities of players, and hence their tactical and technical contributions to the game.

A knowledge of circadian rhythm is very important for optimising the performance of soccer teams, as it can facilitate a reduction in jet lag following long-haul flights that cross multiple time zones. Such flights are common in both international and club competition. Jet lag refers to the feelings of disorientation, light-headedness, impatience, lack of energy, loss of appetite, difficulty in sleeping, poor concentration and co-ordination and general discomfort that follow travel across time zones (Waterhouse *et al.*, 2007). Such feelings may linger for several days after arrival, though there are large inter-individual differences in the extent to which players experience such symptoms and the time course over which such feelings may persist. This change in mental and physiological state clearly has potential to disrupt performance and lead to a failure of teams to progress within competitions that may generate significant prestige and/or prize money. These issues will also affect managerial, coaching and medical staff, and potentially their ability to make key decisions related to both the tactical performance of the team and organisational strategies related to the visit.

The symptoms of jet lag are in part a consequence of the failure of the body's circadian rhythms to adjust to the time at destination. For example, a rapid transition across the time zones that separate the UK and Australia will lead to a 10-h change in time. This may mean that the newly arrived individual may be forced to be awake when they would normally be sleeping if at

**W. Gregson and B. Drust**

home. In the new environment, the time of sunrise and darkness, and activity and social contact, will force the circadian cycles to adjust in time. This re-synchronisation of the important circadian rhythms (such as those of core temperature and arousal) in time lead to a loss of the symptoms of jet lag and a return to the performance levels usually observed at home.

The severity of jet lag is influenced by various factors. Crossing a large number of time zones is more difficult for the majority of people to deal with than shorter flights. This may mean that the travel that is usually typical of European teams in UEFA competitions is more easily tolerated than flights that are more typical within large continents, such as Asia and the Americas. The direction of travel is also an important factor in the severity of jet lag. Research evidence suggests that it is far easier to cope with flying in a westward than an eastward direction (Waterhouse et al., 2007) because the body rhythms can extend their natural time period during westward travel, as opposed to a forcible shortening of the cycle when travelling eastward. Maximal time-zone shifts of around 12 h seem, however, to result in little difference whether travel is either westward or eastward in direction.

A number of strategies can be employed in an attempt to facilitate the re-synchronisation of an individual's circadian rhythms and minimise the impact that travel may have on their performance. An important initial consideration is time of departure and time of arrival, as inappropriate travel strategies on either the outward or the return leg may prevent appropriate levels of re-synchronisation. Exercise can be an especially important factor in such strategies, as physical activity can speed up the adaptation to a new time zone (Waterhouse et al., 2007). Suitable travel arrangements can help players to immediately adopt the phase characteristics of the new environment. For example, the travel schedule could be arranged so that players are able to complete a light training session in the evening upon arrival, which helps to anchor the body temperature rhythm to its new time zone and delays the onset of sleep to a time that is more suitable. Alternatively, training should be avoided if the arrival is scheduled for the morning, when activity could promote the anchoring of the body clock to the departed time zone (e.g., after a long-haul flight to the east).

Irrespective of the timing of the initial training session, the activities included should be adapted for a short time period (2–3 days) following arrival. Skills that require fine co-ordination are likely to be disrupted for a few days in the new environment as a consequence of the de-synchronisation of relevant circadian rhythms. These changes may lead to accidents or injuries as players seek to regain their technical and physical competencies. Reducing the intensity of the initial sessions may help to prevent unsuitable physiological loads on players as they adjust to both the new climate and time zones. This factor may mean that is beneficial to incorporate friendly games during the first week if the travel has been undertaken to play important competitive games in which positive results are required. The timing of sleep is also crucial in any strategy to minimise the effects of jet lag, as napping at an inappropriate time (a time that the player should have been asleep at home) for prolonged periods will only make subsequent sleep more difficult and prolong the adjustment of the biological clock.

## SUMMARY

Soccer is played in a variety of challenging environments, consequently, living, training and competing under such conditions remains an on-going challenge for the elite soccer player. Stresses may include heat, cold, altitude or disruption of the circadian body clock. Some account must be taken of the environment in which competition is scheduled. This may involve a range of physiological and behavioural preparation strategies, and changes in tactics may also be needed to enable players to cope.

Humans are homoeothermic in that they have the capacity to maintain a relatively constant internal body temperature. However, when training or competing under high ambient temperatures, marked increases in physiological strain may arise which impair exercise performance. Similarly, a fall in limb temperature in the cold may reduce motor performance, muscular strength and power output. Care must therefore be taken to reduce the risk of heat injury and preserve limb temperature under extreme cold. In the heat, preparatory measures include acclimation, reducing the intensity of the pre-match warm-up and the application of external cooling modalities. The latter may also be applied during the half-time period. Since the main avenue for heat loss in the heat is sweating, and the resultant body water loss further contributes to heat-induced decrements in performance, it is essential that players also remain hydrated. Cold is less of a problem than heat, in that the body may be protected against exposure to the adverse environmental conditions. Maintaining a high work-rate and choice of appropriate clothing are likely to ensure that players are able to offset the detrimental effects of cold ambient temperatures on performance.

Another important environmental challenge to the modern player is that associated with completing matches at high altitudes. Performing at heights in excess of 1200 m complicates the demands associated with match-play by adding the physiological challenge of a relative lack of oxygen, as compared to games at sea-level. This change in the availability of oxygen may limit the activities completed by players during games, thereby reducing the overall team effort. In addition to the potential for reduced activity are alterations in the technical requirements of the sport as a consequence of changes in air resistance. These two factors may necessitate the coach to change tactics if a suitable acclimatisation period cannot be completed by the squad before competition.

The travel requirements to complete such preparatory periods or actual competitions can also temporarily affect the performance of players, due to the disruption of the circadian rhythms. Circadian rhythms (e.g., core body temperature) that recur around the solar day (with a length of 24 hours) are influenced by both internal mechanisms and external factors such as activity, meals and the light–dark cycle. Such rhythms in physiological functions are important, as they can impact on a number of characteristics that are important for soccer performance. Minimising the effects of such rhythms requires careful organisation of the travel strategies used by teams and the adoption of suitable schedules following the arrival at the final destination.

**W. Gregson and B. Drust**

# REFERENCES

Barr, D., Reilly, T., and Gregson, W. (2010). The impact of different cooling modalities on the physiological responses in firefighters during strenuous work performed in high environmental temperatures. *European Journal of Applied Physiology* 111 (6), 959–967.

Bergh, U., and Ekblom, B. (1979). Influence of muscle temperature on maximal muscle strength and power output in human skeletal muscles. *Acta Physiologica Scandinavica* 107, 33–37.

Bergland, B. (1992). High altitude training aspects of haematological adaptation. *Sports Medicine* 14, 289–303.

Brooks, G., Butterfield, G.A., Wolfe, R.R., Groves, B.M., Mazzeo, R.S., Sutton, J.R., Wolfel, E.E., and Reeves, J.T. (1991). Increased dependence on blood glucose after acclimatization to 4300 m. *Journal of Applied Physiology* 70, 919–927.

Davies, C.T., and Young, K. (1983). Effect of temperature on the contractile properties and muscle power of triceps surae in humans. *Journal of Applied Physiology* 55, 191–195.

de Looy, A., Minors, D., Waterhouse, J., Reilly, T., and Tunstall-Pedoe, D. (1988). *The Coach's Guide to Competing Abroad*. Leeds: National Coaching Foundation.

Drust, B., Rasmussen, P., Mohr, M., Nielsen, B., and Nybo, L. (2005a). Elevations in core and muscle temperature impairs repeated sprint performance. *Acta Physiologica Scandinavica* 183, 181–190.

Drust, B., Waterhouse, J., Atkinson, G., Edwards, B. and Reilly, T. (2005b). Circadian rhythms in sports performance – an update. *International Society for Chronobiology* 22, 21–44.

Edwards, A.M., and Clark, N.A. (2006). Thermoregulatory observations in soccer match play: professional and recreational level applications using an intestinal pill system to measure core temperature. *British Journal of Sports Medicine* 40, 133–138

Ekblom, B. (1986). Applied physiology of soccer. *Sports Medicine* 3, 50–60.

Gant, N., Atkinson, G., and Williams, C. (2006). The validity and reliability of intestinal temperature during intermittent running. *Medicine and Science in Sports and Exercise* 38, 1926–1931.

Gonzalez-Alonso, J., Mora-Rodriguez, R., Below, P.R., and Coyle, E.F. (1997). Dehydration markedly impairs cardiovascular function in hyperthermic endurance athletes during exercise. *Journal of Applied Physiology* 82, 1229–1236.

Gore, C.J., McSharry, P.E., Hewitt, A.J., and Saunders, P.U. (2008). Preparation for football competition at moderate altitude. *Scandinavian Journal of Medicine and Science in Sports* 18, Suppl 1, 85–95.

Gregson, W., Drust, B., Atkinson, G., and Salvo, V.D. (2010). Match-to-match variability of high-speed activities in premier league soccer. *International Journal of Sports Medicine* 31, 237–242.

Gregson, W.A., Drust, B., Batterham, A. and Cable, N.T. (2005). The influence of pre-warming on the physiological responses to soccer-specific intermittent exercise. In T. Reilly, J. Cabri and D. Araújo (eds), *Science and Football V*, London: Routledge, pp. 377–385.

Houmard, J.A., Costill, D.L., Davis, J.A., Mitchell, J.B., Pascoe, D.D., and Robergs, R.A. (1990). The influence of exercise intensity on heat acclimation in trained subjects. *Medicine and Science in Sports and Exercise* 22, 615–620.

Kurdak, S.S., Shirreffs, S.M., Maughan, R.J., Ozgünen, K.T., Zeren, Ç., Korkmaz, S., Yazici, Z., Ersöz, G., Binnet, M.S., and Dvorak, J. (2010). Hydration and sweating responses to hot-weather football competition. *Scand J Med Sci Sports* 20, 133–139.

Levine, B., Stray-Gundersen, J.S., Mehta, R.D. (2008). Effect of altitude on football performance. *Scand J Med Sci Sports* 18 (Suppl.1): 76–84.

Lind, A.R. and Bass, D.E. (1963). Optimal exposure time for development of heat acclimation. *Federation Proceedings* 22, 704–708.

Maughan, R.J., Shirreffs, S.M., Ozgünen, K.T., Kurdak, S.S., Ersöz, G., Binnet, M.S., and Dvorak, J. (2010). Living, training and playing in the heat: challenges to the football player and strategies for coping with environmental extremes. *Scand J Med Sci Sports* 20, 117–124.

McSharry, P.E. (2007). Understanding the effect of altitude on physiological performance using results of international football games: a statistical analysis. *British Medical Journal* 335, 1278–1281.

Millet, G.P., Roels, B., Scmitt, L., Woorons, X., and Richalet, J.P. (2010). Combining hypoxic methods for peak performance. *Sports Medicine* 40, 1–25.

Minett, G.M., Duffield, R., Marino, F.E., and Portus, M. (2011). Volume-dependent response of pre-cooling for intermittent-sprint exercise in the heat. *Medicine and Science in Sports and Exercise*. (Epub ahead of print)

Mohr, M., Mujika, I., Santisteban, J., Randers, M.B., Bischoff, R., Solano, R., Hewitt, A., Zubillaga, A., Peltola, E., and Krustrup, P. (2010). Examination of fatigue development in elite soccer in a hot environment: a multi-experimental approach. *Scand J Med Sci Sports* 20, 125–132.

Montain, S.J., and Coyle, E.F. (1992). Influence of graded dehydration on hyperthermia and cardiovascular drift during exercise. *Journal of Applied Physiology* 73, 1340–1350.

Morris, J.G., Nevill, M.E., and Williams, C. (2000). Physiological and metabolic responses of female games and endurance athletes to prolonged, intermittent, high-intensity running at 30 degrees and 16 degrees C ambient temperatures. *European Journal of Applied Physiology* 81, 84–92.

Nadel, E.R., Cafarelli, E., Roberts, M.F., and Wenger, C.B. (1979). Circulatory regulation during exercise in different ambient temperatures. *Journal of Applied Physiology* 46, 430–437.

Nielsen, B. (1994). Heat stress and acclimation. *Ergonomics* 37, 49–58.

Nybo, L., and Nielsen, B. (2001). Hyperthermia and central fatigue during prolonged exercise in humans. *Journal of Applied Physiology* 91, 1055–1060.

Özgünen, K.T., Kurdak, S.S., Maughan, R.J., Zeren, Ç., Korkmaz, S., Yazıcı, Z., Ersöz, G., Shirreffs, S.M., Binnet, M.S., and Dvorak, J. (2010). Effect of hot environmental conditions on physical activity patterns and temperature response of football players. *Scand J Med Sci Sports* 20, 140–147.

Price, M.J., Boyd, C., and Goosey-Tolfrey, V.L. (2009). The physiological effects of pre-event and midevent cooling during intermittent running in the heat in elite female soccer players. *Applied Physiology, Nutrition and Metabolism* 34, 942–949.

Racinais, S., and Oksa, J. (2010). Temperature and neuromuscular function. *Scand J Med Sci Sports* 20, Suppl 3, 1–18.

Rehrer, N.J. (2001). Fluid and electrolyte balance in ultra-endurance sport. *Sports Medicine* 31, 701–15.

Reilly, T. (2000). Temperature and performance: heat. In M. Harries, G. McLatchie, C. Williams, and J. King (eds), *ABC of Sports Medicine*. London: BMJ Books, pp 68–71.

100

Reilly, T., Maughan, R.J., Budgett, R., and Davies, B. (1997). The acclimatisation of international athletes. In S.A. Robertson (ed.), *Contemporary Ergonomics 1997*. London: Taylor and Francis, pp 136–140.

Ross, M.L., Garvican, L.A., Jeacocke, N.A., Laursen, P.B., Abbiss, C.R., Martin, D.T., and Burke, L.M. (2011). Novel precooling strategy enhances time trial cycling in the heat. *Medicine and Science in Sports and Exercise* 43, 123–133.

Shaffrath, J.D., and Adams, W.C. (1984). Effects of airflow and work load on cardiovascular drift and skin blood flow. *Journal of Applied Physiology* 56, 1411–1417.

Shirreffs, S.M., and Maughan, R.J. (1998). Urine osmolality and conductivity as indices of hydration status in athletes in the heat. *Medicine and Science in Sports and Exercise* 30, 1598–1602.

Waterhouse, J., Reilly, T., Atkinson, G., and Edwards, B. (2007). Jet lag: trends and coping strategies. *The Lancet* 369, 1117–1129.

# PART II

# BEHAVIOURAL
# AND SOCIAL SCIENCES

# CHAPTER 6

## 'GAME INTELLIGENCE'

ANTICIPATION AND DECISION MAKING

A.M. Williams and P.R. Ford

### INTRODUCTION

At the very highest level in soccer the physiological or anthropometrical attributes of players do not differentiate between those who are successful and those who are less successful (e.g., Reilly, Williams, Nevill, and Franks, 2000). For example, consider the 2011 Champions League Final at Wembley, which pitted Manchester United, the champions of England, against Barcelona, the champions of Spain. Barcelona was unlikely to have prevailed over Manchester United because of having larger, stronger or fitter players. At this level there are more compelling arguments that the technical, psychological (e.g., mental toughness, resilience under pressure) and 'game intelligence' (e.g., anticipation and decision making) attributes of the players are the discriminating factors, along with the strategic and tactical plan developed by the coaching staff, and the manner in which it is implemented by players.

In this chapter, we focus exclusively on 'game intelligence', with a particular focus on anticipation and decision making. Anticipation necessitates that players 'read the game' and perceive ahead of the action occurring what opponents and teammates are likely to do in any particular situation. Decision making requires that players plan, select and execute an action or set of actions based on the current circumstances on the field of play and the strategic tactical game plan that is decided ahead of the match and that continuously evolves as events unfold. Researchers (e.g., Roca, Ford, McRobert, and Williams, 2011; Williams and Davids, 1998) have consistently shown that skilled soccer players are more accurate at anticipation and decision making, as compared to their less skilled counterparts. In writing this chapter, we have two main aims. First, we identify the skills, processes and mechanisms underpinning anticipation and decision making in soccer and, in so doing, illustrate how performance may be measured empirically in an applied setting. Second, we examine how players with superior ability to anticipate and to make decisions have acquired this attribute and how training interventions may be used in an applied setting in an effort to develop 'game intelligent' players.

### ANTICIPATION AND DECISION MAKING: SKILLS, PROCESSES AND MECHANISMS UNDERLYING SUPERIOR PERFORMANCE

Over the last three decades there are have been numerous attempts by researchers to identify the perceptual-cognitive skills, processes and mechanisms underpinning anticipation and decision making. Although there is a substantive research base involving other sports (see Williams and Ericsson, 2005; Williams, Ford, Eccles, and Ward, 2011), we focus mainly on research involving adult and youth male soccer players. No research, to our knowledge, has involved female players. However, while this remains an important oversight, it is unlikely that the skills would differ greatly, if at all, as a result of specific gender differences rather than the accumulation of experience/practice. In the first part of this section, we review those skills and processes involved in 'reading the game' through anticipation and situational assessment. In the second part, we review those processes and mechanisms involved in the player 'affecting the game' through the planning, selection and execution of a decision or set of decision/s by the player.

## 'Reading the game': anticipation and situation assessment

### Visual search processes

When observing a soccer match, one can see skilled players consistently moving their heads and eyes to 'look around' the pitch, at the ball, the movements of opponents and teammates and areas of space that may be exploited or exposed. Researchers have demonstrated empirically that skilled soccer players use their visual system in a systematically different manner when compared to less skilled players. One of the earliest studies examining visual search or gaze behaviours in soccer was conducted with goalkeepers when attempting to predict the direction of a penalty kick (Tyldesley, Bootsma, and Bomhoff, 1982; for other examples, see Dicks, Button, and Davids, 2010a, 2010b; Savelsbergh, Williams, van der Kamp, and Ward, 2002; Savelsbergh, van der Kamp, Williams, and Ward, 2005). Players were shown to direct a high proportion of their first fixations (60%) at the hips and almost 30% at the legs, feet and ball. Second fixations tended to be directed at the shoulders. Generally, the skilled players used a more structured search process, with fixations being restricted to the right side of the body and the shooting leg, in the case of a right-footed penalty taker. This study was ahead of its time, given the technical difficulties of recording visual search behaviour data at that time, albeit static images of penalty takers were presented as stimuli and a pen-and-paper response was employed.

Since this early work, numerous research studies have been published involving soccer, with advances in technology leading to a progressive improvement in the methods employed, enabling data to be captured in increasingly more realistic scenarios. Visual search behaviours have been evaluated as soccer players attempt to anticipate the actions of opponents in outfield scenarios involving 1 versus 1 situations, in various micro phases of defensive play involving 3 versus 3 simulations and in more macro phases involving larger groups of outfield players (Roca et al., 2011; Williams and Davids, 1998; Williams, Davids, Burwitz, and Williams, 1994). Similarly, visual search behaviours have been evaluated in situations that require players to make decisions during various phases of play, in offensive situations involving set-plays, and in sequences of play that traverse the length of the playing field and involve numerous interactions between players (Helsen and Starkes, 1999; Roca et al., 2011; Vaeyens, Lenoir, Williams, Mazyn, and Philippaerts, 2007a, 2007b). Figure 6.1 presents an illustration of visual search behaviour being measured as a player responds to an offensive sequence of play acted out on-screen by opponents. The broad conclusions of these studies are that

A.M. Williams and P.R. Ford

typically skilled players look at different areas of the visual display, for varying periods of time, using different search strategies, as compared with less skilled players (for a recent review of this area of work, see Vickers, 2011).

As an illustration, Roca *et al.* (2011) recorded the eye movements of skilled and less skilled soccer players who moved and interacted with life-sized video sequences of 11 versus 11 soccer situations filmed from the perspective of a central defender (see Figure 6.1). The video was occluded in the moment before a key event occurred. Participants were required to anticipate the action of the player in possession of the ball and to decide what course of action they should take. Skilled players were more accurate at anticipation and decision making, as compared to the less skilled players. Skilled players made more visual fixations of shorter duration and on significantly more locations in the display, as compared with the less skilled players. They spent more time fixating the opposing team players and areas of space, as compared to less skilled players who, in contrast, spent more time fixating the player in possession and the ball. The argument is that skilled players use visual processes in a different manner when compared to less skilled players in order to pick up the key information needed to guide their ability to anticipate and make decisions. The research data are not entirely

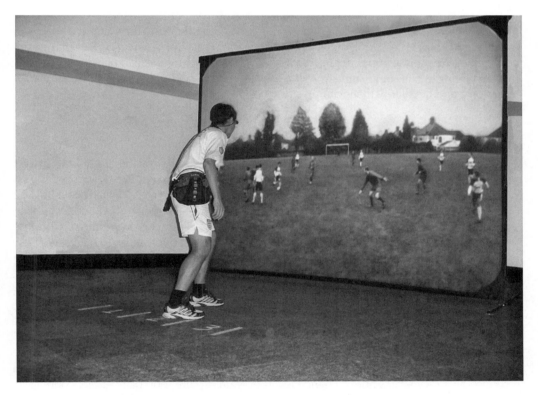

**Figure 6.1** Visual gaze behaviour being recorded as a defender interacts with a filmed simulation of an offensive sequence of play.

*Source*: Roca *et al.* (2011).

consistent across studies and in some instances no differences in gaze characteristics have been reported across skill groups. In these latter instances, variations in performance between skilled and less skilled players are likely due to more effective recognition of information using peripheral vision or differences in the amount or quality of information extracted per fixation (Williams and Davids, 1998).

A more recent progression by researchers has been to focus on identifying how stressors such as anxiety and fatigue influence the visual search behaviours employed (Causer, Holmes, Smith, and Williams, 2011; Vickers and Williams, 2007; Wilson, Wood, and Vine, 2009). Wilson et al. (2009; see also Wood and Wilson, 2011) examined the gaze behaviours of penalty takers as they completed kicks under low- and high-threat conditions. When anxious, in the high-threat condition, the penalty takers made faster first fixations and fixated for longer periods on the goalkeeper, with these changes in gaze behaviour leading to reductions in shooting accuracy and an increased likelihood of placing the ball nearer the goalkeeper, as compared to the low-threat condition. The current evidence suggests that skilled athletes are more robust to the negative effects of stress and fatigue. There remains a notable lack of empirical research to evaluate how stress and fatigue influences visual search strategy in outfield situations in soccer.

Players have information entering their visual system continuously throughout a match or practice. Information entering the visual system varies in its importance. Skilled players are better able to recognise important information, as compared to less skilled players, particularly that pertaining to cues emanating from the movements of other players and those pertaining to patterns and familiarity that occur in situations during play.

### Recognising information from the movements of other players

An extensive body of research exists to show that skilled soccer players are able to extract relevant early-arising advanced information from the postural movements of opponents (and probably teammates) as they, for example, execute a pass or shot at goal. Williams and Burwitz (1993) used a temporal occlusion approach to measure the ability of skilled and less skilled goalkeepers to predict penalty kick direction. A number of players were filmed from the perspective of a goalkeeper facing the penalty. These action sequences were then selectively edited to present varying extents of early and late information relative to foot–ball contact; the video sequences were occluded 120 ms before ball contact, 80 ms before ball contact, at the moment of foot–ball contact, and 120 ms after foot–ball contact. Figure 6.2a presents an illustration of the film sequences presented when using temporal occlusion techniques. Players viewed the action sequences on a near-life-sized screen and were required to indicate using a pen-and-paper response which corners of the goal the penalty kicks were directed towards. Skilled players were more accurate in their decisions than less skilled players only at the earliest (i.e., pre foot–ball contact) occlusion conditions. Moreover, skilled players recorded response-accuracy scores above chance levels even in the pre foot–ball contact conditions, illustrating their ability to process advance information from the penalty taker's run-up and postural movements. The errors in judging the ball's height only reduced significantly after viewing the first portion of ball flight.

A.M. Williams and P.R. Ford

Since this early work, researchers have conducted many studies in which they have identified the key sources of postural information underpinning anticipation. A popular methodological approach has been to record eye movement data as players view film-based simulations (Dicks *et al.*, 2010a; Savelsbergh *et al.*, 2002, 2005) or as they actually perform the task in situ (Dicks *et al.*, 2010a; Piras and Vickers, 2011). Moreover, there have been efforts to describe biomechanically the kinematic information available to the goalkeeper (Dicks *et al.*, 2010b; Lees and Owens, 2011). For example, Savelsbergh *et al.* (2002) used a very similar temporal occlusion methodology to Williams and Burwitz (1993), but in addition they recorded eye movement data. Skilled goalkeepers were more accurate at anticipating penalty direction, making fewer visual fixations of longer duration to a smaller number of locations, as compared with the less skilled goalkeepers. During the early stages of the penalty kick, the skilled goalkeepers spent more time fixating the face of the kicker, which may give them early information as to the direction of the kick. In contrast, less skilled keepers fixated on 'unclassified' regions early on. In the moments before foot–ball contact, the skilled keepers fixated on the kicking leg, non-kicking leg and ball regions, whereas less skilled keepers fixated on the trunk, arm and hip regions. The search strategies used by the skilled goalkeepers and their ability to recognise advance postural cues emanating from the movements of the taker led to their being more successful at saving penalties. Although there have been no direct

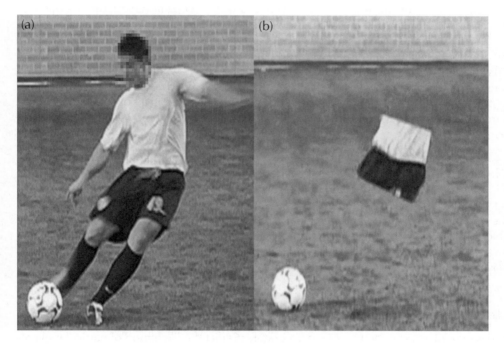

**Figure 6.2** The penalty taker as presented in (a) a temporal-occlusion condition where information is available up to foot–ball contact and (b) a spatial occlusion condition where only the hips are presented.

*Source*: From Causer and Williams (2012).

attempts to examine the ability of players to predict pass destination in situations involving open play, it is likely that the processes employed by outfield players do not differ from those employed by goalkeepers at penalty kicks.

*Recognising patterns and detecting familiarity in sequences of play*

Another skill that appears to be important when 'reading the game' is the ability to recognise familiarity or patterns in evolving sequences of play. The assumption is that skilled players are able to identify familiarity through structures or patterns in play as sequences unfold (e.g., 2 versus 1 situation, triangle or diamond shape forming between players in possession) and that this ability enables them to anticipate the likely outcome of events ahead of time. This skill is usually examined using the recognition paradigm. Players are presented with filmed footage from competitive matches involving either structured (i.e., footage involving a typical offensive move) or unstructured sequences (e.g., players during a break for injury in a match). These sequences last between 3 and 10 seconds. In a subsequent recognition phase, players are presented with a combination of clips in that some were presented in the earlier viewing phase, whereas some where not and were novel. The accuracy with which players are able to recognise previously viewed clips is taken as the dependent measure. Skilled players are more accurate than less skilled players in recognising structured sequences only. A number of published research studies illustrate the importance of this skill in soccer (e.g., North, Williams, Ward, Hodges, and Ericsson, 2009; North, Ward, Ericsson, and Williams, 2011; Williams, Hodges, North, and Barton, 2006). Most recently, there have been efforts to identify the specific sources of information used when recognising structured sequences. A combination of visual search recording, think-aloud verbal reports and different manipulations to the film displays (e.g., occlusion of players, removal of superficial display features) have been used to examine this question (for a review, see Williams and North, 2009).

The proposal is that skilled players initially extract relational information from the positions and movements of players and the ball, and match these stimulus characteristics with their previous knowledge (Dittrich, 1999). Skilled players recognise familiar patterns of play based upon structural relations between features (e.g., teammates, opponents and the ball), as well as the tactical and strategic significance of these relations. In contrast, less skilled players are unable to pick up important relational information and have less knowledge, constraining them to employ more distinctive surface or background features (e.g., pitch condition, colour of playing uniforms) when making such decisions.

*Predicting likely event occurrences*

Skilled soccer players are better able to accurately predict the likelihood of particular events or actions occurring in any given situation, as compared to less skilled players. For example, if a goalkeeper throws the ball to one of his/her full-backs, what are the passing options available to the player as (s)he receives the ball? It is likely that the opposing players will develop expectations as to the pass options that may be chosen by the player in possession of the ball and then try to match up this prediction with the available visual information. Ward

# 110

and Williams (2003) examined the importance of this skill in soccer by showing a series of 10-second duration film sequences of match action to elite and sub-elite soccer players. At the end of the sequence, the final frame of action was frozen on screen. Participants were required to imagine themselves as an opponent and to highlight on a paper copy of the frozen frame the options available to the player in possession of the ball and then rank those in order of threat to the defence. The elite players were better than the sub-elite group at highlighting the key options and were more accurate in ranking those options in order of threat, as determined by an independent panel of expert coaches. In contrast, sub-elite players were less efficient in their selection and ranking of key options (see also, Williams, Bell-Walker, Ward, and Ford, 2012).

Skilled soccer players are able to assign a hierarchy of probabilities to potential events as the action unfolds by weighing up the likely options and their potential of occurring. These probabilities may exist across a broad range of situations, as well as being task, player/opponent and context specific (Williams, 2000). A challenge for researchers examining situational probabilities in the future is to provide evidence that this ability is part of actual soccer performance rather than potentially being a by-product of experience in the sport.

## Interventions 'affecting the game': decision making

Thus far, we have outlined some of the perceptual-cognitive skills and processes that allow skilled soccer players to 'read the game' via assessment of the situation and anticipation of what will happen next. However, an equally important ability is that of deciding what action/s to execute based upon the available information. In this section, we review current under-standing of decision making in soccer.

### Action selection and execution

In any given situation during match-play, one can see that expert players select and execute actions that are more appropriate and successful, as compared to those of less skilled players. Researchers (e.g., Roca et al., 2011; Vaeyens et al., 2007a, 2007b) have provided empirical evidence supporting the observation that expert players make a greater number of accurate decisions in a variety of soccer situations when compared to less skilled players. Other researchers have revealed how the decision-making process functions during performance in sport. McPherson and colleagues (e.g., McPherson and Kernodle, 2003) have detailed two conceptual memory adaptations that guide the interpretation of sensory input and the selection of actions during expert decision making. *Action plan profiles* match the current conditions in the situation with appropriate perceptual and/or motor actions. Current conditions can be player positions and movements, ball placement and patterns/structure in play. *Current event profiles* are contextual information in regard to current, past and future factors. These contextual factors can be situational (e.g., score or time in a match), athlete characteristics (e.g., their age and skill level), phases of play (e.g., team in possession), opponent characteristics (e.g., shot tendencies), and environmental characteristics (e.g., facilities) (McPherson and Kernodle, 2003).

These two conceptual memory structures are thought to function through rule-based procedures that link external conditions to goals, actions and their regulation. As an illustration, during a match a player might find themselves in possession of the ball in a 2 versus 1 situation with a defender approaching them and their teammate in free space. In this situation, the player might decide to select and execute a pass to their teammate, which would involve an action plan profile guiding this process. However, contextual factors from the current situation might change the decision. For example, if the player in possession's team were winning, with limited time left in the match, then the player might turn back to retain possession rather than playing a risky forward pass. In this case, the decision and action would be guided by a current event profile.

## Mechanisms underpinning anticipation and decision making

Researchers are interested in revealing the mechanisms that underpin successful anticipation and decision making. In this section, we briefly review the work of researchers who are beginning to reveal the neurophysiology of the brain during expert anticipation and decision making. We also review the work of other researchers who have described the mechanistic role of memory in expert sports performance.

### The role of the brain

When selecting and executing a decision during match-play, the brain acts upon incoming or sensory information and translates this into motor commands for action. Motor commands are sent through the central nervous system to activate and coordinate muscles, joints, limbs to achieve the identified goal (Magill, 2007). To date, no researchers have examined the neurophysiology of the brain in expert soccer players. Some researchers have examined the brain areas involved in anticipation during racket sports. For example, Wright, Bishop, Jackson, and Abernethy (2011) used functional magnetic resonance imaging (fMRI) to show that players activated brain areas of the mirror-neuron system and visual attention system when anticipating opponent shot types, and the activation was stronger in expert as compared to novice players. It is thought that greater activation of certain brain areas indicates structural and physiological changes in the brain, due to increased cell size or the growth of new neurons in those areas (probably caused through previous experiences) in athletes when compared to the general population (Yarrow, Brown, and Krakauer, 2009). Humans appear to use the same brain areas for perception and action (e.g., Schubotz, Friederici, and Yves von Cramon, 2000) and it is in these areas (and possibly others as yet unidentified) that one might predict adaptation to occur through experience in soccer. In the near future, researchers will examine the neurophysiology of anticipation and decision making in expert soccer players and advances in technology will eventually mean this can be done during actual performance.

**A.M. Williams and P.R. Ford**

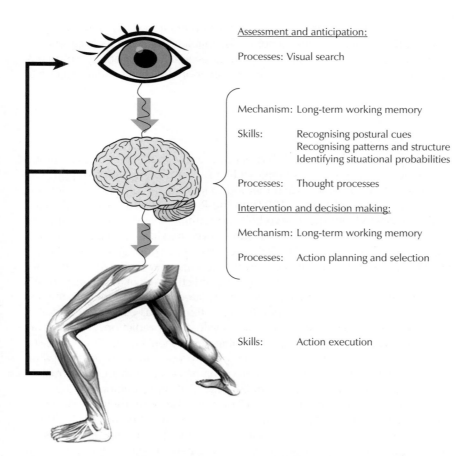

Assessment and anticipation:

Processes: Visual search

Mechanism: Long-term working memory

Skills: Recognising postural cues
Recognising patterns and structure
Identifying situational probabilities

Processes: Thought processes

Intervention and decision making:

Mechanism: Long-term working memory

Processes: Action planning and selection

Skills: Action execution

**Figure 6.3** The mechanisms, processes and skills underpinning anticipation and decision making.

A role for memory

Memory has been put forward by cognitive psychologists as the mechanism within the brain that underpins expert anticipation and decision making (e.g., Williams *et al.*, 2010). They have shown that the classic information-processing conception of memory involving short-term working memory and long-term memory does not explain the performance of experts (e.g., Ericsson and Kintsch, 1995). Long-term working memory theory has been proposed by Ericsson and co-workers (e.g., Ericsson and Delaney, 1999; Ericsson and Kintsch, 1995) to explain expert performance. It holds that experts bypass the limitations of short-term working memory by acquiring the ability to rapidly and reliably encode and retrieve domain-specific information into long-term memory when required. Long-term working memory consists of knowledge structures containing domain-specific information. A central component of long-term working memory theory is that retrieval cues kept in short-term working memory facilitate rapid and reliable access to that domain-specific information stored in long-term working memory. In contrast, classic long-term memory is unreliable and slow at these functions. A further component holds that expert players have stored information in memory in such a way that they can successfully anticipate future retrieval demands, enabling them to effectively encode new domain-specific information. In contrast, in normal everyday life, people are usually unable to anticipate what information from the current situation they will need to encode to memory for later use.

## Memory processes

Another recent development in the research has been to use verbal report or think-aloud protocols to identify the thought-processes employed by soccer players. Verbal reports can in certain conditions and tasks provide a valid method to identify the processes underlying decision making (e.g., Ericsson and Simon, 1993). In the Roca et al. (2011) study detailed earlier, the researchers collected retrospective verbal reports immediately after skilled and less skilled players had made a decision based on the action shown on a video simulation of a short offensive sequence of play (see Figure 6.1). Verbal reports were coded into four different levels of statements: monitoring (recall of current actions and events); evaluations (interpretation or meaning to current actions and events); predictions (what might occur next); and planning (possible alternative actions and outcomes) statements. As predicted, the less skilled players generated significantly more monitoring statements, as compared to skilled players. In contrast, the skilled players verbalised more evaluation, prediction, and planning statements in comparison with less skilled players. Findings have been interpreted as showing that skilled players have a more sophisticated memory representation for soccer when compared to less skilled players. In order to deal with a dynamic, ever-changing performance environment, expert performers are thought to build a detailed representation of the past, current or future events in long-term working memory that supports their performance (Ericsson and Kintsch, 1995; McPherson and Kernodle, 2003; Ward et al., 2011). These situation models are thought to combine the contextual information from the situation in order to guide and regulate behaviour prior to and during performance (McPherson and Kernodle, 2003; Ward et al., 2011).

A number of questions remain unanswered as to the exact nature of memory's role in actual soccer performance. The causal link between memory and anticipation/decision making is yet to be demonstrated by researchers (Yarrow et al., 2009). Ecological psychologists hold that expert athletes do not develop an enriched domain-specific memory that controls decision making. They state that the mechanism controlling skilled decision making is the progressive development of *perceptual attunement* to relevant information sources in the environment that affords and constrains action possibilities (for reviews, see Araújo and Davids, 2011; Araújo, Davids, and Hristovski, 2006; Davids, Button, and Bennett, 2008). Although the mechanism by which 'perceptual attunement' occurs is not clear, we presume that the authors mean that, when making decisions, athletes have greater activation in areas of the brain related to perception (e.g., visual attention system), as compared to those related to memory (e.g., Wright et al., 2011). Moreover, the explicit nature of verbal reports of thought processes collected directly after a trial ends is at odds with concepts of 'flow', 'implicit knowledge' and 'automaticity' that have been observed to characterise or underpin expert performance during actual soccer performance (e.g., Jackson and Csikszentmihalyi, 1999; Masters, 1992). Soccer is a dynamic, time-constrained game, and findings from tasks that do not mimic these same constraints may not apply directly to performance and its underlying mechanisms in this sport. In order to answer some of the outstanding questions, further research is required in the area of neuroscience examining the brain-related mechanisms underpinning anticipation and decision making in soccer.

## THE ACQUISITION OF ANTICIPATION AND DECISION MAKING

### Developmental activities

A key question currently being investigated by researchers is how skilled players acquire their anticipation and decision-making ability. Researchers have examined whether players who exhibit varying levels of anticipation and decision-making competency can be differentiated based on the amount and type of soccer activity they have engaged in during their development. Although initial attempts focused on sports such as field-hockey, netball, basketball, Australian rules football and cricket (Baker, Côté, and Abernethy, 2003a, 2003b; Berry, Abernethy, and Côté, 2008; Ford, Low, McRobert, and Williams, 2010a), there are two recent reports involving soccer. Williams et al. (2012) categorised elite-level soccer players aged 18 years into 'high-performing' and 'low-performing' groups, based on their performance on established tests of perceptual-cognitive expertise involving both an anticipation test and a situational assessment task. A group of non-elite soccer players acted as controls. The Career Practice Questionnaire was completed by all players in order to elicit information about their participation history profiles (see Ward, Hodges, Starkes, and Williams, 2007). The high-performing group had accumulated more hours in soccer-specific play activity over their last six years of engagement in the sport, as compared to their low-performing counterparts and the non-elite controls. No differences were reported for hours accumulated in soccer-specific practice or competition. The mean hours in each type of activity for the different groups and across each age category are presented in Table 6.1. Players who had superior game intelligence skill had accumulated significantly more hours in soccer-specific, non-coach-led play activity (i.e., street soccer).

In a follow-up study, Roca, Williams, and Ford (2012) categorised skilled adult soccer players into 'high-performing' and 'low-performing' groups based on their performance on an interactive test that measured the ability of players to anticipate and make decisions (see Figure 6.1). A group of recreational players acted as controls. The Participation History Questionnaire (Ford et al., 2010a) was used to collect retrospectively recalled developmental

Table 6.1 Average hours per year in three soccer activities for soccer players aged 18 years in the 6 years prior to the perceptual-cognitive test.

| Group | Match-play | Practice | Play |
|---|---|---|---|
| Elite high-performing | 47.64 | 270.55 | 245.91 |
| Elite low-performing | 50.99 | 285.94 | 172.49 |
| Recreational | 78.45 | 222.08 | 92.17 |

Source: Williams et al. (2012).

activity data across participants. During childhood (6–12 years), the high-performing skilled group averaged more hours per year in soccer-specific play, as compared to the other two groups. During adolescence (13–18 years), both skilled groups engaged in more hours in soccer-specific practice and competition, as compared to the recreational group. Statistical analysis showed that 21.8% of the variance in performance on the test was accounted for by the average hours per year accumulated in soccer-specific play activity during childhood, with a further 13.2% of the variance being due to the hours spent in soccer-specific practice during adolescence.

Skill-based differences in game intelligence and in the amount of accumulated hours in soccer activity have been shown to occur as early as 8 years of age in soccer (Ward and Williams, 2003). It is hypothesised that the structure and conditions of soccer-specific play games create the opportunity for players to experiment with different skills and tactics against opponents and with teammates, which likely leads to the acquisition of anticipation and decision making. No evidence has been reported to suggest that engagement in sports other than soccer during the developmental years may lead to perceptual-cognitive expertise in the sport (e.g., players in Roca et al., 2012, only engaged in two other sports). However, some support exists for the notion that perceptual-cognitive skills transfer across sports of a similar nature (Smeeton, Ward, and Williams, 2004), although further research is required, as, contrary to this suggestion, recent reports indicate that these skills may be specific to a particular position (Williams, Ward, Smeeton, and Ward, 2008) or role (Catteeuw, Helsen, Gilis, and Wagemans, 2009).

### Simulation training

An important issue for coaches and practitioners is whether the skills underpinning anticipation and decision making can be acquired through structured training interventions. Certainly, coaches can structure practice in a manner so as to have their players acquire these abilities (for a review, see Ford, Yates, and Williams, 2010b). However, in this section, we show how simulation-based training programmes can be used to facilitate the acquisition of anticipation and decision making. A growing research base now exists examining whether the acquisition of perceptual-cognitive skills may be facilitated using simulation-based training. A detailed review of this broad field of research is available elsewhere (e.g., see Ward, Williams, and Hancock, 2006; Williams and Ward, 2003; 2007) and, consequently, only research involving soccer is reviewed in this section. However, surprisingly, given the popularity of the sport, there is limited research on soccer. A possibility is that researchers have favoured sports that present fewer challenges for creating simulations and measurement.

The majority of researchers have focused on using simulation to train goalkeeper anticipation in the penalty kick in soccer. Williams and Burwitz (1993) used video training to develop anticipation in a group of inexperienced goalkeepers. A number of penalty takers were filmed from the perspective of the goalkeeper and the footage was presented in conjunction with instruction and feedback. The instruction highlighted key postural cues (e.g., orientation of the lower leg in penalty kicks) as well as critical relationships between these display features and subsequent performance. Significant improvements in performance on the anticipation test were observed following 90 minutes of video training. Savelsbergh, Van Gastel, and Van

Kampen (2010) modified the visual search behaviours employed by inexperienced soccer goalkeepers using video training. The goalkeepers were required to anticipate penalty kick direction by moving a joystick in response to the video sequences. An intervention group viewed clips where key information from the run-up was highlighted, whereas a training group watched unedited sequences and a control group completed only the pre- and post-tests. The visual search behaviours of participants in the intervention group changed significantly from pre- to post-test, leading to earlier initiation of joystick movement and significant improvements in anticipation, as compared with the training and control groups.

Williams, Heron, Ward, and Smeeton (2005) attempted to improve the ability of players to use situational probabilities when attempting to predict pass destination in soccer. Novice soccer players were assessed, pre- and post-training, on their ability to identify the passing options available to the player in possession of the ball, and then to determine the relative threat posed to the participant's team for each highlighted option. An intervention group received 45 minutes of video training in which they had received instruction regarding the passing options facing a specific player in possession of the ball, areas of space that could be exploited or exposed, runs made by forward players, and the importance of defensive shape and organisation in the specific context. Participants in a placebo group were instructed on standard defensive soccer techniques for a similar period of time using the video simulation. The training group improved their ability to highlight key passing options over and above that of the placebo group, implying that the ability to use situational probabilities might be amenable to simulation training and instruction.

Although such training interventions have significant potential for performance enhancement in soccer, there are many unanswered questions and considerable scope exists for further empirical work in this area of study (Carling, Reilly, and Williams, 2009). The key, and as yet unanswered, question is whether the improvements found in these simulation training studies transfer to improved performance on the pitch (for an example of this research in tennis, see Williams, Ward, Knowles, and Smeeton, 2002). Thus far, there have been no reported attempts to use simulation-based training to improve the ability of players to recognise patterns of play in soccer or to change the visual search behaviours and thought processes that may be engaged during performance. However, simulation training is currently underused in soccer and has the potential to improve the performance of players.

A major advantage of simulation training is that players can engage in it when injured or when resting and recovering from physical activity. Moreover, players can experience multiple soccer situations in a short space of time, as compared to when physically playing the game. Advances in technology enable performance to be captured relatively easily, offering varied opportunities to use simulation in all its various guises for performance enhancement (e.g., Cave-based Virtual Reality, smart-phones, web-based applications). Research (e.g., Wulf, Raupach, and Pfeiffer, 2005) showing the learning that occurs from observational practice provides strong support for the use of simulation training with players.

## SUMMARY

We have reviewed research that has focused on anticipation and decision making in soccer. We highlight the key perceptual-cognitive processes, skills and mechanisms that differentiate those with exceptional levels of game intelligence skill from those with less of this ability. It appears that those with superior levels of anticipation and decision making are better able to pick up postural information from the orientation of opponents and teammates, identify structure and familiarity in sequences of play and predict more accurately the likely opportunities available during play. These skills are underpinned by more refined visual search behaviours and more forward-thinking rather than reactive thought processes. The ability to anticipate and to make decisions develops progressively through extensive engagement in soccer-specific practice and play activities. Physical and simulation training interventions to facilitate the acquisition of anticipation and decision-making skill were discussed, with the overall aim being to develop players with superior 'game intelligence'.

## REFERENCES

Araújo, D., and Davids, K. (2011). What exactly is acquired during skill acquisition? *Journal of Consciousness Studies* 18, 7–23.

Araújo, D., Davids, K., and Hristovski, R. (2006). The ecological dynamics of decision making in sport, *Psychology of Sport and Exercise* 7, 653–676.

Baker, J., Côté, J., and Abernethy, B. (2003a). Learning from the experts: practice activities of expert decision makers in sport. *Research Quarterly for Exercise and Sport* 74, 342–347.

Baker, J., Côté, J., and Abernethy, B. (2003b). Sport-specific practice and the development of expert decision making in team ball sports. *Journal of Applied Sport Psychology* 15, 12–25.

Berry, J., Abernethy, B., and Côté, J. (2008). The contribution of structured activity and deliberate play to the development of expert perceptual and decision-making skill. *Journal of Sport and Exercise Psychology* 30, 685–708.

Carling, C., Reilly, T.P., and Williams, A.M. (2009). *Performance Assessment in Field Sports*. London: Routledge.

Catteeuw, P., Helsen, W.F., Gilis, B., and Wagemans, J. (2009). Decision-making skills, role specificity, and deliberate practice in association football refereeing. *Journal of Sports Sciences* 27, 1125–1136.

Causer, J., and Williams, A.M. (2012). Sports clothing and disguise: playing tricks on the eyes. Unpublished manuscript.

Causer, J., Holmes, P.S., Smith, N.J., and Williams, A.M. (2011). Anxiety, visual attention, and movement kinematics in elite-level performers. *Emotion* 11(3), 595–602.

Davids, K., Button, C., and Bennett, S. (2008). *Dynamics of Skill Acquisition: A Constraints-led Approach*. Champaign, IL: Human Kinetics.

Dicks, M., Button, C., and Davids, K. (2010a). Examination of gaze behaviours under in situ and video simulation task constraints reveals differences in information pickup for perception and action. *Attention Perception and Psychophysics* 72, 706–720.

Dicks, M., Davids, K., and Button, C., (2010b). Individual differences in the visual control of intercepting a penalty kick in association football. *Human Movement Science* 29, 401–411.

Dittrich, W.H. (1999). Seeing biological motion: is there a role for cognitive strategies? In A. Braffort, R. Gherbi, S. Gibet, J. Richardson, and D. Teil (eds), *Gesture-based Communication in Human–computer Interaction* (pp. 3–22). Berlin, Germany: Springer-Verlag.

Ericsson, K.A., and Delaney, P.F. (1999). Long-term working memory as an alternative to

## 118

capacity models of working memory in everyday skilled performance. In A. Miyake, and P. Shah (eds), *Models of Working Memory: Mechanics of Active Maintenance and Executive Control* (pp. 257–297). New York: Cambridge University Press.

Ericsson, K.A., and Kintsch, W. (1995). Long-term working memory. *Psychological Review* 102, 211–245.

Ericsson, K.A., and Simon, H.A. (1993). *Protocol Analysis: Verbal Reports as Data* (rev. edn). Cambridge, MA: Bradford Books/MIT Press.

Ford, P.R., Low, J., McRobert, A.P., and Williams, A.M. (2010a). Developmental activities that contribute to high or low performance by elite cricket batters at recognizing type of delivery from advanced postural cues. *Journal of Sport and Exercise Psychology* 32, 638–654.

Ford, P.R., Yates, I., and Williams, A.M. (2010b). An analysis of practice activities and instructional behaviours used by youth soccer coaches during practice: Exploring the link between science and application. *Journal of Sports Sciences* 28, 483–495.

Helsen, W.F., and Starkes, J.L. (1999). A multidimensional approach to skilled perception and performance in sport. *Applied Cognitive Psychology* 13, 1–27.

Jackson, S.A., and Csikszentmihalyi, M. (1999). *Flow in Sports: The Keys to Optimal Experiences and Performances*. Champaign, IL: Human Kinetics.

Lees, A., and Owens, L. (2011). Early visual cues associated with a directional place kick in soccer. *Sports Biomechanics* 10(2), 125–134.

Magill, R.A. (2007). *Motor Learning and Control: Concepts and Applications*. New York: McGraw-Hill.

Masters, R.S.W. (1992). Knowledge, knerves and know-how: the role of explicit versus implicit knowledge in the breakdown of a complex motor skill under pressure. *British Journal of Psychology* 83, 343–358.

McPherson, S.L., and Kernodle, M.W. (2003). Tactics, the neglected attribute of expertise: problem representations and performance skills in tennis. In J. Starkes and K.A. Ericsson (eds), *Expert Performance in Sport: Recent Advances in Research on Sport Expertise* (pp. 137–168). Champaign, IL: Human Kinetics.

North, J.S., Ward, P., Ericsson, K.A., and Williams, A.M. (2011). Mechanisms underlying skilled anticipation and recognition in a dynamic and temporally constrained domain. *Memory* 19, 155–168.

North, J.S., Williams, A.M., Ward, P., Hodges, N.J., and Ericsson, K.A. (2009). Perceiving patterns in dynamic action sequences: the relationship between anticipation and pattern recognition skill. *Applied Cognitive Psychology* 23, 1–17.

Piras, A., and Vickers, J.N. (2011). The effect of fixation transitions on quiet eye duration and performance in the soccer penalty kick: instep versus inside kicks. *Cognitive Processing*. DOI 10.1007/s10339-011-0406-z.

Reilly, T., Williams, A.M., Nevill, A., and Franks, A. (2000). A multidisciplinary approach to talent identification in soccer. *Journal of Sports Sciences* 18, 668–676.

Roca, A., Williams, A.M., and Ford, P.R. (2012). Developmental activities and the acquisition of superior anticipation and decision making in soccer players. *Journal of Sports Sciences* Article first published online: 9 July 2012. DOI: 10.1080/02640414.2012.701761.

Roca, A., Ford, P.R., McRobert, A., and Williams, A.M. (2011). Identifying the processes underpinning anticipation and decision-making in a dynamic time-constrained task. *Cognitive Processing*. DOI 10.1007/s10339-011-0392-1.

Savelsbergh, G.J.P., Van Gastel, P.J., and Van Kampen, P.M. (2010). Anticipation of penalty kicking direction can be improved by directing attention through perceptual learning. *International Journal of Sport Psychology* 41, 24–41.

Savelsbergh, G.J.P., van der Kamp, J., Williams, A.M., and Ward, P. (2005). Anticipation and visual search behaviour in expert soccer goalkeepers: A within-group comparison. *Ergonomics* 48, 11–14, 1686–1697.

Savelsbergh, G.J.P., Williams, A.M., van der Kamp, J., and Ward, P. (2002). Visual search, anticipation and expertise in soccer goalkeepers. *Journal of Sports Sciences* 20, 279–287.

Schubotz, R.I., Friederici, A.D., and Yves von Cramon, D. (2000). Time perception and motor timing: a common cortical and subcortical basis revealed by fMRI. *NeuroImage* 11, 1–12.

Smeeton, N., Ward, P., and Williams, A.M. (2004). Transfer of perceptual skill in sport. *Journal of Sports Science* 19, 3–9.

Tyldesley, D.A., Bootsma, R.J., and Bomhoff, G. (1982). Skill level and eye movement patterns in a sport orientated reaction time task. In H. Rieder, K. Mechling, and K. Reischle (eds), *Proceedings of an International Symposium on Motor Behaviour: Contribution to Learning in Sport* (pp. 290–296). Cologne: Hofmann.

Vaeyens, R., Lenoir, M., Williams, A.M., Mazyn, L., and Philippaerts, R.M. (2007a). The effects of task constraints on visual search behavior and decision-making skill in youth soccer players. *Journal of Sport and Exercise Psychology* 29, 156–175.

Vaeyens, R., Lenoir, M., Williams, A.M., Mazyn, L., and Philippaerts, R.M. (2007b) Visual search behavior and decision-making skill in soccer. *Journal of Motor Behavior* 39, 5, 395–408.

Vickers, J.N. (2011). Mind over muscle: the role of gaze control, spatial cognition, and the quiet eye in motor expertise. *Cognitive Processing*. DOI 10.1007/s10339-011-0392-1.

Vickers, J.N., and Williams, A.M. (2007). Why some choke and others don't! *Journal of Motor Behavior* 39(5), 381–394.

Ward, P., and Williams, A.M. (2003). Perceptual and cognitive skill development in soccer: the multidimensional nature of expert performance. *Journal of Sport and Exercise Psychology* 25, 93–111.

Ward, P., Williams, A.M., and Hancock, P. (2006). Simulation for performance and training. In K.A. Ericsson, P. Hoffman, N. Charness, and P. Feltovich (eds) *The Cambridge Handbook of Expertise and Expert Performance* (pp. 243–262). Cambridge, UK: Cambridge University Press.

Ward, P., Hodges, N.J., Starkes, J., and Williams, A.M. (2007). The road to excellence: deliberate practice and the development of expertise. *High Ability Studies* 18, 119–153.

Ward, P., Suss, J., Eccles, D.W., Williams, A.M., and Harris, K.R. (2011). Skill-based differences in option generation in a complex task: a verbal protocol analysis. *Cognitive Processing*. DOI 10.1007/s10339-011-0397-9.

Williams, A.M. (2000). Perceptual skill in soccer: Implications for talent identification and development. *Journal of Sports Sciences* 18, 737–740.

Williams, A.M., and Burwitz, K. (1993). Advance cue utilization in soccer. In T.P. Reilly, J. Clarys, and A. Stibbe (eds), *Science and Football II* (pp. 239–244). London: E. and F.N. Spon.

Williams, A.M., and Davids, K. (1998). Visual search strategy, selective attention, and expertise in soccer. *Research Quarterly for Exercise and Sport* 69(2), 111–128.

Williams, A.M., and Ericsson, K.A. (2005). Some considerations when applying the expert performance approach in sport. *Human Movement Science* 24, 283–307.

Williams, A.M., and North, J.S. (2009). Identifying the minimal essential information underlying pattern recognition. In D. Arajuo, H. Ripoll, and M. Raab (eds), *Perspectives on Cognition and Action* (pp. 95–107). New York: Nova Science Publishing Inc.

Williams, A.M., and Ward, P. (2003). Perceptual expertise: development in sport. In J. L. Starkes, and K. A. Ericsson (eds), *Expert Performance in Sports: Advances in Research on Sport Expertise* (pp. 220–249). Champaign, IL: Human Kinetics.

Williams, A.M., and Ward, P. (2007). Perceptual-cognitive expertise in sport: exploring new horizons. In G. Tenenbaum, and R.C. Eklund (eds), *Handbook of Sport Psychology* (pp. 203–223). New York: John Wiley and Sons.

Williams, A.M., Bell-Walker, J., Ward, P., and Ford, P.R. (2012). Perceptual-cognitive expertise, practice history profiles, and memory recall in soccer. *British Journal of Psychology* 103, 393–411.

Williams, A.M., Davids, K., Burwitz, L., and Williams, J.G. (1994). Visual search strategies of experienced and inexperienced soccer players. *Research Quarterly for Exercise and Sport* 5(2), 127–135.

Williams, A.M., Ford, P.R., Eccles, D., and Ward, P. (2011). Perceptual-cognitive expertise in sport and its acquisition: implications for applied cognitive psychology. *Applied Cognitive Psychology* 25, 432–442.

Williams, A.M., Heron, K., Ward, P., and Smeeton, N.J. (2005). Using situational probabilities to train perceptual and cognitive skill in novice soccer players. In T.P. Reilly, J. Cabri, and D. Araujo (eds), *Science and Football V* (pp. 337–340). London: Taylor and Francis.

Williams, A.M., Hodges, N.J., North, J.S., and Barton, G. (2006). Perceiving patterns of play in dynamic sport tasks: identifying the essential information underlying skilled performance. *Perception* 35, 317–332.

Williams, A.M., Ward, P., Knowles, J.M., and Smeeton, N.J. (2002). Anticipation skill in a real-world task: measurement, training, and transfer in tennis. *Journal of Experimental Psychology: Applied* 8, 259–270.

Williams, A.M., Ward, P., Smeeton, N.J., and Ward, J. (2008). Task specificity, role, and anticipation skill in soccer. *Research Quarterly for Exercise and Sport* 79, 429–433.

Wilson, M.R., Wood, G., and Vine, S.J. (2009). Anxiety, attentional control, and performance impairment in penalty kicks. *Journal of Sport and Exercise Psychology* 31, 761–775.

Wood, G., and Wilson, M.R. (2011). Quiet-eye training for soccer penalty kicks. *Cognitive Processing*. DOI 10.1007/s10339-011-0393-0.

Wright, M.J., Bishop, D.T., Jackson, R.C., and Abernethy, B. (2011). Cortical fMRI activation to opponents' body kinematics in sport-related anticipation: Expert-novice differences with normal and point-light video. *Neuroscience Letters* 500, 216–221.

Wulf, G., Raupach, M., and Pfeiffer, F. (2005). Self-controlled observational practice enhances learning. *Research Quarterly for Exercise and Sport* 76, 107–111.

Yarrow, K., Brown, P., and Krakauer, J.W. (2009). Inside the brain of an elite athlete: The neural processes that support high achievement in sports. *Nature Reviews* 10, 585–596.

# CHAPTER 7

## THE ACQUISITION OF SKILL AND EXPERTISE

### THE ROLE OF PRACTICE AND OTHER ACTIVITIES

P.R. Ford and A.M. Williams

### INTRODUCTION

Winning soccer matches is the main goal of most adult players, teams, coaches and support staff across the world. In the majority of cases to achieve this goal requires consistent and skilled performance from the team and players. Professional soccer clubs pay huge transfer fees to other clubs to acquire the most skilled players in pursuit of these two goals. National, club and private youth-development schemes spend years and large sums of money attempting to develop players that are skilled enough to help their teams achieve these goals (or in some cases at least to gain a financial profit from future transfer fees). Coaches and support staff also spend many years acquiring their skills through education and experience so as to improve the performance of players and teams. Many factors must combine across an extended period of time for expert performance to be attained and maintained in sport (for a review, see Davids and Baker, 2007). In this chapter, we review research showing how engagement in practice and other soccer activities might lead to the acquisition of skill and the attainment of expert performance in players. Moreover, research examining the microstructure of practice activity and its effect on skill acquisition in soccer is reviewed. We begin the chapter with a review of the developmental activities that players engage in during their formative years.

### DEVELOPMENTAL ACTIVITIES AND PATHWAYS

#### The developmental activities engaged in by elite players

The quantity and quality of time spent in soccer-specific activities, such as practice, is likely related to the acquisition of skill and the level of performance attained by players. Players typically engage in three main types of activity during their time in the sport. First, *practice* is formal activity engaged in with the primary aim of improving performance, such as coach-led practice. Second, *competition* is formal activity engaged in with the main intention of winning matches. Third, *play* is informal activity engaged in with the primary aim of fun and enjoyment, such as street or playground soccer. Researchers have examined the amount of engagement in these activities by elite players and how this differs across their time in the sport. The most comprehensive examination of the developmental activities engaged in by elite soccer players was conducted by Ford et al. (2012). A total of 328 elite soccer players aged 16 years from Brazil, England, France, Ghana, Mexico, Portugal and Sweden ($n=50$ for each country, except

Ghana where *n*=28) completed the Participation History Questionnaire (PHQ; Ford, Low, McRobert, and Williams, 2010a). The PHQ records milestones achieved (e.g., start age in soccer, start age in elite training scheme), average hours per year accumulated in the three developmental activities in soccer, and engagement in other sports.

Players started in soccer at 5 years of age. Figure 7.1 shows the average hours per year accumulated in the three soccer activities during childhood and early adolescence. During childhood, they engaged in soccer practice for 186 hrs/yr, play for 186 hrs/yr and competition for 37 hrs/yr. Of the 328 players, 229 engaged in an average of two other sports during this

**(a)**

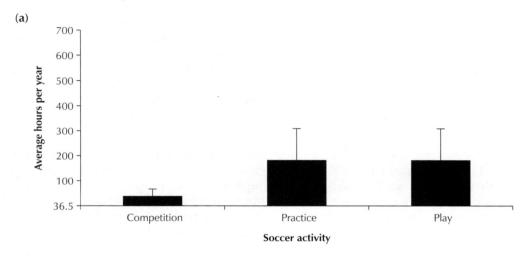

**(b)**

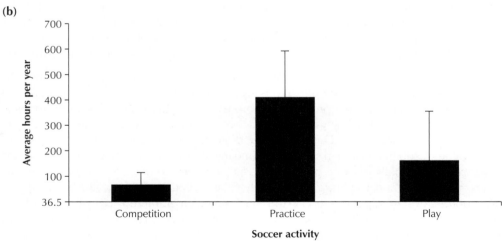

**Figure 7.1** The average hours per year in three soccer activities (competition, practice, play) by 328 elite youth players from around the world during (a) childhood and (b) adolescence.

*Source*: Ford *et al.* (2012).

*effective practice and instruction*

period. Players started their participation in an elite training scheme at 11 to 12 years of age. During adolescence, they engaged in soccer practice for 412 hrs/yr, play for 160 hrs/yr and competition for 67 hrs/yr. During this period, 132 of the players engaged in two other sports. After 10 years of engagement in the sport, they had accumulated 4553 hrs ($s=1749$) in soccer activity.

Some between-country differences in the nature of the engagement in soccer activities were reported. During childhood, players in Brazil engaged in significantly less formal practice and competition activity, as compared to the overall data set. They engaged in soccer-specific play activity for 4 or 5 hrs/wk during this period. They also engaged in meaningful amounts of futsal activity (i.e., 3 hrs/wk for 3 yrs) during childhood, whereas players in other countries did not. The data from the players in Brazil shows that expert performance in soccer can probably be achieved without engaging in high amounts of coach-led practice and competition during childhood. During adolescence, players in Mexico engaged in more, and players in England engaged in less, soccer practice, as compared to the combined data. During this period, players in Brazil and France engaged in less soccer play, whereas players in Portugal engaged in more play, compared to the combined data. Players in Mexico (mean value = 5449 hrs) had engaged in more total soccer activity after 10 years, as compared to the other countries, except for players in Ghana and Sweden.

Ward, Hodges, Starkes, and Williams (2007) used a questionnaire to examine the developmental activities engaged in by 203 elite and recreational male soccer players in England aged between 8 and 18 years. The players started in the sport at 5 years of age. The amount of hours accumulated in team practice was the only activity to consistently discriminate between the elite and recreational players from the under-9 years age group onwards. The elite training programme in England begins at the under-9 years age group and the elite players engaged in significantly more team practice from that point onwards, as compared to recreational players. The hours accumulated in soccer play and competition did not discriminate the skill groups. However, during childhood both groups spent meaningful amounts of time engaging in soccer play activities (i.e., around 7 hrs/wk). The number of other sports in which they engaged did not discriminate groups, with participants engaging in two other sports on average.

Ford and Williams (2011, see also Ford, Ward, Hodges, and Williams, 2009) examined the developmental activities of elite youth players aged 16 years in England. Two groups of players were examined who had either progressed to professional status in late adolescence or were released from the elite training programme between 15 and 16 years of age and did not progress to professional status. During childhood, average hours per year in soccer practice (mean value = 200 hrs/yr) and in soccer play (mean value = 210 hrs/yr) were greater for the players who eventually became professional, as compared to the released players (mean values = 130 hrs/yr and 132 hrs/yr, respectively). Players engaged in four other sports during this period. They started participation in the elite training programme at 10 to 11 years of age. During early adolescence, the average hours per year in soccer practice (mean value = 305 hrs/yr), play (mean value = 180 hrs/yr), and competition (mean value = 60 hrs/yr) did not differentiate the two groups. After 10 years of involvement in the sport, the professional players (mean value = 4840 hrs) had accumulated more hours in soccer activity, as compared to released players (mean value = 3581 hrs). The hours of soccer activity accumulated by the professional players at 15 to 16 years of age did not differ when compared with the approximately 5000 hrs reported for other elite youth players in other studies at the same age (e.g., Ford et al., 2012).

## The developmental pathways of elite players: early engagement

The 'early engagement' model has been proposed by Ford et al. (2009; 2012; Ford and Williams, 2011) as the developmental activity pathway currently followed by elite soccer players. The early engagement pathway involves players participating during childhood in meaningful amounts of soccer play activity. Childhood engagement in soccer practice and competition is dependent on the country the player lives in and the development system within that country. For example, players in Brazil engage in 124 hrs/yr of soccer practice during childhood, whereas players in Mexico engage in 240 hrs/yr (Ford et al., 2012). During childhood, players engage in a relatively low amount of other sports. For example, players engaged in two other sports on average in Ford et al. (2012). During adolescence, they engage in relatively large amounts of soccer practice (e.g., 10 hrs/wk; Ford et al., 2012) and the amount of play activity begins to reduce. The amount of soccer competition activity increases across the years. The developmental pathways that elite players follow might not be the optimal way to develop professional adult players. The pathways and activities they engage in only reflect the current system of talent development in their country (for a review of other developmental pathways from other sports, see Côté, Baker and Abernethy, 2007). Those developmental pathways and activities might not be the optimal way to develop professional adult players.

Other researchers (e.g., Baker, Cobley, and Fraser-Thomas, 2009) have raised concerns about the potentially negative consequences of children engaging in high amounts of sport-specific practice and competition. They advocate the *early diversification pathway*, which involves engagement in a number of different sport activities during childhood and late or delayed specialisation into the primary sport in early adolescence (Côté et al., 2007). There has been evidence showing that this pathway characterises the development of successful athletes in other sports in some countries (e.g., Berry, Abernethy, and Côté, 2008; Carlson, 1988; Côté, 1999; Monsaas, 1985; Soberlak and Côté, 2003). However, these successful athletes have usually engaged during childhood in relatively meaningful amounts of activity, usually play activity, in their primary sport in addition to other sports (e.g., Berry et al., 2008; Carlson, 1988; Côté, 1999; Monsaas, 1985; Soberlak and Côté, 2003).

It is noteworthy that elite players in Brazil engage mostly in soccer-specific play activity and futsal during childhood rather than in coach-led practice and competition (Ford et al., 2012). Players who engaged in greater amounts of play activity in soccer during childhood have been shown to possess superior anticipation and decision-making ability, as compared to those who engaged in less of this activity (Roca, Williams, and Ford, 2012; Williams, Bell-Walker, Ward, and Ford, 2011). Moreover, because engagement in soccer play activity is fun and enjoyable, it likely increases motivation to continue engagement in the sport. This increased motivation may be especially important when players reach adolescence and adulthood and engage in relatively high amounts of soccer practice and competition (Ford et al., 2012). The engagement in meaningful amounts of soccer-specific play activity during childhood may help to protect players against the potentially negative motivational consequences of engaging in too much practice activity, such as burnout or dropout (Baker et al., 2009; Côté et al., 2007).

A concern is that children in the majority of countries do not engage in as much soccer-specific play activity, compared to previous generations. Moreover, children may be engaging in too much practice and competition at a young age, which might lead to negative consequences later in life (e.g., Baker *et al.*, 2009). Therefore, there is a need for adults to provide more opportunities for children to engage in meaningful amounts of soccer-specific play. Some practical solutions include scheduling more soccer-specific play in formal physical education classes and practice sessions, creating school playgrounds and parks that enable children to safely engage in play, and changing the formal match or games programme so that it becomes more play oriented (for an excellent example, see Fenoglio, 2003).

In addition to the type and amount of soccer activity that players engage in during their development, the microstructure of these activities is an important part of skill acquisition. An extensive amount of research exists in the area of motor learning examining the practice structures and instructional strategies that best facilitate learning (for reviews, see Magill, 2007; Schmidt and Lee, 2005). In the next section, we review the main evidence-based principles from this body of research to show how certain practice structures/conditions might lead to skill acquisition in soccer.

## MICROSTRUCTURE OF PRACTICE

### Motor learning research on practice structure

Researchers (e.g., Shea and Morgan, 1979) have shown that the manner in which practice is structured affects whether and how much skill learning takes place. For example, during practice of motor skills, the order in which a number of discrete skills, such as a pass, header and turn, are executed can vary. *Random practice* involves executing a number of discrete motor skills so that a single attempt on one skill is followed by an attempt on a different skill, and so on. In contrast, *blocked practice* involves executing a discrete skill a number of times without interruption from other skills, before a number of attempts at a different skill are undertaken, and so on. The typical finding is that blocked practice leads to better *performance* during the practice phase, as compared to random practice. However, when *learning* is assessed sometime later through retention and/or transfer tests (Schmidt and Lee, 2005), random practice typically results in greater learning, as compared to blocked practice (for a review, see Lee, 2012). No published research exists examining how random and blocked practice affects the learning of soccer skills. The typical finding that blocked practice causes superior performance, whereas random practice results in superior learning, has been shown with other discrete motor skills, such as golf putting (Porter and Magill, 2010), badminton serves (Goode and Magill, 1986) and baseball batting (Hall, Domingues, and Cavazos, 1994). Some researchers (e.g., Porter and Magill, 2010) have shown that the amount of random practice should be progressively increased as learning occurs.

Similar differential effects on the amount of motor skill learning to those caused by random and blocked practice orders have been shown for other combinations of practice structures. *Distributed practice* contains longer rest periods or periods of other activity between each attempt at a motor skill, as compared to *massed practice*. *Variable practice* contains variation in each attempt at a discrete motor skill, such as speed, distance or initial conditions. In contrast, *constant practice* contains no variation in the elements of each attempt at a discrete motor skill. The typical finding in motor learning research is that a distributed or a variable practice order produced better learning than a massed or a constant practice order (for a review, see Schmidt and Lee, 2005). Recently, researchers have shown that *self-selected* or *self-controlled practice orders* lead to superior motor learning, as compared to other practice schedules, including random practice (Hodges, Edwards, Luttin, and Bowcock, 2011; Keetch and Lee, 2007; Wulf, 2007).

## Limitations in the generalisability of motor learning research on practice structure

Motor learning researchers examining practice structure have focused on perceptual-motor skills only, that are executed outside of game-play. For example, Porter and Magill (2010) had participants execute basketball passes that were thrown to a target on a wall. However, soccer is a game played with and against other players. As such, the performance of expert soccer players during match-play is characterised by the need for superior 'game intelligence', which is also termed *perceptual-cognitive skills*, as well as motor skills. These perceptual-cognitive skills include superior: (a) visual search processes; (b) recognition of information from other players' movements; (c) recognition of patterns and familiarity in sequences of play; (d) prediction of likely event occurrences; and (e) action selection and execution. These skills and processes enable players to anticipate what it is that opponents/teammates are likely to do in any given situation and to make decisions as to what action to take. Research evidence has suggested that these 'game intelligence' skills are acquired through soccer-specific activity, particularly play activity (Roca, *et al.*, 2012).

A number of authors (Patterson and Lee, 2008; Vickers, 2007; Williams and Ford, 2009) have detailed the correct practice structure required for learners to acquire the perceptual, cognitive and motor skills needed during matches. These authors have suggested practice should be organised or structured around the competition decision-making processes of the athlete such that practice has the same underlying structure as competition. That is, the perceptual-cognitive processing of the athlete during the practice should be the same as in the environment in which the athlete must apply the skills learnt in practice, which in soccer is the match. When processing in practice is the same as in the transfer environment, the practice contains *transfer-appropriate processing* (Lee, 1988). In the next section, we review research examining the proportion of activity undertaken during practice that presents players with the opportunity to develop perceptual, cognitive and motor skills under transfer-appropriate conditions.

## Microstructure of youth practice sessions

Ford, Yates, and Williams (2010b; see also Partington and Cushion, 2011) analysed the microstructure of practice activities employed by 25 youth soccer coaches across 70 different practice sessions in England. The coaches worked at the under-9, 13 and 16 years age groups and at elite, sub-elite and non-elite skill levels. Practice sessions were video recorded and a time-use analysis was undertaken to identify the specific activities that coaches had players engage in during each session. The activities across all the sessions were coded into two categories, termed *Training Form* and *Playing Form*. Training Form activity was defined as activities that did not have a game-play context, such as opponents, and consisted of work on fitness, technique and skills practices. Playing Form activity was defined as activities that replicated game-related conditions containing teammates and opponents. It consisted of small-sided games, conditioned games and phase-of-play activities. Playing Form activity was judged to be more similar to the structure of competition and therefore the activity from which greater transfer of perceptual, cognitive and motor learning to match-play would occur, as compared to Training Form activity. The proportions of time spent in the two different activities are presented in Table 7.1. Overall, the proportion of time spent in Training Form and Playing Form activity was 65% and 35%, respectively. Only minor variations in these proportions were noted across the different age and skill groups.

It appears that coaches use the part-practice activities or 'drills' that we categorised as Training Form activity in an attempt to lessen the demands of the game for learners (Patterson and Lee, 2008). Moreover, they use practice activities that contain blocked, constant and massed practice structures because players make few mistakes and performance appears to be good during the practice activity itself (e.g., repetitive executions of a short pass). Although the use of these types of activity is well intended, and broadly speaking repetition is an important part of practice, such widespread use would not be supported by empirical research. The possibility exists that Training Form activities present fewer opportunities for players to develop the perceptual-cognitive skills that are important during match-play at higher levels of the sport. In contrast, Playing Form activities, such as small-sided and possession games, are engaged in to a lesser extent by players during practice, albeit researchers have identified that this type of activity promotes the development of perceptual-cognitive skills, such as anticipation and decision making (Ford *et al.*, 2010b; Roca *et al.*, 2012; Williams *et al.*, 2011). Ford *et al.* (2010b) raised concern as to whether coaches are providing players with sufficient opportunity to engage in activities containing transfer-appropriate processing.

**Table 7.1** The percentage (%) of session duration spent in Training Form and Playing Form activity by youth soccer players in England, as a function of skill and age.

| Comparison | Training Form | Playing Form |
| --- | --- | --- |
| Total | 64.37 | 35.63 |
| *Skill group* | | |
| Elite | 59.41 | 40.59 |
| Sub-elite | 64.67 | 35.33 |
| Recreational | 72.25 | 27.75 |
| *Age group* | | |
| 9 years of age | 69.38 | 30.62 |
| 13 years of age | 59.02 | 40.98 |
| 16 years of age | 64.50 | 35.50 |

*Source*: Ford *et al.* (2010b).

**P.R. Ford and A.M. Williams**

Training Form activities can be designed to centre on the competition decision-making processes of the athletes by including opposition and/or teammates who force the player to process information and make decisions in the manner they would do in a match. However, there was no evidence of this type of activity being employed by coaches in the study by Ford *et al.* (2010b). Coaches may require education from specialists in skill acquisition on how best to design this type of activity and practice environments in general (Williams and Ford, 2009).

## Reducing the demands of Playing Form activity

Coaches use low amounts of the activity that Ford *et al.* (2010b) categorised as Playing Form, probably because they perceive it as too demanding for learners. When an aspect of an activity is too demanding for learners, this is known as a *rate limiter*. Rate limiters are most often thought of as an individual characteristic, such as height or muscle strength, that is holding back the progression of learning and development (Haywood and Getchell, 2001; Horn and Williams, 2004). However, rate limiters can exist within characteristics of the task or environment and can hold back the progression of learning. For example, in soccer, opponents tackling the player in possession and reducing time/space makes the game very difficult for relatively novice players and acts as a key rate limiter, reducing the opportunity for them to learn to manipulate the ball and move around opponents.

A number of scientific principles can be applied to ensure that Playing Form activity is appropriately demanding for young players. *Task simplification* (Renshaw, Chow, Davids, and Hammond, 2010; Davids, Button, and Bennett, 2008) involves lowering the difficulty of the task to an appropriate level for the learner while maintaining the natural performance of the task (e.g., small-sided games in Playing Form activity). The *challenge point framework* presented by Guadagnoli and Lee (2004) is a similar idea to that of 'task simplification'. Practice activities present differing levels of difficulty that are dependent on the skill level of the performer and the practice conditions. *Nominal task difficulty* includes only the constant difficulty of the task, irrespective of the person performing it, whereas *functional task difficulty* includes the task and how challenging it is to the individual. The *optimal challenge point* occurs around the point of functional task difficulty that a performer at a specific skill level would need in order to optimise perceptual, cognitive and motor learning. When a practice task is too easy or too difficult for a performer either no or minimal learning may occur. Coaches typically schedule high amounts of Training Form activities to lower the functional task difficulty for learners. However, the key is to schedule greater amounts of Playing Form activity for young players and to adapt it so as to set the optimal challenge point for the participating players, which will be dependent on their skill level. The *constraints-led approach* (Davids et al., 2008) reviewed in the next section provides a framework to guide such activity.

## The constraints-led approach

The constraints-led approach detailed by Davids *et al.* (2008), among others, presents a framework for designing environments for skill acquisition in sport. In this framework, constraints are defined as boundaries that shape and bring order to behaviour and its emergence in humans (Newell, 1986). Three types of constraints have been identified: (i) *individual constraints*, such as leg strength or aerobic capacity; (ii) *environment constraints*, such as the ground surface and light; and (iii) *task constraints*, such as the rules, goals and conditions of soccer. Coaches can manipulate these constraints so that behaviour emerges and learning occurs during the practice task. Task constraints are the easiest for coaches to manipulate and many coaches already do this intuitively. Davids *et al.* (2008) have termed manipulating task constraints as 'bending the rules' so that key player behaviour and learning emerges during the practice task. Some examples of how a coach can manipulate task constraints so as to lower the challenge point of small-sided games to an appropriate level of functional difficulty for the skill level of the learners are presented in Table 7.2. Another potential reason why coaches schedule high amounts of Training Form activities is so that they can focus their learners on practising specific motor skills. However, the key is to schedule more Playing Form activity and to adapt it so as to increase the repetitions of players' practising specific motor skills. Table 7.3 presents examples of how a coach can manipulate the task constraints of small-sided games so as to have their players execute greater amounts of soccer-specific motor skills and tactics.

However, the constraints-led approach takes the idea of manipulating key constraints further, and in doing so provides an underlying framework for designing practice environments (Davids *et al.*, 2008). All three types of constraints can be manipulated by the coach in order for the required player behaviour to emerge and learning to occur. Moreover in this framework, *functional variability* plays an important role in skill acquisition. Traditionally, in most learning environments variability is viewed as negative, and the concept of variability's being positive is often difficult for coaches to comprehend. In this framework, variability of factors that are inherent in the task and environment enables the learner to explore the various opportunities afforded by that task and environment, so that flexible behaviour and learning emerge. Playing Form activity provides an ideal activity to harness and manipulate this variability in order to develop 'adaptive' rather than 'routine' expertise (Holyoak, 1991).

Table 7.2 Some examples of manipulations to the rules of small-sided games (e.g., 3 vs. 3) that may reduce the 'challenge point' of Playing Form activity (i.e., task simplification) for learners.

1  Increase the size of the pitches
2  Reduce the number of players on each team
3  Include extra players who play for whichever team is in possession of the ball during the game (i.e., 'floaters')
4  Ban tackling – allowing only blocks of passes and pressure
5  Ban tackling in the middle half of the pitch only – allowing only blocks of passes and pressure in that area
6  Use unidirectional games in which there are more teammates than opposition (e.g., 2 vs. 1; 3 vs. 1; 4 vs. 2)

P.R. Ford and A.M. Williams

**Table 7.3** Some examples of manipulations to the rules of small-sided games (e.g., 4 vs. 4) so that players practise specific perceptual-motor skills.

| Motor skill | Adaptation |
|---|---|
| Dribbling | Remove goals and have players score by dribbling across their opposition's goal touchlines. |
| Passing | All small-sided games contain a lot of passing, although to encourage one- and two-touch passing, the coach can limit touches (e.g., '2-touch'). |
| Long passing | Make the pitch very long but not too wide. Alternatively, have two very small goals with no goalkeepers and a 'no go' penalty area. |
| Forward passing | Remove goals and replace with two relatively large American Football-style 'end zones'. Players score by passing the ball into the path of a teammate, who runs into the opposition's end zone. Use the touch line that marks the start of the 'end zone' as an 'offside line'. |
| Switch-play passing | Make the pitch wide but short. Plus, remove goals and replace with two smaller goals at each goal line, which are placed on the goal lines extending in from both corners. Players must score by dribbling the ball through one of the two small goals. |
| Turning | Allow both teams to score at either end of the pitch. |
| Shooting | Place large goal nets at either end of the pitch. |
| Crossing | Place corridors along the touchlines from which players who play for whichever team is in possession can cross the ball without opposition. Limit the number of players allowed in the 'penalty area'. |
| Attacking heading | Place corridors along the touchlines from which players who play for whichever team is in possession can cross the ball without opposition. Limit the number of players allowed in the 'penalty area'. Goals can be scored only from headers. |
| Defensive heading | Make the pitch very long but not too wide. |

## Deliberate practice

The 'power law of practice' holds that in the early stages of learning a new task or domain, performance improvement is rapid, whereas later in the process the rate begins to slow or plateau (Newell and Rosenbloom, 1981). For many performers, the plateau occurs because they are competent at the task and are satisfied to remain at that level of performance. However, Ericsson (2003; 2007) has termed this plateau in performance 'arrested development'. He holds that expert performers are not satisfied with being merely competent and, as a consequence, they engage in an activity termed *deliberate practice*, with the intention of improving performance beyond its current level. The engagement in deliberate practice is physically and mentally effortful, is highly relevant to improving performance and may not be enjoyable. The motivation to engage in deliberate practice is not necessarily because it is enjoyable during the activity, but because it improves future performance. The amount of domain-specific deliberate practice engaged in by an individual has been shown to be positively correlated to their attained level of performance (Ericsson, Krampe, and Tesch-Römer, 1993). Deliberate practice is designed to improve a specific aspect/s of current or

131

future player/team performance and, as such, what aspect is focused on and activity engaged in appears to be specific to the individual or team and their needs at that time.

Childhood engagement in the type of frequent and intense training that characterises deliberate practice has been linked to a number of negative consequences, such as burnout and dropout (Baker et al., 2009). Moreover, the 'power law of practice' suggests that early in learning a sport such as soccer it may not be necessary to engage in high amounts of intense deliberate practice because performance improvement should occur from correctly structured activity regardless of its intent, such as play activity. However, at some later stage, when a performance plateau occurs, performers must engage in deliberate practice activity to further improve their performance (Ericsson, 2003; 2007). It appears that adolescent and adult players should be engaging in meaningful amounts of deliberate practice (e.g., centred on tactical knowledge acquisition, McPherson and Kernodle, 2003), rather than or as well as in 'maintenance' or fun activities. For example, in our recent study, expert adult Gaelic football players practising free kicks self-selected to engage in deliberate practice in which they focused on and improved their weaknesses, experienced less enjoyment from the activity itself and put in more effort when compared to intermediate players (Coughlan, Williams, and Ford, in review).

## INSTRUCTIONAL STRATEGIES

### Motor learning research on instructional strategies

Researchers have shown that the type and amount of augmented information provided during practice, such as verbal instruction, verbal feedback and visual demonstrations, influences whether and how much motor skill learning occurs. Verbal instruction and feedback that is either explicit, movement focused, immediate, negative or very frequent has generally been shown to be worse for motor learning, as compared to feedback that encourages implicit learning, is action-effect focused, delayed, positive or reduced in frequency (Masters, 1992; Wulf, McConnel, Gärtner, and Schwarz, 2002; Wulf, Chiviacowsky, and Lewthwaite, 2010; Swinnen, Schmidt, Nicholson, and Shapiro, 1990; Sherwood, 1988). When participants who have learnt a motor skill through explicit instruction are put into stressful conditions their explicit knowledge interferes with movement processes that normally function automatically, and performance decreases (Masters, 1992). A similar hypothesis has been forwarded to explain the benefit of external- over internal-focus instructions (Wulf et al., 2002). Moreover, immediate augmented feedback is thought to disrupt the intrinsic and automatic feedback processes of learners, as compared to delayed feedback (Swinnen et al., 1990).

### Instructional strategies in youth practice sessions

Based on the literature presented above, coaches would be advised to provide relatively low and delayed amounts of instruction and feedback to players learning the game. Ford et al. (2010b; see also Partington and Cushion, 2011) analysed the instructional strategies used by 25 youth soccer coaches during 70 different practice sessions in England. Practice sessions

132

were video recorded and a version of the Arizona State University Observation Instrument (ASUOI, Lacy and Darst, 1985) was used to analyse the instructional behaviours. The behaviours across all the sessions were coded into four categories termed Instruction, Support and Encouragement, Management, and Silence. Instruction was defined as verbal or visual information explaining how to perform a skill, play, tactic, assignment, strategy and so forth, which was provided before, during or after the skill, play, tactic, assignment or strategy. Support and Encouragement was defined as verbal or non-verbal compliments (i.e., praise), dissatisfactions (i.e., scold), or intensifications (i.e., hustle). Silence was defined as a deliberate period of 5 s or greater when the coach was silent. Management was defined as verbal statements about the organisation of the practice, not related to skill, play, tactic, assignment or strategy.

Ford et al. (2010b) reported that approximately 30% of all behaviours were instruction, 22% were management, 25% were support and encouragement, 20% were silence, with the remainder being uncoded. Moreover, the rate per minute of all behaviours except silence was greater than 1. The data showed that the coaches provided instruction and feedback very frequently, along with behaviours that managed the practice session. There were only minor variations reported between practice type, player age or skill level. Although Ford et al. did not measure the nature of the verbalisations of the coaches they examined (Jolly, 2010), it is assumed that the instruction and feedback were mainly explicit in nature, with at least some of those verbalisations internally focused toward the movements completed by learners. The high frequency of verbalisations contradicts the motor learning research on instructional strategies, and suggests that learning may be degraded by some of these coaching behaviours.

## Limitations in the generalisability of motor learning research on instructional strategies

Motor learning researchers examining instructional strategies have focused on perceptual-motor skills that are executed outside of game-play. For example, in Beilock, Carr, MacMahon, and Starkes (2002) participants were required to dribble a soccer ball through a slalom course. However, as detailed earlier, expert soccer performance requires perceptual-cognitive as well as perceptual-motor skills. Moreover, the research has mainly focused on the early stages of motor skill learning by using short acquisition phases (e.g., 4 practice sessions, Masters, 1992), albeit some have examined skilled participants (e.g., Beilock et al., 2002), whereas players spend many years rather than a few hours in practice before reaching professional level. Much of the research on instructional strategies focuses on the development of automaticity in motor skill, or at least not disrupting automatic movement processes. In the early stages of learning, such as a child player in soccer, the research suggests that acquiring automaticity in motor skill may be important. Later in learning, when some level of automaticity is reached in motor skill, it is expected that attention, which can be thought of as a capacity or resource, becomes free to focus on other tasks. In games like soccer, it may be that those tasks are goal directed or tactical in nature, since focusing on the movements themselves is likely to be disruptive.

Ericsson and Towne (2010) contend that 'expert performers counteract automaticity by developing increasingly complex mental representations to attain higher levels of control of their performance' (p. 405). These mental representations are used to plan and engage in deliberate practice to improve aspects of future performance. This type of self-regulatory activity occurring outside of physical activity is underresearched in elite adolescent and adult athletes. However, Toering, Elferink-Gemser, Jordet, and Visscher (2009; see also Jonker, Elferink-Gemser, and Visscher, 2010) have shown that elite adolescent soccer players in the Netherlands scored higher on the reflection and effort aspects of self-regulation, as compared to less skilled players. Moreover, elite netball players in Great Britain enhanced aspects of their decision making, tactical knowledge, and the associated on-court performance through a structured, deliberate, explicit, thought-out, planned and discussed off-court process involving coaches and players (Richards, Colllins, and Mascarenhas, 2012). Similarly, North American Olympic champions in a variety of sports state that they conduct thorough post-competition evaluations in order to improve their future performance (Durand-Bush and Salmela, 2002). It may be that during performance professional players experience total absorption in the task or 'flow' (Jackson and Csíkszentmihályi, 1999), whereas between performances some are explicitly and cognitively involved in trying to improve that performance beyond its current level.

## SUMMARY

The engagement in practice and other soccer activities is one of the necessary factors for the acquisition of skill in players. Typically, elite players start playing soccer at 5 years of age and by the age of 15 have accumulated approximately 5000 hours of soccer activity (Ford et al., 2012). The activities of elite players across their development tend to follow what has been termed the 'early engagement' pathway (Ford et al., 2009; 2012). Players engage in greater amounts of soccer-specific play activity during childhood, as compared to adolescence, whereas during adolescence they engage in greater amounts of practice, as compared to childhood. However, in certain countries children engage in high amounts of soccer-specific practice and competition (Ford et al., 2012). Such data present descriptive rather than causal or optimal accounts, and what elite players currently do during childhood may not be optimal in terms of developing expert performance.

Research from the areas of skill acquisition and motor learning can be used to design optimal learning environments for players. For children, our research suggests that players should engage in meaningful amounts of soccer-specific play activity that contains the same underlying structures as match-play, such as small-sided games. Those games should be adapted to an appropriate level of functional difficulty for learning to occur (i.e., challenge point, Guadagnoli and Lee, 2004) and adapted so that various tactics and skills are explored by the players (e.g., Davids et al., 2008). Adult and adolescent players should engage in meaningful amounts of practice designed to improve or maintain their performance (e.g., tactical) and in competition in which the intention is to win. When designing practice sessions and learning environments for players, coaches should seek to use the research-based principles that are reviewed in this chapter, rather than or alongside the traditional emulation of other coaches, historical precedence or intuition (Williams and Hodges, 2005).

# REFERENCES

Baker, J., Cobley, S., and Fraser-Thomas, J. (2009). What do we know about early sport specialization? Not much! *High Ability Studies* 20, 77–89.

Beilock, S. L., Carr, T. H., MacMahon, C., and Starkes, J. L. (2002). When paying attention becomes counterproductive: impact of divided versus skill-focused attention on novice and experienced performance of sensorimotor skills. *Journal of Experimental Psychology: Applied* 8, 6–16.

Berry, J., Abernethy, B., and Côté, J. (2008). The contribution of structured activity and deliberate play to the development of expert perceptual and decision-making skill. *Journal of Sport and Exercise Psychology* 30, 685–708.

Carlson, R. (1988). The socialization of elite tennis players in Sweden: an analysis of the players' backgrounds and development. *Sociology of Sport Journal* 5, 241–256.

Côté, J. (1999). The influence of the family in the development of talent in sport. *The Sport Psychologist* 13, 395–417.

Côté, J., Baker, J., and Abernethy, B. (2007). Play and practice in the development of sport expertise. In G. Tenenbaum and R. C. Eklund (eds), *Handbook of Sport Psychology*, 3rd edn (pp. 184–202). New York: Wiley.

Coughlan, E. K., Williams, A. M., and Ford, P. R. (in preparation). A test of deliberate practice theory and its predictions: how experts learn.

Davids, K., and Baker, J. (2007). Genes, environment and sport performance: why the nature–nurture dualism is no longer relevant. *Sports Medicine* 37, 961–980.

Davids, K., Button, C., and Bennett, S. (2008). *Dynamics of Skill Acquisition: A Constraints-led Approach*. Champaign, IL: Human Kinetics.

Durand-Bush, N., and Salmela, J. H. (2002). The development and maintenance of expert athletic performance: perceptions of world and Olympic champions. *Journal of Applied Sport Psychology* 14, 154–171.

Ericsson, K. A. (2003). The development of elite performance and deliberate practice: an update from the perspective of the expert-performance approach. In J. Starkes and K. A. Ericsson (eds), *Expert Performance in Sport: Recent Advances in Research on Sport Expertise* (pp. 49–81). Champaign, IL: Human Kinetics.

Ericsson, K. A. (2007). Deliberate practice and the modifiability of body and mind: toward a science of the structure and acquisition of expert and elite performance, *International Journal of Sport Psychology* 38, 4–43.

Ericsson, K. A., and Towne, T. J. (2010). Expertise. *WIREs Cognitive Science* 1, 404–416.

Ericsson, K. A., Krampe, R. T., and Tesch-Römer, C. (1993). The role of deliberate practice in the acquisition of expert performance. *Psychological Review* 100, 363–406.

Fenoglio, R. (2003). The Manchester United 4 v 4 pilot scheme for U9s. *Insight: The FA Coaches Association Journal* 6(3), 18–19.

Ford, P. R., and Williams, A. M. (2011). The developmental activities engaged in by elite youth soccer players who progressed to professional status compared to those who did not. *Psychology of Sport and Exercise* 13, 349–352.

Ford, P. R., Yates, I., and Williams, A. M. (2010b). An analysis of practice activities and instructional behaviours used by youth soccer coaches during practice: exploring the link between science and application. *Journal of Sports Sciences* 28, 483–495.

Ford, P. R., Low, J., McRobert, A., and Williams, A. M. (2010a). Developmental activities that contribute to high or low performance by elite cricket batters when recognizing type of delivery from bowlers' advanced postural cues. *Journal of Sport and Exercise Psychology* 32, 638–654.

Ford, P. R., Ward, P., Hodges, N. J., and Williams, A. M. (2009). The role of deliberate practice and play in career progression in sport: the early engagement hypothesis. *High Ability Studies* 20, 65–75.

Ford, P. R., Carling, C., Garces, M., Marques, M., Miguel, C., Farrant, A., Stenling, A., Moreno, J., Le Gall, F., Holmström, S., Salmela, J. H., and Williams, A. M. (2012). The developmental activities of elite soccer players aged 16 years from Brazil, England, France, Ghana, Mexico, Portugal and Sweden. *Journal of Sports Sciences*. Article first published online: 12 July 2012. doi: 10.1080/02640414.2012.701762.

Goode, S., and Magill, R. A. (1986). Contextual interference effects in learning three badminton serves. *Research Quarterly for Exercise and Sport* 57, 308–314.

Guadagnoli, M. A., and Lee, T. D. (2004). Challenge point: a framework for conceptualizing the effects of various practice conditions in motor learning. *Journal of Motor Behavior* 36, 212–224.

Hall, K. G., Domingues, D. A., and Cavazos, R. (1994). Contextual interference effects with skilled baseball players. *Perceptual and Motor Skills* 78, 835–841.

Haywood, K., and Getchell, N. (2001). *Life Span Motor Development*. Champaign, IL: Human Kinetics.

Hodges, N. J., Edwards, C., Luttin, S., and Bowcock, A. (2011). Learning from the experts: gaining insights into best practice during the acquisition of three novel motor skills. *Research Quarterly for Exercise and Sport* 82, 178–187.

Holyoak, K. (1991). Symbolic connectionism: toward third generation theories of expertise. In K. A. Ericsson and J. Smith (eds), *Toward a General Theory of Expertise* (pp. 301–336). Cambridge: Cambridge University Press.

Horn, R., and Williams, A. M. (2004). Rate limiters in the development of football skills. *Insight: The FA Coaches Association Journal* 7(1), 59–62.

Jackson, S. A., and Csíkszentmihályi, M. (1999). *Flow in Sports: The Key to Optimal Experiences and Performances*. Champaign, IL: Human Kinetics.

Jolly, S. (2010). An analysis of practice activities and instructional behaviours used by youth soccer coaches during practice: exploring the link between science and application. *Journal of Sports Sciences* 28, 1625.

Jonker, L., Elferink-Gemser, M. T., and Visscher, C. (2010). Differences in self-regulatory skills among talented athletes: the significance of competitive level and type of sport, *Journal of Sports Sciences* 28, 901–908.

Keetch, K. M., and Lee, T. D. (2007). The effect of self-regulated and experimenter-imposed practice schedules on motor learning for tasks of varying difficulty. *Research Quarterly for Exercise and Sport* 78, 476–486.

Lacy, A. C., and Darst, P. W. (1985). Systematic observation of behaviours of winning high school head football coaches. *Journal of Teaching in Physical Education* 4, 256–270.

Lee, T. D. (1988). Transfer-appropriate processing: A framework for conceptualizing practice effects in motor learning. In O. G. Meijer and K. Roth (eds), *Complex Movement Behaviour: The Motor-action Controversy* (pp. 201–215). Amsterdam: Elsevier.

Lee, T. D. (2012). Contextual interference: generalizability and limitations. In A. M. Williams and N. J. Hodges (eds), *Skill Acquisition in Sport: Research, Theory, and Practice* (pp. 79–93). London: Routledge.

Magill, R. A. (2007). *Motor Learning and Control: Concepts and Applications* (9th edn). New York: McGraw-Hill.

Masters, R. S. W. (1992). Knowledge, knerves and know-how: the role of explicit versus implicit knowledge in the breakdown of a complex motor skill under pressure. *British Journal of Psychology* 83, 343–358.

McPherson, S. L., and Kernodle, M. W. (2003). Tactics, the neglected attribute of expertise: problem representations and performance skills in tennis. In J. Starkes and K. A. Ericsson (eds), *Expert Performance in Sport: Recent Advances in Research on Sport Expertise* (pp. 137–168). Champaign, IL: Human Kinetics.

Monsaas, J. A. (1985). Learning to be a world-class tennis player. In B. S. Bloom (ed.), *Developing Talent in Young People* (pp. 211–269). New York: Ballantine.

Newell, A., and Rosenbloom, P. S. (1981). Mechanisms of skill acquisition and the law of practice. In J. R. Anderson (ed.), *Cognitive Skills and Their Acquisition* (pp. 1–55). Hillsdale, NJ: Erlbaum.

Newell, K. M. (1986). Coordination, control, and skill. In D. Goodman, R. B. Wilberg, and I. M. Franks (eds), *Differing Perspectives in Motor Learning, Memory and Control* (pp. 295–317). Amsterdam: Elsevier.

Partington, M., and Cushion, C. J. (2011). An investigation of the practice activities and coaching behaviours of professional top-level youth soccer coaches. *Scandinavian Journal of Medicine and Science in Sport*. Article first published online: 13 September 2011. doi: 10.1111/j.1600-0838.2011.01383.

Patterson, J. T., and Lee, T. (2008). Organizing practice: the interaction of repetition and cognitive effort for skilled performance. In D. Farrow, J. Baker, and C. McMahon (eds), *Developing Sports Expertise: Researchers and Coaches Put Theory into Practice* (pp. 119–134). London: Routledge.

Porter, J. M., and Magill, R. A. (2010). Systematically increasing contextual interference is beneficial for learning sport skills. *Journal of Sports Sciences* 28, 1277–1285.

Renshaw, I., Chow, J. Y., Davids, K., and Hammond, J. (2010). A constraints-led perspective to understanding skill acquisition and game play: a basis for integration of motor learning theory and physical education praxis? *Physical Education and Sport Pedagogy* 15, 117–137.

Richards, P., Collins, D., and Mascarenhas, D. R. D. (2012). Developing rapid high-pressure team decision-making skills. The integration of slow deliberate reflective learning within the competitive performance environment: A case study of elite netball. *Reflective Practice* 13, 407–424.

Roca, A., Williams, A. M., and Ford, P. R. (2012). Developmental activities and the acquisition of superior anticipation and decision making in soccer players. *Journal of Sports Sciences*. Article first published online: 9 July 2012. doi: 10.1080/02640414.2012. 701761.

Schmidt, R. A., and Lee, T. D. (2005). *Motor Control and Learning: A Behavioural Emphasis*, 5th edn. Champaign, IL: Human Kinetics.

Shea, J. B., and Morgan, R. L. (1979). Contextual interference effects on the acquisition, retention, and transfer of a motor skill. *Journal of Experimental Psychology: Human Learning and Memory* 5, 179–187.

Sherwood, D. E. (1988). Effect of bandwidth knowledge of results on movement consistency. *Perceptual and Motor Skills* 66, 535–542.

Soberlak, P., and Côté, J. (2003). The developmental activities of professional ice hockey players. *Journal of Applied Sport Psychology* 15, 41–49.

Swinnen, S., Schmidt, R. A., Nicholson, D. E., and Shapiro, D. C. (1990). Information feedback for skill acquisition: instantaneous knowledge of results degrades performance. *Journal of Experimental Psychology: Learning, Memory and Cognition* 16, 706–716.

Toering, T. T., Elferink-Gemser, M. T., Jordet, G., and Visscher, C. (2009). Self-regulation and performance level of elite and non-elite youth soccer players. *Journal of Sports Sciences* 27, 1509–1517.

Vickers, J. N. (2007). *Perception, Cognition, and Decision Training: The Quiet Eye in Action.* Champaign, IL: Human Kinetics.

Ward, P., Hodges, N. J., Starkes, J., and Williams, A. M. (2007). The road to excellence: deliberate practice and the development of expertise. *High Ability Studies* 18, 119–153.

Williams, A. M., and Ford, P. R. (2009). Promoting a skills-based agenda in Olympic sports: the role of skill-acquisition specialists. *Journal of Sports Sciences* 27, 1381–1392.

Williams, A. M., and Hodges, N. J. (2005). Practice, instruction and skill acquisition in soccer: challenging tradition. *Journal of Sports Sciences* 23, 637–650.

Williams, A. M., Bell-Walker, J., Ward, P., and Ford, P. R. (2011). Perceptual-cognitive expertise, practice history profiles, and memory recall in soccer. *British Journal of Psychology* 103, 393–411.

Wulf, G. (2007). Self-controlled practice enhances motor learning: implications for physiotherapy. *Physiotherapy* 93, 96–101.

Wulf, G., Chiviacowsky, S., and Lewthwaite, R. (2010). Normative feedback effects on learning a timing task. *Research Quarterly for Exercise and Sport* 81, 425–431.

Wulf, G., McConnel, N., Gärtner, M., and Schwarz, A. (2002). Feedback and attentional focus: enhancing the learning of sport skills through external-focus feedback. *Journal of Motor Behavior* 34, 171–182.

# CHAPTER 8

## SOCIOLOGICAL AND CULTURAL INFLUENCES ON PLAYER DEVELOPMENT

D. Richardson, H. Relvas and M. Littlewood

### INTRODUCTION

Soccer is undoubtedly the most popular sport in the world, and subsequently an important aspect of popular culture. The need for professional clubs to operate as more of a business entity has never been greater. The soccer industry is one that embraces a service of performance, entertainment and financial profit (Bourke, 2003; Vaeyens, Coutts, and Philippaerts, 2005). At the highest level, soccer involves a frenzied environment more commonly associated with the entertainment business, while ensuring the continuation of the high financial rewards that success at, or progress to, the higher echelons of European competitions brings. At lesser levels, the game is about the continued delivery of a quality product to an audience with hope, aspiration and expectation. Both ends of the spectrum require the continual delivery of a team that can perform, remain financially stable, avoid relegation and possibly even progress through the leagues. The level and status of any of these professional clubs will dictate the aspirations and expectations of its supporters. Similarly, each club is a hostage to its own values, traditions and culture. Clubs will function at a particular level or operate in a particular way because it is an expected part of the club's identity. However, a prerequisite of attaining all these aspirations is the need for the club to operate as effectively as possible. At this juncture it is pertinent to establish that soccer clubs, at whatever level, need to reflect on their purpose and function in order to establish clear organisational aims and subsequent (relative) success (De Knop, Van Hoecke and De Bosscher, 2004; Slack and Parent, 2006; Zink, 2005).

With finances at a premium, it is natural for soccer clubs, as most businesses, to look inwardly to establish a sound, robust and effective model that ensures the long-term proliferation of the work-force. Subsequently, more systematic development plans such as the English Football Association's (FA) 'Football Education for Young Players: A Charter for Quality' (1997) have emerged. In essence, the Charter's purpose was to provide a more structured approach to player development. The FA was, in effect, encouraging (or challenging) the clubs to be responsible for developing players from within. In France, the French Football Federation (FFF), together with the Ligue du Football Professionnel (LPF), implemented a similar 'quality' model through the adoption of the 'Charte du Football Professionnel' (2007). The Charte is a document updated and released every season to regulate the Academies of professional clubs in France. As in England, the FFF defines requirements for the Academies, including facilities, staff, players and quality criteria. More recently, the governing bodies of football in Belgium, Finland and Germany (DBF), as well as the Professional Football League (DFL) in Germany,

## 139

have recognised the lack of 'home-grown' players and the dearth of individuals progressing from the Academy environment to the professional teams, and the subsequent effect on the future success of professional clubs. Such developments have seen an increase in the numbers of coaches and expert support practitioners that typically furnish these entities. The sport now offers an array of credible and tangible careers for exercise physiologists, strength and conditioning coaches, sports psychologists, performance analysts and education and welfare practitioners. The purpose and structure of the youth academy has been well documented (see Richardson et al., 2005) and it would appear that such Academies have now been well established for over a decade. Given the presence of youth development programmes and the proliferation of expert practitioners to assist and guide player development, it could be argued that young players today have never had it so good. However, both empirical and anecdotal evidence has continued to question the productivity and effectiveness of football Academies at the elite level and, as such, there are a number of issues that need to be considered that are central to this topic.

The aim of this chapter is to critically explore the broader external (i.e., birthdate and birthplace effect, labour migration patterns) and specific internal (i.e., organisational culture of clubs, management of career transitions) sociological and cultural factors that permeate the identification and development of talented players. The chapter also seeks to explain how practitioners can, with an enhanced understanding and appreciation of such factors, better manage, and ultimately develop, talented players to progress to higher levels in professional soccer.

## THE RELATIVE AGE EFFECT: IGNORANCE OR EDUCATION?

The relative age effect (RAE) has been recognised as a key factor in the development of academic and sporting talent (Musch and Grondin, 2001). It refers to the notion that children born immediately after a cut-off date are advantaged by a difference of up to 12 months in age between themselves and their peers in the same age classification (Vaeyens, Coutts and Philippaerts, 2005). For example, in English youth soccer, where the selection period runs from 1 September to 31 August, children born in September possess a near 1-year age advantage over children born in August of the following year. Chronological age is a measure of time, not of physical and cognitive maturity (Boucher and Mutimer, 1994), and therefore different developmental stages may lead to maturational differences of more than 2 years (Malina and Bouchard, 1991). This phenomenon was first researched in academic settings. Dickinson and Larsen (1963) found that the academic 'early bird' was less likely to suffer problems at school. This was supported by Pidgeon and Dodds (1961), who suggested that children born in the months of June, July and August are exposed to less infant schooling and are therefore immediately at a disadvantage relative to their peers.

Although competitive sport employs a similar cut-off criterion to academia, education is, by comparison, compulsory, which prevents age-disadvantaged children dropping out (Musch and Grondin, 2001). One of the first studies to relate this skewed birth distribution in a sporting context was Grondin et al. (as cited in Musch and Grondin, 2001: 148), who observed the effect in both youth and professional players in the North American Hockey League (NHL). They showed that four times more players were born in the first quarter of the competition

140

year, as compared to the final quarter. Other researchers showed the phenomenon in competitive minor ice hockey (Boucher and Halliwell, 1991; Boucher and Mutimer, 1994), indicating that the RAE was evident across playing standards. Researchers have conclusively shown a similar effect in cricket (Edwards, 1994), tennis (Dudink, 1994), swimming (Baxter-Jones et al., 1995), American football (Glamser and Marciani, 1992) and baseball (Grondin and Koren, as cited in Musch and Grondin, 2001: 152).

The earliest study in football was by Dudink (1994), who tabulated the birth dates of all players at English league clubs across four divisions for the 1991–92 season. More players were born in the months immediately after the September cut-off date than at any other period during the year. Musch and Grondin (2001) suggested that the phenomenon exists worldwide. For example, Musch and Hay (1999) reported two key conclusions in the analysis of the birth dates of players in the top national leagues of Australia, Brazil, Germany and Japan. First, by observing an RAE within countries with distinct cultures and climates it was concluded that the cut-off date and not socio-cultural or climatic factors was the cause. For example, Japan's competition year begins on 1 April and the bias is observed in May–July, whereas in Germany and Brazil similar distributions were observed in the months after the 1 August starting date. Moreover, the analysis showed that when the cut-off date in Australia changed from January to August, the distribution of birthdates shifted accordingly.

Other researchers have looked at the RAE from different perspectives. Edgar and O'Donoghue (2005) observed the distribution of 736 players from the 2002 FIFA World Cup and provided no evidence of a relationship between the season-of-birth bias and team success based on FIFA world rankings. They suggested that a season-of-birth bias within a squad might be to the detriment of the team's performance. A limitation of the study was that it used an August cut-off date, as proposed by FIFA in 1988; however, this cut-off would not have been applicable to any of the participating players, as they would have already progressed to senior level under previously used cut-off dates. This arguably led to the conclusion that there was no significant season-of-birth bias for World Cup squads from Europe, whose member countries predominantly operate a January cut-off. Research by the Association of Football Statisticians (cited in Owen, 2005) also looked at team success, highlighting that Liverpool's 2005 Champions League-winning starting 11 contained 6 players born in the first quarter of the English selection year. However, these 6 players were from countries that operate a January cut-off date and therefore this contradicts the idea that they would have been the oldest in their year and benefited from being physically more mature.

The most researched area within the relative age literature is the distribution of birth date within youth international players. Brewer et al. (1992) examined whether junior international soccer squads contained disproportionately large numbers of individuals born in the early part of the selection year and whether this is related to physical growth. The findings indicated a birth-date bias for the Swedish Under-17 squad and that these players tended to be above average height and weight. A number of other researchers have made an association between date of birth and selection into junior international squads (Baxter-Jones, 1995; Brewer, Balsom and Davis, 1995; Helsen, Starkes and van Winckel, 1998; Simmons and Paull, 2001; Helsen et al. 2005). It was suggested that players selected in elite junior squads were exposed to higher standards of training and were therefore more familiar to the selectors and the pressures of competition, improving their chances of success in later years (Brewer et al., 1995). The comparison by Brewer et al. (1995) between the birth dates of 103 players who were resident

# 141

at the Football Association National School over a 5-year period with those of 1,722 senior professionals at English clubs provided further evidence for the RAE in both adult and youth players.

Vaeyens, Renaat and Malina (2005) also found asymmetries in the distribution of birth dates of semi-professional and amateur soccer players, indicating that the phenomenon is present across a number of different playing standards. However, more importantly, it was revealed that players born in the first quarter received more minutes on the pitch and an increased number of selections. This indicated that birth date alone might not accurately reflect competitive soccer participation. As the RAE was evident in semi-professional and amateur soccer, it can be inferred that those players that drop out at a young age never return to the game at any level.

The evidence is extremely powerful in support of the bias evidenced towards early-born individuals in soccer, and the trends have not deviated significantly over time. These studies have continually questioned the procedures and practices employed by talent recruiters (or scouts) to identify talented players, given the dominance to acquire older, and perhaps taller, stronger, more physically advanced players. Clearly, the ability to identify talented players who can progress through to a club's first team can save a club significant funds transfer fees. Yet, it may be argued that clubs may be missing such talented players, due to the identification constraints that they are operating under. The propensity to 'spot' players with enhanced physical qualities, over and above technical markers of talent, may be influenced by the philosophy and culture that is present within a youth development system. Qualitative research examining the perceptions of talent recruiters on this issue is sparse and we suggest that there is a greater need for researchers to explore this particular concept. Until then, we are unsure whether such practices are simply down to ignorance, or due to a lack of education regarding the RAE on the part of those individuals responsible for identifying young talented players.

## BIRTHPLACE EFFECT: THE IMPORTANCE OF POPULATION SIZE

A further environmental factor that has started to receive attention in the literature is the birthplace effect. This concept suggests that 'where' one is born can influence the opportunities to engage in a particular sport at an early age, and subsequently, the practice opportunities to achieve expert status (Côté et al., 2006). Côté et al. (2006) suggest that individuals born and raised in smaller cities may have greater access to facilities and sports that may not be as easily accessible to individuals residing in larger urban areas. There are also thought to be structural differences in actual practice activities between urban and rural areas. For example, sports practised by individuals in urban areas are described as having greater monitoring processes from coaches, and specific time and game constraints in contrast to rural areas. Furthermore, less densely populated areas are considered to promote the integration of players of different ages, sizes and abilities, whilst larger populated areas structure competition based on age and size restrictions. The former point is advocated by Côté et al. (2003), who contend that individuals who have more opportunities to play with older children (and adults), and to experiment with a range of sports and physical activities, might enhance the development of expertise.

142

From an empirical perspective, there is a dearth of academic research into the birthplace effect, especially in professional soccer. The few studies that have explored this effect (see Carlson, 1988; Curtis and Birch, 1987), in Swedish elite tennis players and Olympic and National Hockey League (NHL) players, respectively, found evidence to suggest that players born in rural areas (or with a population size between 1,000 and 500,000) were more represented than regions with different population sizes. Côté and colleagues' (2006) research involving players in the National Hockey League (NHL), National Basketball Association (NBA), Major League Baseball (MLB) and Professional Golfers Association (PGA) showed a birthplace bias towards those individuals born in cities of less than 500,000. The authors speculate that the physical environment and psychosocial properties of such areas may positively promote the encountering of early sporting experiences by such individuals. Important factors to consider in this regard include the amount of social support provided and the self-efficacy, and ultimately personal identity, of the individual participating in the sport (perhaps as a function of support, feedback and opportunities to play).

A requirement exists to better understand the experiences of athletes residing in both urban and rural areas so as to complement the data. Such research would serve to expand the knowledge about safety concerns, access to open spaces and sources of leisure time by children in both areas, which Côté et al. recognise as important contextual factors that mediate their findings. Moreover, the quantitative nature of the birthplace research is somewhat limited, as it is difficult to accurately determine if athletes resided in specific cities and areas for the duration of their childhood and adolescence. A more robust monitoring and tracking process would enhance current knowledge. In summary, a fundamental feature of any talent pathway is the environment that is created by significant others (especially the coach) and the relational dynamic that exists, whether that be in rural or urban areas. We contend that more research in this area would serve to better understand the experiences of athletes within the context of their childhood and developing years in adolescence.

## COMMERCIALISATION AND LABOUR MIGRATION IN PROFESSIONAL FOOTBALL: IMPACT ON PLAYER DEVELOPMENT

Gammelsæter and Jakobsen (2008) suggest that the game is obsessed with commercialisation and a subsequent need to win and survive (at all costs). We contend that the notion of financial profit and/or sustainability has influenced the recruitment of players to the first team. More and more, clubs appear to favour bringing high-profile players into the club in order to obtain immediate results. These trends are particularly evident in the top leagues within (European) professional soccer, and the English Premier League is a prime example of where such player acquisition activity has been a constant feature since its inception in 1992 (see Littlewood, 2005). This activity has been fuelled by the substantial television rights negotiated by the Premier League with BSkyB on behalf of the clubs within the league. The relationship between these organisations has gone from strength to strength and has seen revenue sharply increase, from £49m in 1996/97 to £957.4m in 2009/10. At the time, this was the highest figure in the English Premier League's history, and is shared equally amongst all professional clubs (Football Economy, 2009). More recently this figure has been surpassed by another record-breaking deal spanning three Premier League seasons. The deal, split between BSkyB and British Telecom (BT), is reportedly a 70% increase on the last rights deal and incorporates a promise to extend

**Table 8.1** FIFA confederational region, frequency and percentage of players acquired by clubs that remained consistently in the FA Premier League (1992–2008).

| FIFA regional affiliation | Frequency | % |
|---|---|---|
| UEFA | 645 | 85.1 |
| CONCACAF | 13 | 1.7 |
| CONMEBOL | 37 | 4.9 |
| CAF | 49 | 6.5 |
| AFC | 7 | 0.9 |
| OFC | 7 | 0.9 |
| Total | 758 | 100% |

the current internet TV services (Fielden, 2012). The Premier League deal followed similar record-breaking deals announced in both the Bundesliga and Italy's Serie A by Sky Deutschland and Sky Italia, respectively. The pressure on clubs to remain in the Premier League has intensified as the financial rewards have increased, reflecting the proliferation in player acquisition trends. Littlewood, Richardson and Elliot (2011) examined the player acquisition strategies by 7 clubs that had consistently remained in the English Premier League over an 18-year period (1992–2008). The findings illustrated that players were acquired predominantly from within the UEFA confederation of FIFA (85% of total acquisitions), followed by players from the African confederation (6.5%).

More specific analysis of the UEFA confederation revealed that the number of players originating from the United Kingdom and Republic of Ireland had decreased in frequency over time, at the expense of an increase in players from Scandinavia, Western and Eastern European nations (Figure 8.1).

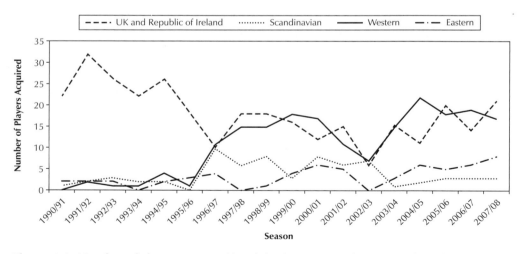

**Figure 8.1** Number of players acquired by clubs that remained consistently in the FA Premier League (1992–2008), as a function of UEFA sub-group.

# 144

Supporting these observations, there has been an explosion in movement of foreign players across Europe in recent years. Littlewood, Mullen and Richardson (2011) explored the player acquisition trends of the 'big five' European professional football leagues (i.e., English Premier League, Ligue 1, Bundesliga, Serie A and La Liga) between 2004/5 and 2008/9. The study differentiated between the presence and impact of indigenous home-grown players, non-indigenous home-grown players and foreign players within the respective leagues. Table 8.2 shows that the Spanish La Liga and Italian Serie A have the largest presence of indigenous home-grown players in their leagues, with 64.3% and 66.6%, respectively. The only league where foreign players outnumbered home-grown players (both indigenous and non-indigenous), was the German Bundesliga, with 52.7%. Such findings would appear to suggest that the philosophy and culture in terms of progressing young talented players in both Spain and Italy is focused internally. Further research is needed to determine the precise rationale of these observations.

The prevalence of clubs and leagues acquiring foreign players has largely been enabled by European Union (EU) legislation, which enabled 'freedom of player movement' within the EU, and the Bosman judgment in 1995, which allowed players to move freely to another club at the end of their contract with their current team. However, administrators did not foresee that such legislation would hinder the development of young players from within their own clubs and countries. The perceived need to invest in more typically 'finished' or complete players (i.e., a talented young player who may have been more exposed to high-level, meaningful competitive soccer), such as those evidenced in Table 8.1 and Figure 8.1 (Richardson, Littlewood and Gilbourne, 2005), suggests a lack of readiness and/or even willingness to prepare the indigenous youth Academy players for the elite level. The apparent lack of emerging young talent in the Union of European Football Associations (UEFA) federations and the perceived reluctance to invest in youth development programmes by some clubs (Richardson *et al.*, 2005) has become an increasing concern for the game's governing bodies. Some measures to rectify this situation have recently been taken by national and international organisations. For example, UEFA proposed that, by the 2008/9 season, each club participating in UEFA competitions should include in its squad four players from its own academy and four others from clubs of the same national association (UEFA, n.d.). It was anticipated that these new measures, and the increased values of young players, would encourage professional clubs to begin to invest more in youth academies, talent identification and development (Williams

Table 8.2 Cumulative player types across all five European Leagues.

|  | English Premier League | Spanish La Liga | French Ligue 1 | German Bundesliga | Italian Serie A |
|---|---|---|---|---|---|
| Indigenous home-grown | N=883 (49.8%) | N=1144 (64.3%) | N=977 (54.7%) | N=691 (43.4%) | N=1233 (66.6%) |
| Non-indigenous home-grown | N=92 (5.2%) | N=14 (0.8%) | N=100 (5.6%) | N=63 (3.9%) | N=37 (2%) |
| Foreign | N=799 (45%) | N=622 (34.9%) | N=709 (39.7%) | N=838 (52.7%) | N=582 (31.4%) |

*Source*: Adapted from Littlewood, Mullen and Richardson (2011: 795).

and Reilly, 2000; Reilly, Williams and Richardson, 2003; Vaeyens, Renaat and Malina, 2005). However, although some talented young players (i.e., playing in youth programmes and national youth squads) are often labelled as future stars, frequently, when they progress to the professional environment, they do not perform or achieve the level expected of them.

We have just sketched a scene that suggests that investment in youth development programmes is crucial. These programmes offer young players a rich resource of expert practitioners who cover an array of support roles ranging from fitness and conditioning to sports psychology. However, concerns remain over a lack of progression of indigenous home-grown talent. It would appear that the attention given to players' development has been mainly focused on their athletic career (e.g., physical condition and technical ability). More recently, research has begun to explore the non-athletic aspects that may affect an athlete's sports career. While the contribution of sports psychology is becoming more evident within the game, we contend that the youth player's development pathway from youth to the professional environment, subsequently culminating in first team playing experiences, is a highly complex journey. This journey includes physical, technical and psychological development. However, it can be shaped and dictated by an array of more subtle sociological, organisational and cultural issues as players progress through their careers. Typically, the cultural distance that exists between youth environments (and their aligned practitioners) and the professional environment (and its aligned practitioners) makes for one of the most challenging and critical periods of transition for any young player. The next section of the chapter explores how an organisation's culture can influence the player development process.

## ORGANISATIONAL CULTURE

In seeking to ascertain how the culture of a sport and/or the associated sports organisations may affect a player's transition from the youth environment through to the professional environment and ultimately to making and sustaining a place in the first team, it is important to recognise that culture itself is an extremely complex phenomenon. Culture is typically referred to as a series of, or patterns of, behaviour that form a durable and robust template through which behaviour is transferred from one generation to the next or from one group to another (Wilson, 2001). Wilson (2001) explains that the transfer of behaviour is not genetic, but occurs more through social interaction between members of the group. Furthermore, Kotter and Heskett (1992: 4) considered that 'at the deeper and less visible level, culture refers to values that are shared by the people in a group and that tend to persist over time even when group membership changes. At the more visible level, culture represents the behaviour patterns or style of an organisation that new employees are automatically encouraged to follow by their fellow employees. Each level of culture has a tendency to influence the other.' The definition makes reference to two levels of culture that might exist within an organisation, namely the visible level, such as observed behaviours, the physical and social environment or the spoken language, and the deeper level, which is usually related to aspects that we cannot observe just by looking but that exist (written or not) and that can influence the organisational culture. Some of these aspects include norms, values and goals of the organisation; both visible and deeper levels of culture interact with and influence each other.

Similarly, we can assume that organisational practices that have become entrenched have typically been passed down through the generations. Such practices are extremely powerful, as 'newcomers' to such environments can become socialised in, and through, such cultural norms in order to 'fit in' to their new surroundings. It is highly contentious for individuals to contest any of these practices that *appear*, to those inside the organisation or the group, to work. When they do work, then organisational socialisation is not such a bad thing. However, when they don't work, practices become so entrenched, outdated and/or flawed that poor practice is allowed to continue. Such practices tend to be endured, as the template (good or bad) that has evolved has been validated and approved by generations; any challenge to such practices must be highly credible, and pitched on sound and tangible sources. However, even if 'new' practices are presented in a cogent and coherent way, they can still be dismissed with 'we don't do that sort of thing here, we do it like this!' Unfortunately, our experiences suggest that soccer suffers from such an entrenched and robust culture. The typical organisation of a club includes the youth environment and the professional environment. Within these environments, an array of distinct practitioners are observed, including the coaches, the physiologist, the strength and conditioning coach, the scouts, the doctor, the physiotherapist, the psychologist and the education and welfare practitioners. As within any organisation, each 'set' of practitioners has the potential to form sub-groups, and subsequently sub-cultures, within the organisation.

The formation of such sub-cultures was evident in the work of Relvas and colleagues (2010), where distinct cultural distance was reported to exist between the youth environment and the professional environment. In reality, every organisation is a hostage to the formation of distinct sub-cultures within the fabric of the global organisation. Wilson (2001) also suggests that such sub-cultures can co-exist in harmony with, in conflict with or even indifference to each other. The key would appear to be the management, co-ordination and coherency that would need to exist, especially in soccer, to allow for a smooth transition from the youth to the professional environment.

## PLAYER TRANSITIONS

The topic of athlete transitions and talent development has received considerable attention in the literature. Wylleman and colleagues (2004: 8) defined a transition as the 'occurrence of one or more specific events that brings about a change in assumptions about oneself, but also a social disequilibrium that goes beyond the ongoing changes of everyday life'. Stambulova (2000) identified two types of transitions; normative, characterised by events that are predictable and expected to happen (e.g., transition from youth to senior environment of a talented player), and non-normative, referring to those events that are unpredictable and unexpected (e.g., injuries or unexpected success). Much of the research within this area has tended to concentrate on career termination or (normal) retirement (a normative transition) and the psychological adjustment difficulties associated with this event. There has been a growing requirement for researchers to explore the 'within-career' transitions that many athletes and players undoubtedly experience in sport. Both individuals experiencing career termination and those undergoing within-career transitions require considerable personal adjustment, and a number of theoretical perspectives and models have been proposed to better understand these processes.

Lavallee and Wylleman (2000) brought together a comprehensive collection of career transitional literature in sport. Theoretical perspectives (e.g., social gerontology and thanatology) and research on career transitions have mainly focused on the understanding of and preparation for career termination or retirement (Pummell, Harwood and Lavallee, 2008). Social gerontology, or the study of the aging process, has been aligned with post-sport career transitions and the process of retirement from the labour force. Thanatology is associated with the study of death and the process of dying and has been used to help understand post-sport career transitions, in that athletes (and practitioners) may be better able to mourn the loss of their athletic identity by understanding that behaviours and experiences may be similar to those of bereavement or social death (Lavallee and Wylleman, 2000). While these theoretical perspectives offer some useful points in relation to the career-termination stage, they are limited in their application and contextualisation to the daily transitional experiences that players face. Neither of the perspectives has a sport-specific focus and both perceive the career termination as a singular and negative event (see Sinclair and Orlick, 1993).

The model of human adaptation to transition developed by Schlossberg (1981) and Charner and Schlossberg (1986) has characterised retirement as a process and examined the interaction of the retiring athlete and the environment. Three major factors were suggested to be critical in this process: the characteristics of the individual; their perception of the particular transition; and the characteristics of the pre- and post-transition environment. Empirical work exists to support the efficacy of the model, yet the model affords limited flexibility to the practitioner (Taylor and Ogilvie, 1994). Taylor and Ogilvie (1998) offered a more comprehensive model of career transition that considered factors associated with the entire course of transition (including causal factors, developmental factors, coping resources, quality of adjustment and treatment issues for distressful reactions). After viewing career termination or retirement as a singular, all-ending event, researchers then re-appraised this event as a transitional process of the athletic career (Wylleman et al., 2004). This perspective of career termination as a transitional process shifted the focus of career-transitions research from career end and termination to a more holistic life-span perspective, where athletes encounter distinct phases and transitions (Wylleman et al., 2004).

This shift in focus recognised the transitions that occur in other domains of the athlete's life and was represented in the developmental model of transitions produced by Wylleman, Alfermann and Lavallee (2004). The model represents transitions at four levels: athletic; psychological; psychosocial; and academic/vocational interactions across the life span. The athletic level includes the three stages defined by Bloom (1985) (initiation, development, mastery), plus a discontinuation phase. The second level represents the psychological changes through childhood, adolescence and adulthood, while the third is focused on the psychosocial interrelationships developed during the athletic career. The interaction with key stakeholders throughout the athletic career is outlined and includes relations with parents, siblings, peers, coaches and family and other relevant relations to the athlete. The fourth level outlines the progression through the academic/vocational level (primary through to higher education). While the model acts as a useful framework to appreciate the developmental, interactive and interdependent nature of transitions and stages faced by athletes, it lacks the contextual detail and specificity that is critical in better understanding the unique social and cultural features within many sports, and, in this case, in professional soccer. In professional soccer, we argue that there is a need to consider additional levels and stages of player development that may be aligned with Wylleman, Alfermann and Lavallee's (2003) developmental model. Specifically, we have identified the critical post-academy development phase that exists in

## 148

professional soccer (i.e., when players receive a 1- or 2-year professional contract but do not necessarily belong to, nor indeed play for, the first team). Furthermore, we recognise that an array of more socio-cultural factors exist that may play a significant role in shaping a player's successful or unsuccessful navigation through to the higher echelons of professional soccer (Table 8.3).

The model identifies the post-Academy or 'developing mastery' phase. We contend that this phase is possibly the most critical period of time for a young soccer player. As players exit the Academy setting, they become recognised as professional players. At an athletic level, in the traditional transition model, they would have progressed through the development phase and into the mastery phase. However, at this stage of development, many young players are not the 'finished' or 'polished' article. These players typically lack the many key attributes and/or experiences that would enable them to evidence mastery. In this regard, the post-Academy phase is still a period of development. We have termed this 'developing mastery'. Relvas and colleagues (2010) report the need to recognise this additional stage of development in soccer. Specifically, (most) young players still require continued and focused developmental work after their Academy experience. Typically, these players are not ready for the first team, yet there is an expectation for them to function and survive within the new 'mastery' environment. We believe that a significant number of young players are ill prepared and/or ill equipped for this (apparently) normative transition, with a deficiency in the requisite skills, knowledge and experience to cope, survive and perform within this environment. These players have been embedded (in some cases since the age of 9 years) in the Academy environment. At a socio-cultural level, the Academy environment is associated with *softer* cultural practices (Nesti, 2010), a more process-oriented and caring culture that allows considerably more time for development to occur. The Academy players tend to be surrounded by a range of 'supportive' practitioners (e.g., full and part-time coaches and heads of education and welfare). The softer cultural markers are reflected in their relationships with the players. These more caring, nurturing and empathic features of the Academy environment are in stark contrast to the

Table 8.3 Socio-cultural model of elite player development in professional soccer at Academy, post-Academy and first team level.

| Athletic level | Academy (16-19s) Development | Post-Academy Developing Mastery | First team Mastery |
|---|---|---|---|
| **Psychological level** | Adolescence | Social insecurity & comparison | (young) Adulthood Limelight stardom |
| **Psycho-social level** | Peers, parents, coach, sports psych, Ed & welfare | Partner New coach(es) Family | Manager New coach(es) |
| **Environmental and cultural level** | Process oriented Nurturing Caring Empathic | Uncompetitive Lonely Isolated Uncertain Stagnant | Outcome oriented Ruthless Masculine macho Heightened competition Team |
| **Nature of support** | Highly supportive | Bereft of social support | (Typically) crisis management, sophist |

often brutal, ruthless, hyper-macho and outcome-oriented environment that exists within the first-team world (Nesti, 2010; Nesti and Littlewood, 2011). In this regard, young players are expected to make this 'critical' transition to a new and 'harder' culture (i.e., a culture of 'first team') on their own. Young players will often find themselves in new surroundings, with new teammates. Additionally, they will be required to 'prove their worth' amongst established senior professionals. Unquestionably, some players will thrive. However, most will struggle to cope with this 'newness' alongside their diminished social status. No longer are they the best player or the most promising player in the environment. They are now coming to a realisation that they are part of the first team squad and they have to *prove their worth* over and above the established hierarchy (e.g., senior professionals, internationals, home and foreign stars). During this exciting yet rather daunting phase of their development, they find an environment that is *typically* bereft of social support, and ultimately a ruthless 'survive or die' culture. The two counter sub-cultures exist within one organisation, some all housed at the same training venue, others on separate sites. It is these socio-cultural features that are some of the most critical challenges that many professional soccer clubs and aligned practitioners face in the pursuit of developing and successfully progressing home-grown talent.

## SUMMARY

This chapter has addressed the importance of understanding a number of sociological and cultural factors that exist within the development of young soccer players. These factors are both externally and internally situated and can indirectly and directly influence the development process engaged in by players. We contend that many of the messages presented within this chapter can be addressed and managed more appropriately by practitioners and agencies involved in the identification and development of talented young players. Whilst such a message may seem quite clear and straightforward, the education of practitioners responsible for identifying and developing talented soccer players needs to be embraced by clubs and associated national governing bodies. This shift will undoubtedly take time and requires a greater appreciation, and embracement, of the contemporary evidence that exists within this area. There is a real danger that the sociological and environmental problems associated with player identification and development will continue to surface if the key messages are not fully embraced and discussed by relevant individuals (who have clear strategic influence) and organisations within the sport.

## REFERENCES

Baxter-Jones A. (1995). Growth and development of young athletes. Should competition levels be age related? *Sports Medicine* 20, 59–64.

Baxter-Jones, A., Helms, P., Maffull, N., Baines-Preece, J., and Preece, M. (1995). Growth and development of male gymnasts, swimmers, soccer and tennis players: a longitudinal study. *Annals of Human Biology* 22, 381–394.

Bloom, B.S. (1985). *Developing Talent in Young People*. New York: Ballantine.

Boucher, J., and Halliwell, W. (1991). The novem system: a practical solution to age grouping. *Canadian Association for Health, Physical Education and Recreation* 57, 16–20.

# 150

Boucher, J.L., and Mutimer, B.T.P. (1994). The relative age phenomenon in sport: a replication and extension with ice-hockey players. *Research Quarterly for Exercise and Sport* 65(4), 377–381.

Bourke, A. (2003). The dream of being a professional soccer player: insight on career development options of young Irish players. *Journal of Sport and Social Issues* 27, 399–419.

Brewer, J., Balsom, P., and Davis, J. (1995). Seasonal birth distribution amongst European soccer players. *Sports Exercise and Injury* 1, 154–157.

Brewer, J., Balsom, P., Davis, J., and Ekblom, B. (1992). The influence of birthdate and physical development on the selection of male junior international soccer squad. *Journal of Sports Sciences* 10, 561–562.

Carlson, R.C. (1988). The socialization of elite tennis players in Sweden: an analysis of the players' backgrounds and development. *Sociology of Sport Journal* 5, 241–256.

Charner, I., and Schlossberg, N.K. (1986). Variations by theme: the life transitions of clerical workers. *The Vocational Guidance Quarterly* 34(4), 212–224.

Côté, J., Baker, J., and Abernethy, B. (2003). From play to practice: a developmental framework for the acquisition of expertise in team sports. In J. Starkes and K.A. Ericsson (eds), *Expert Performance in Sports: Advances in Research on Sport Expertise* (pp. 89–110). Champaign, IL: Human Kinetics.

Côté, J., Macdonald, D.J., Baker, J., and Abernethy, B. (2006). When 'where' is more important than 'when': birthplace and birthdate effects on the achievement of sporting expertise. *Journal of Sports Sciences* 24(10), 1065–1073.

Curtis, J.E., and Birch, J.S. (1987). Size of community of origin and recruitment to professional and Olympic hockey in North America. *Sociology of Sport Journal* 4, 229–244.

De Knop, P., Van Hoecke, J., and De Bosscher, V. (2004). Quality management in sports clubs. *Sport Management Review* 7, 57–77.

Dickinson, D.J., and Larsen, J.D. (1963). The effects of chronological age in months on school achievement. *Journal of Educational Research* 56, 492–493.

Dudink, A. (1994). Birthdate and sporting success. *Nature* 368, 592.

Edgar, S., and O'Donoghue, P. (2005). The distribution of season of birth among the players of the 2002 FIFA World Cup. In T. Reilly, J. Cabri and D. Araújo (eds), *Science and Football V* (pp. 626–631). Abingdon: Routledge.

Edwards, S. (1994). [Letter to the Editor]. Born too late to win? *Nature* 370, 186.

Fielden, J. (2012). Premier League TV rights. *FC Business* 62, 12–14.

Football Economy (2009). English Premier League TV Broadcast Rights – 2007–2010. Retrieved February 14 2011 from http://www.footballeconomy.com/content/english-premier-league-tv-broadcast-rights-2007-2010.

Gammelsæter, H., and Jakobsen, S. (2008). Models of organization in Norwegian professional soccer. *European Sport Management Quarterly* 8(1), 1–25.

Glamser, F.D., and Marciani, L.M. (1992). The birthdate effect and college athletic participation: some comparisons. *Journal of Sport Behaviour* 15, 227–238

Helsen, W.F., Starkes, J.L., and van Winckel, J. (1998). The influence of relative age on success and dropout in male soccer players. *American Journal of Human Biology* 10, 791–798.

Helsen, F.W., van Winckel, J., and Williams, M. (2005). The relative age effect in youth soccer across Europe. *Journal of Sports Sciences* 23(6), 629–636.

Kotter, J.P., and Heskett, J.L. (1992). *Corporate Culture and Performance*. New York: The Free Press.

Lavallee, D., and Wylleman, P. (2000). *Career Transitions in Sport: International Perspectives*. Morgantown, WV: Fitness Information Technology.

Littlewood, M. (2005). 'The impact of foreign player acquisition on the development and progression of young players in elite level English professional football.' Unpublished PhD thesis, Liverpool John Moores University, UK.

Littlewood, M., Mullen, C., and Richardson, D. (2011). Football labour migration: an examination of the player recruitment strategies of the 'big five' European football leagues 2004–5 to 2008–9. *Soccer and Society* 12(6), 788–805.

Littlewood, M., Richardson, D., and Elliot, C. (2011). Player recruitment strategies in English Premier League football 1990–2008: progression of home-grown players. VIIth World Congress in Science and Football, Nagoya, Japan, May 2011.

Malina, R.M., and Bouchard, C. (1991). *Growth, Maturation and Physical Activity*. Champaign, IL: Human Kinetics.

Musch, J., and Grondin, S. (2001). Unequal competition as an impediment to personal development: a review of the relative age effect in sport. *Developmental Review* 21, 147–167.

Musch, J., and Hay, R. (1999). The relative age effect in soccer: cross cultural evidence for a systematic discrimination against children born late in the competition year. *Sociology of Sport Journal* 16, 54–64.

Nesti, M. (2010). *Psychology in Football*. London: Routledge.

Nesti, M., and Littlewood, M. (2011). Making your way in the game: boundary situations within the world of professional football. In D. Gilbourne and M. Anderson (eds), *Critical Essays in Sport Psychology*. Champaign, IL: Human Kinetics.

Owen, G. (2005). Born to win. *Mail on Sunday* 29 May, p. 11.

Pidgeon, D.A., and Dodds, E.M. (1961). Length of schooling and its effect on performance in the junior school. *Educational Research* 3, 214–221.

Pummell, B., Harwood, C., and Lavallee, D. (2008). Jumping to the next level: a qualitative examination of within-career transition in adolescent event riders. *Psychology of Sport and Exercise* 9, 427–447.

Reilly, T., Williams, A., and Richardson, D. (2003). Identifying talented players. In T. Reilly, and A.M. Williams (eds), *Science and Soccer* (pp. 307–326). London: Routledge.

Relvas, H., Littlewood, M., Nesti, M., Gilbourne, D., and Richardson, D. (2010). The structure, philosophy and working mechanisms of youth development in elite football clubs: a pan European perspective. *European Sport Management Quarterly* 10, 165–187.

Richardson, D., Littlewood, M., and Gilbourne, D. (2005). Homegrown or home nationals? Some considerations on the local training debate. *Insight Live*. Retrieved 20 September 2005 from https://ice.thefa.com/ice/livelink.exe/fetch/2000/10647/466509/477135/477257/Homegrown_or_Home_Nationals._The_Case_for_the_Local_Training_Debate.?nodeid-675785&vernum-0.

Schlossberg, N. (1981). A model for analyzing human adaptation. *The Counselling Psychologist* 9(2), 2–18.

Simmons, C., and Paull, G.C. (2001). Season-of-birth bias in association football. *Journal of Sports Sciences* 19, 677–686.

Sinclair, D.A., and Orlick, T. (1993). Positive transitions from high-performance sport. *The Sport Psychologist* 7, 138–150.

Slack, T., and Parent, M. (2006). *Understanding Sport Organizations: The Application of Organization Theory* (2nd edn). Champaign, IL: Human Kinetics.

Stambulova, N. (2000). Athlete's crises: a developmental perspective. *International Journal of Sport Psychology* 31, 584–601.

Taylor, J., and Ogilvie, B.C. (1994). A conceptual model of adaptation to retirement among athletes. *Journal of Applied Sport Psychology* 6, 1–20.

Taylor, J., and Ogilvie, B.C. (1998). Career transition among elite athletes: is there life after sports? In J.M. Williams (ed.), *Applied Sport Psychology: Personal Growth to Peak Performance*, 3rd edn (pp. 429–444). Mountain View, CA: Mayfield.

UEFA (n.d.). Home-grown Players. http://www.uefa.com/uefa/keytopics/kind=65536/index.html (accessed 10 October 2009).

Vaeyens, R., Coutts, A., and Philippaerts, R. (2005). Evaluation of the 'under-21 rule': do young adult soccer players benefit? *Journal of Sports Sciences* 23, 1003–1012.

Vaeyens, R., Renaat, M.P., and Malina, R.M. (2005). The relative age effect in soccer: a match related perspective. *Journal of Sports Sciences* 23(7), 747–756.

Williams, A.M., and Reilly, T. (2000). Talent identification and development in soccer. *Journal of Sports Sciences* 18, 657–667.

Wilson, A. (2001). Understanding organisational culture and the implications for corporate marketing. *European Journal of Marketing* 35(3/4), 353–367.

Wylleman, P., Alfermann, D., and Lavallee, D. (2004). Career transition in sport: European perspectives. *Psychology of Sport and Exercise* 5, 7–20.

Zink, K. (2005). Stakeholder orientation and corporate social responsibility as a precondition for sustainability. *Total Quality Management and Business Excellence* 16(8), 1041–1052.

# CHAPTER 9

## STRESS, COPING AND THE
## MENTAL QUALITIES OF ELITE PLAYERS

M. Pain and C. Harwood

## INTRODUCTION

Over the last decade, research into the psychology of soccer has increased considerably, especially when compared to sports of a similar standing. An illustration of the number of journal articles in sport psychology across three different sports is presented in Figure 9.1. Coaches and players appear more open than ever, and this may stem from a willingness amongst researchers to address the questions of direct relevance to coaches and players themselves. For example, in England the Football Association's psychology strategy, launched in 2002, has attracted over 10,000 people to courses and conferences and has played a role in bringing coaches and psychologists together. However, while this growth certainly represents good progress, the majority of research has focused on youth players, with few studies with adult, elite-level players. It appears that barriers to psychology, identified by Pain and Harwood (2004), are still present in areas of the game.

The overriding theme of the new research conducted with elite youth players is stress. This focus reflects the increasing demands on the modern professional and the decreasing opportunity for youth players to gain a senior contract. For example, in England, on average only 25–30 English players aged 23 years or under regularly represent Premier League sides. The 2007 'Lewis Review' of the Academy system in England reported that youth players face a particularly stressful time when challenging for a first-team place and that a 'climate of fear' exists in the game. All across Europe, teams are spending more money than ever before on talent from abroad, which, alongside extended playing careers, has resulted in fewer places for home-grown players. In addition, the transition from full-time schooling and part-time soccer to the physically intensive programme of an academy player (with education scheduled around training and matches) is often a shock to players who are entering the 'world of work' for the first time. It appears that fuelling many of these stressors is globalised competition for attractive professional contracts.

Senior players are not immune from stress. Arsene Wenger reflected on the failure of high-profile players and teams at the 2010 World Cup: 'The biggest teams who have the highest level of expectation cannot express that talent yet. One reason is caution, fear of failure, response to huge demands. There are so many demands in the modern game, too much pressure, too many expectations and sometimes too much inhibition' (Reuters, 2010).

In this chapter, we review the applied research in elite soccer conducted since the last edition of this book was published in 2003. We first review research on stress in soccer, particularly

## 154

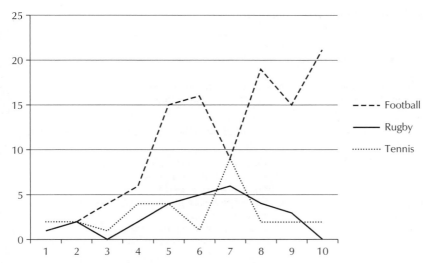

**Figure 9.1** Sport psychology research from three major sports published across 11 major journals from 2001–10.*

*Note: * European Journal of Sport Science, International Journal of Sport and Exercise Psychology, International Review of Sport and Exercise Psychology, Journal of Applied Sport Psychology, Journal of Clinical Sport Psychology, Journal of Sport and Exercise Psychology, Journal of Sport Sciences, Psychology of Sport and Exercise, Research Quarterly for Exercise and Sport, Sport and Exercise Psychology Review, The Sport Psychologist*

concerning the sources of stress. A second strand of research in the chapter focuses on the mental qualities required of professional players today: coping skills and mental toughness. We conclude with a brief look at other factors that can help to mitigate stress, including psychological, parental and social support. Although it is impossible to remove the pressure of the modern game, we feel that much can be done to help players to cope more effectively. Note that, as the research base with elite players is very limited, we review each study in detail.

## STRESS AND COPING IN INTERNATIONAL PLAYERS

Early research suggested a link between competitive anxiety and match performance in players (Rodrigo, Lusiardo, and Pereira, 1990; Maynard, Smith, and Warwick-Evans, 1995). Holt and Hogg (2002) broadened the discussion and examined sources of stress and coping strategies in an international female team during a 6-week preparation camp for the 1999 World Cup Finals. The study set the scene for much of the research that followed in the next decade and signposts many of the themes considered within this review.

Seven players were interviewed during the training camp regarding factors that influenced their psychological readiness and how they dealt with them. Four coping strategies to mediate the impact of these stressors emerged and were related to cognitive, behavioural and social resources (Tables 9.1 and 9.2).

**Table 9.1** Sources of stress for international players.

| Sources of stress | Notes |
| --- | --- |
| *Coaches' communication* | |
| Coach–player interactions in training | Negative and punitive feedback |
| Coach–player interactions in games | Too vocal and distracting |
| *Pace of the game* | |
| Demands of international football | Players doubt whether they can cope with extra pace |
| *Competitive stressors* | |
| Pre-game anxiety | Butterflies a few hours before games |
| Game anxiety | High expectations and pressure |
| Making mistakes | 'I think I have to be perfect' |
| Coming off the bench | Coach emphasising players must 'make an impact'. Negative body language |
| Fear of being dropped | 'Always competing for position' |
| Performance evaluation | 1–10 rating of each player posted in locker room |
| *Distractions* | |
| Fatigue | Cumulative effect of 2 practices a day plus games. Lose intensity and focus |
| Opponent | Physical intimidation |

**Table 9.2** Coping strategies to mediate the impact of stressors.

| Coping strategy | Notes |
| --- | --- |
| *Reappraising (emotion-focused)* | |
| Positive self-talk | |
| Problem solving | After a mistake 'What did I do wrong?' |
| Remembering past successes | |
| *Use of social resources (emotion-focused)* | |
| Encouragement from teammates | |
| Family support | |
| Support from significant others | |
| *Performance behaviours (problem-focused)* | |
| On-field task communication | Between players. Helps maintain focus |
| Good warm-up/start | Sets the 'tone' for the game |
| *Blocking (avoidance)* | |
| Blocking irrelevant stimuli | |
| Blocking coaches | |

Coaches frequently proved to be a source of stress, but rarely a coping resource for players. Gould, Guinan, Greenleaf, Medbery, and Peterson's survey of Olympic athletes (1999) also revealed that for over a third of athletes the coach relationship was perceived to have a strong negative effect on performance. In conclusion, Holt and Hogg (2002) discussed the importance of players' being taught coping strategies associated with the particular team culture and the unique stressors within that environment.

156

Pensgaard and Duda (2002) provided additional insights into the stressors associated with senior international competition. Using an ethnographic methodology, they investigated the experience of a soccer player at the 2000 Olympic Games in Sydney. 'Tina', who played in the Norwegian team, wrote a journal throughout the pre-camp and at the Games themselves. The team sport psychologist (who was also the researcher) corroborated these experiences with daily field reports. Data analysis focused on identifying stressors and coping strategies.

Having previously earned a bronze medal at an earlier Olympic Games, the team's goal at Sydney was to win a gold medal. The team lost its first group game (of three) – a result that Tina put down to overconfidence, with the psychologist also citing the 96,000 capacity crowd. Tina 'offloaded' this frustration by contacting a former coach back home and talking to the sport psychologist. This represented emotion-focused coping.

Before the second game, the 'unique team atmosphere' reportedly began to develop. Pensgaard and Duda (2002) felt that the team began to bond following a training game where 'everybody ends up crying with laughter . . . and are not afraid to make fools of themselves'. The team won the second game, but Tina was still not happy with her own performance. She then revealed in her diary an insight that she felt critical to the overall success. This was the belief that to win the tournament they had to 'WORK HARD ALL THE TIME!' (p. 229, original emphasis). The title of the paper, 'If we work hard, we can do it,' is based on this quote. The team won the third game, to reach the semi-finals with its and Tina's best performance to date.

The authors cite the day before the final as a key turning-point. The following factors emerged: 'Tina is extremely satisfied with the last training session', she has 'renewed belief in her own abilities', in the Olympic village, 'the spirit is very high . . . laughter is everywhere', and 'everybody is full of joy and energy and excitement' (p. 231). The Norwegian team won the match in extra-time, beating the USA, who had beaten them in the very first game of the tournament. The final was seen as the best match the team played, with Tina one of the dominant players, driven by what the authors described as an 'approach oriented way of coping' during the extra-time period.

Tina experienced various stressors during the tournament, including doubts about her own abilities, dissatisfaction with her performance and discontent with the team's philosophy of play, especially after the first game. In response to these stressors, Tina employed both problem-focused (e.g., working hard in training and preparation) and emotion-focused (e.g., venting frustrations to a previous coach and sport psychologist) coping strategies to deal with such issues as lack of self-confidence and coach–player conflicts during the tournament.

Table 9.3 Summary of coping strategies

| Coping strategy | Description |
| --- | --- |
| Problem-focused | Behaviours and thoughts aimed at confronting the source of the problem (e.g., information seeking, working hard in training, preparation) |
| Emotion-focused | Strategies that try to manage the emotional consequences of the problem (e.g., relaxation exercises, emotional support, positive re-interpretation) |
| Avoidance | Disengaging from the stressor (e.g., not talking about the problem, withdrawal, seeking distractions) |

Pain and Harwood's (2007) study of the England youth football teams also highlighted the influence of stress and anxiety on players at tournaments. They interviewed national coaches, players and sport scientists regarding factors that had a positive or negative effect on performance. The analysis covered all aspects of the performance environment, including physical and mental preparation, coaching and planning and organisation. Of the 155 factors listed as impacting on performance, team cohesion clearly emerged as the most frequently cited positive factor. On the negative side psychologically, player anxiety was most frequently cited. The following player quote illustrates how pre-match nerves impacted on performance:

> When I started with the U15s I was nervous before games. Especially the first game. But now, I don't get too excited if I've prepared for the games. I still get a little bit nervous, but nothing like it was. Now I just try to relax and get on with the game. That's helped me. In the Euro Champs I was the only player to play every minute of every game. I think that was the best I've played.
>
> (Pain and Harwood, 2007: 1316)

In the following examples, high expectations were seen by the coach as creating anxiety:

> Of course psychology has a big part. I think the first two and a half games they didn't perform as well as they could. So you could argue that they weren't quite relaxed, some people were saying they were a little bit tense, a little bit nervous. That did come out. Because everyone had so many good things to say about this squad, we were expecting amazing football, and the comment was made by one or two people that we haven't seen the best of you yet. They said that to the players quite a bit.
>
> (Pain and Harwood, 2007: 1316)

> I think the problem they have is a little anxiety, in that 'we're England, we shouldn't lose.' They paint that picture for themselves. And even the staff believe that. You know 'I see a lot of good players in this dressing room.' Unknowingly we create a little bit of anxiety there as well. I've heard it in a lot of dressing rooms, at different levels.
>
> (Pain and Harwood, 2007: 1316)

These findings mirrored those reported by Holt and Hogg (2002) in relation to coach stressors. It was noted, however, that with the younger age groups, coaches tried to de-emphasise the importance of winning and, looking at the overall motivational climate, it was coaches who were more task and process focused than players, who often emphasised outcomes. Pain and Harwood's (2008) follow-up quantitative study revealed team cohesion and leadership as having the most positive reported impact on tournament performance and, alongside team meetings, these were seen as crucial in shaping individual mental responses to the demands of international competition. To date, these four studies are the only ones to include international players in the sample. Although general conclusions can be drawn from them, a unique set of demands exists within club football, and the increasing professionalisation at a young age (Roderick, 2006) appears to underpin many stressors and fears.

## STRESS AND COPING IN ELITE YOUTH PLAYERS

Reeves, Nicholls, and Mckenna (2009) examined stress and coping in 40 male Premier League academy players aged between 12–14 years (early adolescents) and 15–18 years (middle adolescents). The key stressors reported by early adolescents were making errors, the opposition they were playing against, the performance of the team and pressure applied by family members.

> My parents and other peoples' parents shouted quite a lot. There was a lot of criticism and there was nothing helpful about it. I was close to the parents and my dad started shouting at me and it got me down and it was annoying because I had my coaches going 'don't listen to your mum and dad' and I had my dad saying 'don't listen to my coaches' and I didn't know what to do.
>
> (p. 39)

Middle adolescents also reported making errors as the most common stressor, followed by team performance, pressure applied by coaches, pressure associated with being selected for the team or squad, and opposition.

> I gave the ball away three times on the trot and people were on my back. When the ball came back to me I was just thinking, praying that I gave the next pass to a teammate. I was under pressure and thought if I give it away again then the manager's going to be on my back or I might get taken off.
>
> (p. 36)

The following quote illustrates the strategy the player used to deal with the above stressor:

> I made sure I stayed focused on my next movement and the next time I got it I checked my shoulder and tried to think positively and make a good pass. I didn't listen to the manager [coach] and tried not to let him get to me. I forgot about the mistakes and focused on doing good things, I focused on my next movement and next passes. I made sure I kept it simple and gave the ball to a teammate. I kept concentrating on the game.
>
> (p. 37)

Middle adolescents didn't highlight family-related stress as being so much of a problem, as compared to players in the early adolescence age group. They did, however, highlight the stress they were under regarding contractual issues and associated with performing at a higher level, whereas no players aged 12–14 cited these:

> I was with the first team during pre-season and it was horrible because none of the coaches would speak to me. I would train everyday and then play and I'd never get any feedback, there was never a review or a talk. I was there for 4 weeks training with them and at the end of it they were like; right you're back down to the academy. They never said why or what was going on or what I needed to improve or what they thought.
>
> (p. 42)

159

As in previous studies, players reported using problem-focused, emotion-focused and avoidance coping strategies. Reeves *et al.* (2009) found that early and middle adolescents used similar coping strategies, but important differences in dealing with stress were found. Early adolescents used more avoidance coping strategies, whereas middle adolescents favoured emotion-focused coping strategies. Consistent with previous adolescent sport research, cognitive avoidance was more commonly employed than behavioural avoidance. The authors argue that sport psychologists should educate players on effective coping strategies to ensure that they do not become dependent on avoidance coping strategies: 'For example, young players who have just given the ball away should be taught to work hard to win the ball back, focus on their next touch, think rationally about making one mistake, and relax on the ball the next time they have it, rather than trying to avoid the ball' (p. 46).

## FEAR OF FAILURE

A closely related study looked at fear of failure in academy players. Fear of failure has been associated with increased stress, reduced performance, cheating, dropout and unstable self-esteem. Using Conroy's (2008) model, Sagar, Busch and Jowett (2010) evaluated the prevalence of the five main aversive consequences of failure: (a) experiencing shame and embarrassment; (b) devaluing one's self-estimate; (c) having an uncertain future; (d) upsetting important others; and (e) important others losing interest. A total of 81 male footballers aged 16–19 years from four English academies completed the fear of failure questionnaire. As illustrated in Figure 9.2, results showed that shame and embarrassment was the most pronounced fear, followed by upsetting important others, having an uncertain future, important others losing interest and finally devaluing one's self-estimate.

In the second phase of the study, Sagar, Busch and Jowett interviewed the players with the highest-rated fears to see how they defined success and failure, what they saw as the consequences of these and how they coped with fear of failure. The players saw six negative consequences of failure:

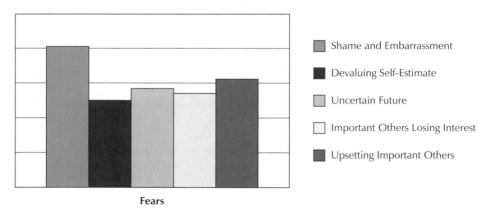

**Fears**

Figure 9.2 Fear of failure in English academy players.

160

1   *emotional cost* – which related to feeling embarrassed 'to talk to people', disappointed and dejected after failure;

2   *diminished perception of self* – related to perception of one's sporting ability after failure, 'I felt I was worst player in the world';

3   *reduced social status and interaction* – related to losing others' respect (teammates and coaches – 'The coach would lose respect for you 'cos he'll think "all this work I've done with him and he's, kinda, thrown it at my face"'), impaired communication with others, 'For a week after that game [failure] . . . I walked past them [coaches and teammates] and said nothing, complete silence', 'I felt embarrassed speaking to my teammates';

4   *punitive behaviour from others* – related to receiving criticism from teammates, coaches and parents after failure, 'If you play bad or lose, people are shouting, hollering all sorts of abuse at you', and to withdrawal of parental love, 'He [dad] was so annoyed we lost, he just left me there [at game venue] . . . and I didn't get any dinner later at home'; 'You go home after [losing] and you're in the dog house with your parents and my dad doesn't talk to me';

5   *uncertain future* – related to the possibility of 'getting dropped from the first team' or from the academy after failure; and,

6   *letting down important others* – related to parents and coaches.

Fear of failure was found to affect the players in three distinct ways. First, it had a negative effect on their performance. When fearing failure, players stated that they felt they were less likely to take the sort of risks in a match that they usually would and tended to play it safe: 'I'd stay back more and wouldn't come out for a catch and shout "keeper's", I'd just leave it to the defenders.' It also had a negative effect on their social interactions, leaving them more argumentative and shorter with other people. The final effect was on the general well-being of the players, for example, becoming more moody and suffering reduced quality of sleep. Factors contributing to a player's fear of failure include bad performances, the score, time on their own, pressure to succeed (from parents, coaches and themselves), opponent reputation and making future plans.

The final part of this study examined the coping strategies that players used to deal with their fear of failure. As with Reeves *et al.* (2009), the most frequent strategy was avoidance – that is, disengaging from the source of stress. This disengagement included pushing thoughts of failure away, not talking about their fears and trying to think about other things. Although this disengagement has some potential short-term advantages, as it allows performers to block out any negative thoughts and focus on the task at hand, it has long-term negative consequences, as it does not address the root of the problem, nor the stress that follows. Emotion- and problem-focused strategies included talking about their worries with family members and training harder, respectively. Also echoing Reeves *et al.* (2009), the authors encouraged coaches and parents to introduce players to a more positive coping style that incorporates both problem- and emotion-focused strategies. This approach included questioning the rationale/logic of their fears and then working on a way to address the problem. Coping strategies are important because, if left unattended, these fears, which are often underpinned by perfectionist traits, can result in burnout in elite youth players, especially if self-worth is low (Hill, Hall, Appleton, Kozub, 2008).

## BALANCING THE DEMANDS OF SCHOOL AND SOCCER

A final yet important stressor to consider for elite youth players is coping with the dual demands of school and soccer. Christensen and Sørensen (2009) conducted interviews with 25 elite Danish players aged 15–19 years and found that many struggled with this balancing act, given that the underlying assumption of elite soccer was, 'you have to go for it 100 percent'. Although players living close to school and training could cope, those who had to travel long distances were particularly at risk:

> Last year I was diagnosed with stress. I was unhappy with myself and with the place. That lasted six months. Over the first months it went well, but then it started going downhill. Then everything went down and I was good for nothing. It's only now after the summer holidays that I've got back on top again.
>
> (p. 124)

The authors concluded that, despite well-considered initiatives, the 'inner logic of the sport' (Bourdieu, 1986) meant that many players in this position were at risk of lower exam results, stress and a feeling of being torn between two options, dropping out of school and, in extreme cases, mental breakdown. They felt that the globalised competition for attractive professional contracts lay behind this potentially damaging situation.

## PENALTY SHOOTOUTS

Jordet's (2009) insightful analysis of the penalty kick provides an appropriate conclusion to this section and clearly illustrates how public appraisal, stress and fear of failure can undermine performance. Selecting the eight most merited European nations, he analysed all 200 penalty kicks from two major international tournaments (World Cup and European Championships). The results showed significant relationships between team status, self-regulation strategies and performance. Players from countries that, at the time of the penalty shootout, either had many international club titles or featured many internationally decorated players, spent less time preparing their shots and were less successful from the penalty spot than were players from countries with lower public status. Specifically, English players, who had the worst record in international tournaments, engaged in the most escapist self-regulation strategies of all teams – they had the lowest response times (median = 0.28 s) and the highest percentage of avoidance looking (56.7% of the English players turned their back to the goalkeeper as they backed up to prepare their shots). He concluded that English players, who represented the most successful club sides and had the highest media profiles, had the most to lose by missing penalties (greatest ego-threat) and therefore unwittingly employed avoidance strategies that hindered performance.

## THE MENTAL QUALITIES OF ELITE PLAYERS

Holt and Dunn's (2004) study of talent development in elite youth soccer provided an insight into the qualities players may need in order to cope with the demands and pressures of the

## 162

modern game. They interviewed 20 adolescent male Canadian international youth players, 14 male Premier League academy players in England, and 6 academy coaches. A combination of four psychosocial competencies were needed to secure a professional contract. A psychosocial competency was defined as a psychological skill which the athlete recognised and knew how/when to make use of it. The four competencies were discipline, commitment, resilience and social support. The latter two are particularly pertinent to coping with stress and are described in more detail.

Resilience was defined as players' ability to bounce back after adversity. Players had to be resilient in order to overcome obstacles such as parental pressure and (for the UK-based players) overseas players coming to the UK who might take their spot. They found that successful players had developed coping strategies to manage the demands of elite soccer. They had learned about the importance of making positive responses to mistakes and criticism and were also learning about having the confidence to thrive on pressure.

With respect to social support, although parents could occasionally put their children under too much pressure, in general they found that successful players learned how to use parental support to help them develop resilience. In particular, mothers and fathers provided emotional support, which was shown when players were able to turn to their parents for comfort, moral support and security during times of stress.

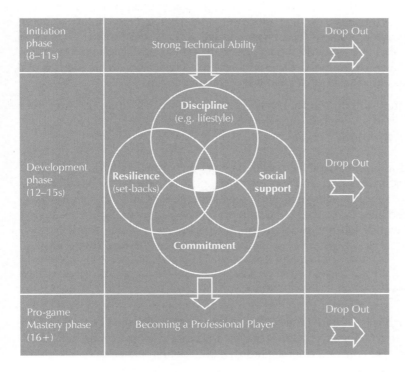

**Figure 9.3** A model of psychosocial competencies associated with success in soccer.

*Source*: Adapted from Holt and Dunn (2004: 206).

Holt and Dunn's (2004) model predicts that by possessing all four of the psychosocial competencies (i.e., discipline, commitment, resilience and social support) players give themselves the best chance of making it as a professional:

> In short, if a player maintains a disciplined lifestyle, makes the necessary sacrifices, develops a strong commitment, is able to rebound from setbacks, and receives adequate support, he potentially increases his chances of moving on to the next level [of professional football]. If not, it is more likely that he will (a) stay where he is until these conditions prevail, (b) be released from his club (in which case he may re-enter the sport at a lower level), or (c) drop out.
>
> (Holt and Dunn, 2004: 216)

Van Yperen (2009) also set out to identify psychological factors that predict career success, adopting in this case a quantitative approach. Predictor variables, including coping skills, were measured in the initial phase of the career of a unique group of highly skilled adolescent youth players from a soccer academy in the Netherlands. Career success was defined as actually playing for a premier soccer team in a European competition for at least 10 years in the 15-year period following data collection.

Altogether, 84.6% of the adolescent youth players were correctly classified as successful or unsuccessful, based on the predictor variables. The findings suggest that psychological factors are vital for career success in soccer. On the basis of the three significant psychological factors alone (i.e., goal commitment, problem-focused coping and seeking social support), 72.3% of the participants were correctly classified. Coping skills were seen as especially important: 'The ultimately successful players may have had a better ability to recover from training activity and cope with the demands and stresses of academy soccer generally' (p. 319).

Tangentially, it was interesting to see that, relative to the unsuccessful group, successful participants had more siblings, were more often of non-white (or non-Dutch) ethnic origin and more often had divorced parents:

> In speculating about these remarkable results, siblings may form a kin group bound by strong ties of trust and support, and may increase social skills which may be helpful to progress in team sports in particular. And being a member of an ethnic minority and having divorced parents may help to develop coping skills and attitudes that are helpful in dealing with all kinds of problems or drawbacks.
>
> (Van Yperen, 2009: 326)

## MENTAL TOUGHNESS

In a study of mental toughness in senior professionals, Thelwell, Weston, and Greenlees (2005) discussed how exposure to difficult situations can help players to learn coping skills. Their starting-point was Jones, Hanton, and Connaughton's (2002) definition of mental toughness:

> Mental toughness is having the natural or developed psychological edge that enables you to:

# 164

- Generally, cope better than your opponents with the many demands (competition, training, lifestyle) that sport places on the performer
- Specifically, be more consistent and better than your opponents in remaining determined, focused, confident, and in control under pressure.

Thelwell *et al.* (2005) used this description as a stimulus for interviews with 6 professional players. The themes from these interviews generated a preliminary definition that consisted of 10 key attributes. They then asked a further 43 professionals to rank order these attributes. The final outcome of the analysis was the list below, which they felt captured what it means to be a mentally tough player:

1  Having total self-belief at all times that you will achieve success;

2  Wanting the ball at all times (when playing well and not so well);

3  Having the ability to react to situations positively;

4  Having the ability to hang on and be calm under pressure;

5  Knowing what it takes to grind yourself out of trouble;

6  Having the ability to ignore distractions and remain focused;

7  Controlling emotions throughout performance;

8  Having a presence that affects opponents;

9  Having everything outside of the game in control;

10  Enjoying the pressure associated with performance.

Players felt that key formative experiences throughout their developmental and early career stages contributed to the development of these qualities. Situations described within the interviews included being dropped, being selected when not expecting it, lacking parent/school support, having to gain respect from the manager, being sent out on loan to another club and training with the senior squad. Thelwell *et al.* (2005) argued that these challenges are likely to occur throughout a player's career and, if managed correctly, exposure to similar situations as a young player can have benefits later on.

## SELF-REGULATION SKILLS

Jonker *et al.* (2010) argued similarly that a rise in the demands of soccer in recent decades might be a driver for improved self-regulation skills. Their study compared the academic level (pre-university or pre-vocational) and self-regulation skills (planning, self-monitoring, evaluation, reflection, effort and self-efficacy) of 128 elite youth soccer players aged 12–16 years with those of 164 age-matched controls (typical students). Countering existing stereotypes, the results demonstrated that the elite youth soccer players were higher academic achievers and had an increased use of self-regulatory skills, in particular self-monitoring, evaluation, reflection and effort, than the typical students. They concluded that the relatively stronger self-regulatory skills reported by the elite youth soccer players may be essential for performance at the highest levels of sport competition and in academia.

Whether the elite youth soccer players in Jonker et al.'s (2010) study inherently possessed these skills or if they were developed from participation in elite soccer is impossible to say, but the suggestion was that environmental factors were likely to play a significant part. In support of this latter notion, Toering and colleagues (Toering, Elferink-Gemser, Jordet, and Visscher, 2009) showed that elite youth soccer players reported using self-regulatory skills more frequently than youth players who were only involved in the sport as a leisure activity. The results revealed that the aspects of reflection and effort were especially associated with performance level. Almost half of the elite players scored high on reflection and effort, whereas only a fifth of the non-elite players did so. Furthermore, just a few of the elite players scored low on reflection and effort. The authors argue that reflection is the key process of expert learning, which translates knowledge into action, making it possible to gain strategy knowledge from specific activities. In the same vein as studies of coping, the authors of these studies conclude that players should be supported to use their self-regulatory skills within and between performance domains to help balance the demands they face and facilitate their achievements.

## PSYCHOLOGICAL, PARENTAL AND SOCIAL SUPPORT

Although the stress management literature is broad and covers many sports, to date it has had little impact on elite soccer. Maynard et al. (1995) reported how pre-match anxiety in semi-professional players can be reduced through cognitive and behavioural interventions, but researchers have yet to address the broader sources of stress discussed in this chapter. With this limitation in mind, we conclude with a brief look at the applied research showing how elite players can cope better with the demands they face.

The first study providing positive direction is Harwood's (2008) 5Cs intervention at a Football League academy in England. Based on a positive youth development model, the study focused on educating players, parents and coaches on the 5Cs of football: commitment, communication, concentration, control and confidence. At its core was an educational and behavioural coaching intervention related to integrating the 5Cs in on-pitch training and practice situations. The 4-month programme aimed to specifically enhance a coach's efficacy in shaping positive psychological and interpersonal skills in young players ranging in age from 9 to 14 years. Six coaches responsible for the development of 95 young players were involved in the programme. The programme appeared to be successful in integrating and developing psychological skills within the normal technical/tactical practices of the coach. By promoting the developmental–psychological role of coaches and their practices, a wider psychological skill climate was encouraged and coaches were positive about this working strategy. As shown by Maynard et al. (1995), psychological skills can certainly help players to cope better with game-specific demands. Thelwell, Greenlees, and Weston (2006) demonstrated that a psychological skills package, including relaxation, improved player performance on a number of position-specific measures. Likewise, Pain, Harwood, and Anderson (2011) show positive effects on flow and performance for an intervention using pre-performance music and imagery scripts.

Parents are also vital when considering stress and coping in young players. Early research suggested how parental support acted as a buffer against the stressful impact of poor performance in elite youth players (Van Yperen, 1995). The parents of non-elite players have also been shown to be a source of support, as well as stress (Holt, Tamminen, Black, Sehn, and Wall, 2008). On-going research suggests this is also the case in youth academy football in England. Harwood, Drew, and Knight (2010) conducted an in-depth qualitative investigation into the stressors experienced by soccer parents within the early (9–12 years) and later specialising phases (13–16 years) of academy football. Their results reinforced the heavy emotional investment that parents experience within academies as well as revealing the personal, social, coaching and organisational demands that parents cope with in their role as the parent of an elite soccer player. It is inevitable that parental stress will, consciously or unconsciously, transfer itself onto the player. Stress management strategies to help players should therefore include the role of parents, and equally professional clubs should focus on induction, education and communication programmes to assist parents in their coping skills.

Returning to the starting-point of this chapter with Holt and Hogg (2002), coach behaviours and the motivational climate will also play a key role. The findings of Pain and Harwood (2007; 2008) highlight how the team environment is important in shaping individual responses in pressure situations. In international tournaments, team meetings were seen by players as the main contributor to their individual mental preparation. In both studies, team cohesion emerged as the variable perceived to have the most positive impact on performance. Pain and Harwood's (2009) team-building intervention also showed the positive impact of an open and supportive team environment. Following the personal disclosure and mutual sharing (PDMS) guidelines of Holt and Dunn (2006), they facilitated a series of meetings in which team functioning was openly discussed between the players and coaching staff. Players reported improvements in cohesion, trust and confidence in teammates, training quality, self-understanding, player ownership and team performance. The intervention appeared to promote a more autonomy-supportive climate, in which social support helped players cope better with the demands placed upon them.

## SUMMARY

Stress is a live issue within elite soccer. A highly competitive and pressured environment for youth players can also cause a fear of failure. We have seen how these issues can affect players in a number of harmful ways, including reduced well-being, anxiety, performance issues and, over the long term, potential burnout. With little education at the present time, players often appear to be implementing unhelpful avoidance coping strategies that do nothing to address the root cause of the issues, which may include coach and parental pressure, and the demands of balancing multiple life demands. Stress management research is also urgently needed within soccer to help inform appropriate intervention strategies.

Players who are mentally tough and have good coping skills are those most likely to succeed in this increasingly demanding environment. Yet, few clubs provide systematic support for developing these skills and more needs to be done in this area. Although growth can occur from negotiating difficult career situations (e.g., Thelwell et al., 2005), players would benefit further from a proactive strategy for developing mental toughness. As we have seen with the 5Cs programme (Harwood, 2008), much of this work can be integrated within normal training sessions by coaches with a willingness to address mental development.

In the meantime, coaches and parents, and others involved in elite soccer, need to be more aware of the stressors that players face and to do what they can to act as a buffer against these.

Social support is often a critical factor in helping players to cope with the demands placed on them and they should be encouraged to seek this out. A comprehensive support system should also include sport psychologists who can provide players and coaches with additional specialist help.

## REFERENCES

Bourdieu, P. (1986). The forms of capital. In J. Richardson (ed.) *Handbook of Theory and Research for the Sociology of Education*. New York: Greenwood.

Christensen, M.K., and Sørensen, J.K. (2009). Sport or school? Dreams and dilemmas for talented young Danish football players. *European Physical Education Review* 1, 115–133.

Conroy, D.E. (2008). Fear of failure in the context of competitive sport: a commentary. *International Journal of Sports Science and Coaching* 3, 179–183.

Gould, D., Guinan, D., Greenleaf, C., Medbery, R., and Peterson, K. (1999). Factors affecting Olympic performance: Perceptions of athletes and coaches from more and less successful teams. *The Sport Psychologist* 13, 371–394.

Harwood, C.G. (2008). Developmental consulting in a professional soccer academy: The 5C's coaching efficacy program. *The Sport Psychologist* 22, 109–133.

Harwood, C.G., Drew, A., and Knight, C.J. (2010). Parental stressors in professional youth football academies: a qualitative investigation of specialising stage parents. *Qualitative Research in Sport and Exercise* 2, 39–55.

Hill, A.P., Hall, H.K., Appleton, P.R., and Kozub, S.A. (2008). Perfectionism and burnout in junior elite soccer players: the mediating influence of unconditional self-acceptance. *Psychology of Sport and Exercise* 9, 630–644.

Holt, N.L., and Dunn, J.G.H. (2004). Toward a grounded theory of psychosocial competencies and environmental conditions associated with soccer success. *Journal of Applied Sport Psychology* 16, 199–219.

Holt, N.L., and Dunn, J.G.H. (2006). Guidelines for delivering personal-disclosure mutual-sharing team building interventions. *The Sport Psychologist* 20, 348–367.

Holt, N.L., and Hogg, J.M. (2002). Perceptions of stress and coping during preparations for the 1999 women's soccer world cup finals. *The Sport Psychologist* 16, 251–271.

Holt, N.L, Tamminen, K., Black, D., Sehn, Z., and Wall, M. (2008). Parental involvement in competitive youth sport settings. *Psychology of Sport and Exercise* 9, 663–685.

Jones, G., Hanton, S., and Connaughton, D. (2002). What is this thing called Mental Toughness? An investigation with elite performers. *Journal of Applied Sport Psychology* 14, 211–224.

Jonker, L., Elferink-Gemser M.T., Toering T.T., Lyons J., and Visscher, C. (2010). Academic performance and self-regulatory skills in elite youth soccer players. *Journal of Sports Sciences* 28, 1605–1614.

Jordet, G. (2009). Why do English players fail in soccer penalty shootouts? A study of team status, self-regulation, and choking under pressure. *Journal of Sports Sciences* 27, 97–106.

Maynard, I.W., Smith, M.J., and Warwick-Evans, L. (1995). The effects of a cognitive intervention strategy on competitive state anxiety and performance in semi-professional soccer players. *Journal of Sport and Exercise Psychology* 17, 428–446.

Pain, M., and Harwood, C. (2004). Knowledge and perceptions of sport psychology within English soccer. *Journal of Sport Sciences* 22, 813–826.

Pain, M., and Harwood, C. (2007). The performance environment of the England youth soccer teams. *Journal of Sport Sciences* 25, 1307–1324.

Pain, M., and Harwood, C. (2008). The performance environment of the England youth soccer teams: A quantitative study. *Journal of Sport Sciences* 26, 1157–1169.

Pain, M., and Harwood, C. (2009). Team building through mutual sharing and open discussion of team functioning. *The Sport Psychologist* 23, 523–542.

Pain, M., Harwood, C., and Anderson, R. (2011). Pre-competition imagery and music: the impact on flow and performance in competitive soccer. *The Sport Psychologist* 25, 212–232.

Pensgaard, A.M., and Duda, J.L. (2002). 'If we work hard, we can do it' – a tale from an Olympic (Gold) medallist. *Journal of Applied Sport Psychology* 14, 219–236.

Reeves, C., Nicholls, A.R., and Mckenna, J. (2009). Stress and coping among academy footballers: age-related differences. *Journal of Applied Sport Psychology* 21, 31–48.

Reuters (2010). Fear of failure hampering big teams, says Wenger. Retrieved from http://www.reuters.com/article/2010/06/19/us-soccer-world-wenger-idUSTRE65I2DZ20100619.

Roderick, M. (2006). *The Work of Professional Football. A Labour of Love?* London: Routledge.

Rodrigo, G., Lusiardo, M., and Pereira, G. (1990). Relationship between anxiety and performance in soccer players. *International Journal of Sport Psychology* 21, 112–120.

Sagar, S.S., Busch, B.K., and Jowett, S. (2010). Success and failure, fear of failure, and coping responses of adolescent academy football players. *Journal of Applied Sport Psychology* 22, 213–232.

Thelwell, R.C., Greenlees, I.A., and Weston, N. (2006). Using psychological skills training to develop soccer performance. *Journal of Applied Sport Psychology* 18, 254–270.

Thelwell, R.C., Weston, N.J.V., and Greenlees, I.A. (2005). Defining and understanding mental toughness within soccer. *Journal of Applied Sport Psychology* 17, 326–332.

Toering, T.T., Elferink-Gemser, M.T., Jordet, G., and Visscher, C. (2009). Self-regulation and performance level of elite and non-elite youth soccer players. *Journal of Sports Sciences* 27, 1509–1517.

Van Yperen, N.W. (1995). Interpersonal stress, performance level, and parental support: a longitudinal study among highly skilled young soccer players. *The Sport Psychologist* 9, 225–241.

Van Yperen, N.W. (2009). Why some make it and others do not: identifying psychological factors that predict career success in professional adult soccer. *The Sport Psychologist* 23, 317–329.

# PART III

# PERFORMANCE ANALYSIS, BIOMECHANICS AND COACHING

# CHAPTER 10

## MATCH AND MOTION ANALYSIS

C. Carling and M. Court

## INTRODUCTION

Objective, accurate and pertinent data on performance are essential to aid coaches and practitioners in making informed judgements and decisions and to provide players with the feedback necessary for skill learning and performance enhancement (Franks, 2004). The dynamic nature of soccer can lead to incomplete or inaccurate recollection of various aspects of game-play, as observers are unable to view and assimilate all the actions taking place on the pitch. The primary function of match analysis (Figure 10.1) is to provide a factual and permanent record of events on individual and team playing performance during competition (James, 2006). Match analysis can be used to collect data on several areas of performance, including physical, technical and tactical factors. Match-related data provides an opportunity to critically appraise how players perform in competition, indicate areas in which performance can be improved, and are the foundation for providing feedback. However, before feedback can be provided, observation and analytic methods must be reliable, accurate and valid to create an objective account of match performance (Drust, Atkinson and Reilly, 2007). In addition, interpretation of information obtained on match performance must always take into account the numerous intrinsic and extrinsic factors that affect how players perform in competition. After assessment and interpretation of information, feedback on collective and individual performance can be provided during team-talks and/or on an individual basis. In coach-led feedback presentations, various techniques are frequently employed including edited video sequences, two-dimensional animated representation of match-plays and graphical information. Finally, decisions on the types of practice necessary for enhancing strategy, tactics, technique and physical condition can be subsequently made on the basis of the coach's evaluation.

Over the last decade or so, match analysis has gained widespread acceptance across the elite soccer community (Carling and Williams, 2008). At the highest levels of play, efficient exploitation of match analysis techniques might occasionally be the fine line between success and failure. Many professional clubs and institutions employ specialist consultants or scientific support staff, known as performance analysts, with specific expertise in this area. These analysts often exploit the very latest in state-of-the-art video and computer technology to record, analyse and evaluate their own team's performance to help coaches identify strengths that can be built upon and weaknesses to be remedied during practice. Data profiling and bench-marking provide an essential means for identifying key trends in performance across games and seasons. Performance analysts are also frequently involved in the analysis of opposition play, with the aim of helping their team to prepare more effectively for upcoming matches. Video and match-related data can be used as a means to identify and exploit weaknesses and draw up plans to counter opposition strengths. Most recently, match analysis is heavily influencing the process of player recruitment. Many professional clubs now employ specialist staff to provide detailed video and statistical data on competitive performance in order to make better-informed decisions on player trading.

In this chapter, the techniques used to collect information on performance are highlighted, including manual-based game analysis and the computer and video technologies currently employed at elite levels. Some examples of published data on physical, technical and tactical performance are provided, along with practical implications for application in training and match preparation.

## MATCH AND MOTION ANALYSIS TECHNIQUES

### Manual techniques

Up to the last two decades or so, pen and paper notation systems were generally employed for the analysis of soccer performance. This process often involves a manual coding system designed to record information on four key factors: the player; the type of action; the outcome of the action; and the time at which the action took place. Spatial information, notably the location (position) of the action, can also be recorded using a coded zone system or via graphical pitch representations divided into zones. Hand notation systems often used analogue video cassette recordings as means for visualising match-play. While video provides a useful medium for collecting, evaluating and presenting information on playing performance, manual

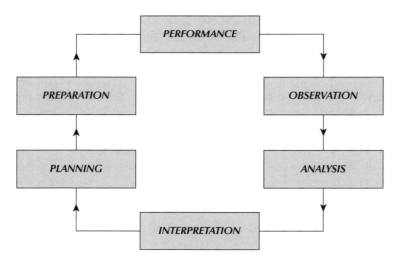

**Figure 10.1** The coaching cycle, highlighting the importance of observation and analysis.

*Source*: Adapted from Carling, Williams and Reilly (2005).

C. Carling and M. Court

searching (rewinding and fast forwarding) through analogue cassettes took time. In addition, analogue video had limited possibilities for producing edited sequences of selected areas of performance. Overall, data collection via analogue video combined with hand-based coding methods was generally labour intensive and time consuming. Efficient analysis and archiving of data for future analysis were also difficult, as records were generally kept on sheets of paper. Furthermore, some of the data collection methods were inaccurate, notably when recording information on positions of actions and running movements.

In contrast, manual analysis systems are relatively cheap and provide pertinent data sets for dissemination. These systems are within the reach of standard coaches and readily provide answers to many of the questions posed on performance, particularly at lower levels of the game. Two definitive studies using manual data coding techniques to collect data on physical and tactical performance, respectively, were developed by Reilly and Thomas (1976) and Reep and Benjamin (1968). The former employed a subjective assessment of distances and exercise intensities recorded manually or onto an audiotape recorder. For additional information on the workings, advantages and limitations of manual coding processes, the reader is referred to Carling, Williams and Reilly (2005).

## Computerised and digital techniques

The use of digital video and computer technology to collect data and provide feedback on play has become prominent in contemporary training and competition. Innovations in technology have streamlined the entire match analysis process, notably the collection and analysis of all forms of performance-related data. Advanced user-friendly data recording interfaces combined with high-quality digital video footage and automatic event indexing are now routinely employed. The use of touch screens and voice recognition systems to input data is commonplace and interfaces can be customised to the specific needs of the analyst. Digital video footage can be accessed, observed, replayed, edited, re-edited and archived at the simple touch of a button. Digital video also allows opportunities for high-quality slow-motion play back combined with special effects such as synchronised split-screen visualisation or image blending to compare actions. In addition, database technologies provide possibilities to create performance benchmarks and undertake trend analysis by comparing data for teams and individual playing positions over any course of time. Data on any aspects of performance (physical, technical and tactical) can be compared, cross-tabulated and displayed in forms such as time (e.g., total time spent in possession in opponents' half), distances (e.g., distance run at high intensities), speeds (e.g. peak sprinting speed), counts (e.g., total number of corners won), percentages (e.g., proportion of completed passes) and ratios (e.g., ratio of corners to goals scored). Contemporary computer analysis software and databases provide seamless graphical output and unlimited possibilities for data presentation. Attractive table and graph formats as well as spatial pitch representations of information are readily available.

Nowadays, a plethora of commercial computerised performance analysis systems and software exist for soccer. A non-exhaustive list of these technologies is presented in Table 10.1. Additional information on systems can be obtained by visiting each company's website. For additional information on the area, the reader is referred to recent reviews (Barris and Button,

175

2008; Carling, Reilly and Williams, 2009; Carling, Bloomfield, Nelsen and Reilly, 2008). Nevertheless, whatever computer system is adopted, it must comply with four basic quality control specifications: accuracy; reliability; objectivity; and validity (Drust, Atkinson and Reilly, 2007). Also, while the cost of computer and video technology has generally fallen over the last decade, many of these systems remain expensive and are therefore inaccessible to practitioners at lower levels of the game.

The Sportscode match analysis software has been embraced by the elite soccer community (see http://www.sportstec.com/). It is frequently used at both senior and youth levels to provide advanced statistical analysis of technical and tactical performance and edited digital video sequences of play (Figure 10.2). More recently, online systems accessible throughout the world have been developed to directly aid in player recruitment using databases of technical and tactical data combined with digital video sequences (for examples, see http://www.pro zonesports.com; http://www.sport-universal.com; http://info.scout7.com/). Detailed statistical information on a potential recruit can be compared against benchmark data for one's own players or against League averages worldwide and for players in the same positional role. This facility is especially useful if a club is looking for a specific type of player to strengthen its

**Table 10.1** Some examples of commercial match and motion analysis systems frequently used in contemporary professional soccer.

| Company | Country | System | Website |
|---|---|---|---|
| *Digital video-editing/statistical analysis* | | | |
| Dartfish | Switzerland | Dartfish | http://www.dartfish.com |
| Elite Sports Analysis | UK | Focus X2 | http://www.elitesportsanalysis.com/ |
| MasterCoach Int | Germany | MasterCoach | http://www.mastercoach.de |
| Prozone | UK | Matchviewer/ Recruiter | http://www.prozonesports.com/ |
| Scanball | France | Scanfoot | http://www.scanball.com/ |
| Sportstec | Australia | SportsCode | http://www.sportstec.com/ |
| Sport-Universal | France | Videopro/ Recruiter | http://www.sport-universal.com |
| *Player tracking technologies* *Digital video* | | | |
| Prozone | UK | Prozone 3 | http://www.prozonesports.com/ |
| Sport-Universal | France | AMISCO Pro | http://www.sport-universal.com/ |
| STATS | Israel | SportVU | http://www.sportvu.com/ |
| Tracab | Sweden | Tracab | http://www.tracab.com/ |
| *Electonic transmitter* | | | |
| Cairos Technologies | Germany | Cairos | http://www.cairos.com |
| Inmotio Object Tracking | Holland | LPM Soccer 3D | http://www.inmotio.nl/ |
| ZXY Sport Tracking AS | Norway | ZXY | http://www.zxy.no/ |
| *Global Positioning System* | | | |
| Catapult Innovations | Australia | MinimaxX | http://www.catapult innovations.com/ |
| GPSports | Australia | SPI | http://www.gpsports.com/ |
| Real Track Football | Spain | Real Track Football | http://www.realtrackfutbol.com |

# 176

squad and for an objective assessment of how the player might perform and adapt to the demands of a new league.

The numerous difficulties encountered when using original manual motion analysis techniques to measure physical performance in match-play (see Reilly and Thomas, 1976; Bangsbo, Nørregaard and Thorsøe, 1991) led to the development in the late 1990s of automated and semi-automated video-based player tracking systems. AMISCO Pro and Prozone 3 (Table 10.1) are considered to be the pioneer player tracking systems. These semi-automatic systems track the movements of all players simultaneously on digital video footage obtained from fixed multiple cameras positioned strategically to cover the entire pitch. This non-intrusive tracking analysis is done semi-automatically post-match, but requires some manual intervention by an operator, with results generally available 12–24 hours after competition. The Prozone system has been shown to be an accurate, reliable and valid means for quantifying physical performance (Di Salvo, Gregson, Atkinson, Tordoff and Drust, 2009). A further development on these systems is Spinsight's K2 Camera System (see http://www.spinsight.com/). This portable system reportedly provides real-time player tracking using a portable camera configuration with three video images being merged into one to provide a panoramic view of the match. The advantage of real-time analysis is the availability of objective performance-related data upon which coaching staff can base their half-time 'team talk' and make tactical changes and/or substitutions over the course of a match.

In recent times, Global Positioning Technology (GPS) has impacted on the measurement of physical performance in team sports (Coutts and Duffield, 2010). GPS receivers can be used to collect real-time data on distances run and movement speeds, and can also provide physiological information (heart-rate). A tri-axis accelerometer can be used to record information on the frequency and intensity of accelerations and impacts such as tackles and collisions. These systems are generally limited to measuring work intensity in training, but are sometimes used in friendly matches and youth competitions, as players must be equipped with electronic material which is currently forbidden at professional and international level. The increased sample rate of more recent models (>5 HZ) has generally improved the validity and reliability of these devices for measuring movement speeds (Jennings, Cormack, Coutts, Boyd and Aughey, 2010), especially for high-intensity activities.

Finally, the development of electronic tracking systems using small, lightweight microchip transmitters worn by players enables real-time data acquisition and analysis. Systems such as the Local Positioning Measurement monitoring system (LPM) accurately collect information on the movements and positions of every player and the ball up to several hundred times per second (Frencken, Lemmink and Delleman, 2010). The LPM system also permits the collection of heart-rate data in response to exercise, but usage is again generally restricted to training, friendly matches and youth competitions.

## ANALYSIS OF TECHNICAL AND TACTICAL PERFORMANCE

The vast majority of practitioners at elite levels use analyses of technical and tactical performance in some form or other to aid in preparing strategy and tactics and in player selection. These aspects of performance can be analysed both quantitatively (e.g., frequency of actions, percentage completion rates) or qualitatively (edited video sequences, animated game

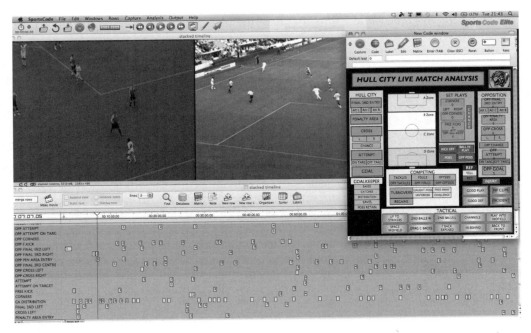

**Figure 10.2** The Sportscode match analysis software (reproduced with permission from Sportstec, Australia).

reconstructions, spatial representations). While the personal philosophy of the coach, his/her prior defined objectives and previous performances of the team can drive the choice of analysis, quantitative match analysis is generally invaluable in that it can help to create an objective, unbiased view of events and provide a solid platform upon which to make informed decisions regarding successful strategy and tactics. Nevertheless, complementary qualitative analyses from video footage are extremely useful, as statistical information may not always paint a true picture of a player's performance or effort. However, coverage of qualitative aspects of match analysis is beyond the scope of this chapter and the reader is referred to Carling, Williams and Reilly (2005) for additional information.

In general, soccer has two basic but principal phases to the game that need to be analysed; these are attacking play to create scoring chances and goals and defensive play to recover possession and prevent opposition scoring chances and goals. While the following sections are mainly concerned with attacking play, implications for defensive strategy and tactics may be drawn via inference. Beforehand, however, it is important to briefly mention the need for match analysts and coaches to consider the potential independent and interactive effects of factors such as match location, quality of opposition, and match scoreline when assessing tactical and technical components of performance. Further information on these respective features of play can be obtained in articles by Taylor, Mellalieu, James and Shearer (2008) and Lago (2009).

C. Carling and M. Court

## Key performance indicators

A performance indicator is a selection or a combination of action variables that aim to define some or all aspects of a performance and often relate to the outcome of events (Hughes and Bartlett, 2002), notably, successful (e.g., number of shots on target) or unsuccessful (e.g., number of shots off-target) actions. When match analysis is employed to study tactical and technical play, performance is usually described and defined using a general set of statistical indicators based on frequencies and/or percentage success rates. In elite soccer, these indicators are frequently referred to as Key Performance Indicators (KPIs). A KPI can be analysed in isolation at team or individual level. Analysis of the team as a whole provides a global idea of how well it performed. These data can then be analysed further to determine the contributions of separate team units and individuals. Primary analysis might involve examining the total time spent in possession by a team, the number of attacking entries into the opponent's penalty area and the number of scoring opportunities created. Secondary analysis could break this information down further to see which players were responsible for gaining possession, how and where possession was won and the types of action preceding the goal attempt. Where possible, tactical and technical performance should be analysed relative to averages observed for previous games and compared to data from the opponents. A list of 20 KPIs commonly used to analyse elite soccer play is presented in Table 10.2.

Whilst the performance of a team may ultimately be judged on the number of goals scored and chances created, the analysis of other match-related actions can provide helpful information on individual and team performance. The overall number of challenges won or

**Table 10.2** Commonly used key performance indicators for analysing tactical and technical attacking play.

| Key performance indicators: attacking play |
| --- |
| Number of goals scored |
| Number of goal attempts |
| Percentage of goal attempts on target |
| Strike rate for goal attempts (ratio goal attempts to goals) |
| Number of set-plays won |
| Number of corners won |
| Number of free-kicks won |
| Number of goal attempts and goals scored from set-plays |
| Strike rate for set-plays (ratio set-plays to goals) |
| Percentage of time in ball possession |
| Percentage of time in ball possession in opponent's half |
| Number of passes |
| Percentage of pass completion |
| Percentage of forward pass completion |
| Number of final third and/or penalty area entries |
| Strike rate for final third and/or penalty area entries (ratio to goals scored) |
| Number of crosses |
| Percentage of cross completion |
| Number of goal attempts / goals scored from crosses |
| Strike rate for crosses (ratio crosses to goals) |

lost, interceptions or turnovers, passes, goal attempts, goals scored from crosses, penalty area entries and free-kicks won or conceded can give a good initial impression of team performance and/or the contributions of individual players. The total number of actions should be combined where possible with the corresponding percentage of success (or completion rates) and failure for each action, to enable an objective evaluation of performance. For example, teams winning games in the group stage of the UEFA Champions League competition (from 2007 to 2010) not only passed the ball more than losing teams but completed substantially more passes (Lago-Peñas, Lago-Ballesteros and Rey, 2011).

Information on the origin and types of key (or final) actions preceding goals or scoring opportunities can have useful implications for attacking and defensive play. In elite soccer, the majority of goals are preceded by actions such as passes and crosses. These actions accounted for around 70% of goals scored in the 2006 World Cup (Breen et al., 2007). Research has also demonstrated an upward trend across World Cup winners in the importance of dribbling as a key event preceding goal attempts and goals scored (Yates et al., 2007).

In soccer, the ability to score when presented with an opportunity is important. Coaches are therefore interested in calculating the strike rate or scoring efficiency of players and teams, that is, the ratio of goal attempts to goals. Winning teams generally have a better 'goal scored' to 'attempt on goal' ratio (Lago-Peñas, Lago-Ballesteros, Dellal, and Gómez, 2010), highlighting the importance of having players who can take full advantage of goal-scoring opportunities. During the 2007/8 Premier League season, clubs ranked at the end as top-four, middle and bottom-four were differentiated not only by the total number of scoring opportunities created but by the percentage of shots on target (Oberstone, 2009). Bell-Walker, McRobert, Ford and Williams (2007) showed that successful teams at the 2002 and 2006 soccer World Cup finals had significantly more attempts at goal compared to unsuccessful teams at the 2002 tournament and, more importantly, demonstrated greater efficiency at converting those attempts into goals scored (Table 10.3). Finally, the majority of goals in elite soccer are scored from a one-touch finish, indicating a need for players to be able to finish quickly and efficiently.

### Analysis of attacking set-plays

In international soccer, teams have been reported to obtain an average of 12 in-direct free-kicks, 2 direct free-kicks, 17 throw-ins and 5 corner kicks in the attacking third per game, with

**Table 10.3** Ratios for the number of attempts at goal to goals scored from open play and set-plays at World Cup 2002.

|  | Successful teams | Unsuccessful teams |
| --- | --- | --- |
| Open-play | Ratio | |
| World Cup 2002 | 7:1 | 22:1 |
| Set-plays | | |
| World Cup 2002 | 10:1 | 14:1 |

Source: Adapted from Bell-Walker et al. (2007).

C. Carling and M. Court

these set-plays playing a substantial part in scoring goals (Carling, Williams and Reilly, 2005). Analyses of the frequency of goals and scoring chances created directly or indirectly from set-plays are therefore pertinent. Breen, Iga, Ford and Williams (2007) reported that set-plays accounted for approximately 36% of all goals scored in the 2006 World Cup (Table 10.4). Indirect free-kicks and corners made up ~30% of the set-play goals. However, successful soccer teams are generally more efficient than less successful opponents at scoring or creating chances from set-plays. Analysis of play in the 2006 World Cup reported a set-play to goal ratio of 1:7.5 for teams who reached the semi-finals, as compared to 1:14 for opponents eliminated before this stage (Bell-Walker, McRobert, Ford and Williams, 2007). In 2002, the same pattern was observed (see Table 10.3) and Brazil, the eventual winner, had an even lower ratio of goals to set-plays: approximately 1:6 (Taylor and Williams, 2002).

Match analyses have attempted to identify strategies that can increase the possibility of scoring from set-plays. The location and outcome of all free-kicks taken directly at goal in the 2007 women's World Cup were assessed to identify areas with the most goal-scoring potential (Alcock, 2010). All free-kicks that resulted in a goal were taken from a central area within 7 m of the penalty circle, placed in the corner of the goal (approximately 1 m from the goalpost), and had an average flight time of 1.09 s, which was significantly faster than that for shots that were saved. Analysis of the men's European Championships in 2000 showed that direct shots from free-kicks in central areas were more effective than a short pass followed by a shot at goal (Ensum, Williams and Grant, 2000). Scoring a goal is generally more likely from in-swinging free-kicks delivered into the central goal region and to the near post regions and in-swinging corners appear to be a more effective attacking ploy than out-swinging corners (Carling Williams and Reilly, 2005). These results have consequences for the design and prescription of training drills to improve the chances of scoring, notably by working on the accuracy and quality of set-play delivery and the movements and positioning of attacking players.

Information on the most efficient methods that lead to winning set-plays is also beneficial. In the 2002 World Cup, the highest proportion of free-kicks in the attacking third was awarded after a player was fouled when running or dribbling the ball past a defender, particularly in central areas of the pitch (Ensum, Taylor and Williams, 2002). This finding highlights the importance of having players who can commit defenders into making challenges by running or dribbling with the ball in attacking areas. Identification and subsequent targeting of opposition players more likely to concede free-kicks or penalties might be warranted.

**Table 10.4** Source of goals in the 2006 soccer World Cup.

| Source of goals | Total (%) |
| --- | --- |
| Open play | 90 (61) |
| Set play | 40 (27) |
| Penalty | 13 (9) |
| Own goals | 4 (3) |
| Total | 147 |

*Source*: Adapted from Breen *et al.* (2007).

## Analysis of attacking from open play

The ability to maintain possession of the ball enables teams to control the structure and tempo of the game but is not always an effective gauge of performance. Teams can either favour a more direct style where the ball is played quickly forwards using a small number of actions or a possession-oriented game using longer 'build ups' in which possession is maintained until a suitable attacking opportunity arises. Whilst coaches might be interested in information on which team dominated possession, they are often keen to know in which zones their team was able to maintain possession (e.g., in opposition half) and if this was used to good effect (e.g., number of scoring chances created). Similarly, information on the effectiveness of a team in regaining possession and subsequently turning defence into attack can have important tactical implications for creating chances and scoring goals. Teams may endeavour to increase their chances of scoring by playing a high-pressure game in an attempt to win back possession in the opponent's half or defending third. In the 2006 World Cup, 90% of all goals scored by Italy, the eventual winner, came about after possession was regained in the opponent's half (Yates, North, Ford and Williams, 2007). Alternatively, winning back possession in one's own defensive areas and then utilising fast counter-attacking play involving a minimum of passes may be productive in creating scoring occasions.

Over the last 50 years, match analyses of competition have consistently produced contrasting results on the different styles of play and their effectiveness in creating potential goal-scoring opportunities, scoring goals and winning games. The definitive piece of work by Reep and Benjamin (1968) provided comprehensive statistical information that generally advocated a direct playing strategy to increase the chance of scoring goals. Additional information can be obtained in a short historical review of this research (see James, 2006). Recent analyses of Premier League matches have shown that teams who were more able to maintain ball possession (using longer passing sequences) than the opposition were far less likely to lose the match, particularly if the difference in possession rates between teams was greater than 8% (Carling, Williams and Reilly, 2005). While global ball possession is important, more successful teams may be the ones that can effectively employ different styles of play. Recent findings in professional soccer in Norway are partly supportive of this theory, as results showed that a combination of quick counter-attacks to take advantage of imbalances in the opponent's defence and the use of sequences of play with five passes or more were both effective in producing goals, scoring opportunities and score box possessions (Tenga, Ronglan and Bahr, 2010). Whatever the playing style of teams, the majority of scoring opportunities and goals scored follow short sequences of play involving one to four consecutive passes. In World Cup tournaments (1998, 2002, 2006), the majority of the attempts on goal and goals from open play by the eventual winners were scored following sequences of four passes or fewer. In addition, goals at the elite level are frequently scored from zero passing sequences (e.g., 'snap shot' following a clearance or rebound) or from a single pass.

## ANALYSES OF PHYSICAL PERFORMANCE IN MATCH-PLAY

Strength and conditioning coaches aim to design fitness programmes to equip players with the optimal physical skills required for competition. These skills refer to a number of charac-teristics that are essential to assist players in competing for possession of the ball, reacting

182

maximally to continually changing game situations and maintaining high performance levels throughout the duration of games and across the entire season. A primary step in the conditioning process is the monitoring of exercise intensity during competition in order to quantify the performance demands of the sport (Reilly, 2003). Institutional rules and regulations often forbid the wearing of electronic devices to measure movement and the sampling of physiological responses during official competition. This ban partly contributed to the development of a process for indirectly classifying and coding match activities according to the intensity of movements, known as motion analysis. Data obtained on running movements can be translated into distances or velocities or the frequency of time spent in a variety of movement activities. Information on the time spent in, and the intensity of recovery between, high-intensity actions is also pertinent. Exercise-to-rest ratios or low- to high-intensity exercise ratios can be calculated to accurately represent the demands of the sport and provide objective guidelines for optimising the conditioning elements of training programmes (Reilly, 2007).

Match performance profiling can highlight individual deficiencies such as a susceptibility to fatigue, shown up by an inability to repeat high-intensity efforts over the course of games. The incapacity to recover after an intense bout of exercise or a general drop-off in performance towards the end of games may suggest a need for supplementary or more individualised conditioning work. Information from motion analyses can be used to a certain extent to determine the effects of fitness training interventions on subsequent physical performance in match-play. In an intense period of training or competitive fixtures, physical profiling may give objective confirmation of the coach's diagnosis that some players are coping well and others are failing to do so, when performance is compared to benchmark data. Results have implications for the different recovery strategies employed by fitness and medical staff between matches. In this section we visit data on physical performance profiles in soccer competition published over the last decade or so. Information on fatigue in soccer match-play is also presented, as well as key factors that affect physical performance. Finally, practical implications of this information are provided.

## Overview of general and position-specific demands

The total distance covered during match-play provides a global representation of the intensity of exercise, since this feature determines the energy expenditure, irrespective of the speed of movement (Reilly, 2003). The total distance run by male professional outfield players playing in the top division in England increased substantially with the inception of the Premier League (Strudwick and Reilly, 2001). On average, contemporary male professional outfield soccer players cover distances ranging from 10–13 km (Carling et al., 2008). At the higher end, outfield players can attain 14 km, while goalkeepers tend to cover 4–6 km. Analyses in top-class and high-level female soccer players have reported distances of 9–11 km (Mohr, Krustrup, Andersson, Kirkendal and Bangsbo, 2008). Youth soccer players aged around 12 years have been reported to run around 6 km for a 60-minute match (Castagna, D'Ottavio and Abt, 2003).

The total distance covered in a game can be broken down into discrete movement activities. The distance covered and/or time spent in these activities, as well as their frequency, are generally determined according to the intensity (determined by the speed) of movement. The main movement categories are classed into walking (and standing), jogging, moderate- and high-intensity and sprinting activities. No consensus exists for the definitions of movement categories according to running speed, resulting in problems in objectively comparing results. In addition, recent work suggests that speed thresholds used to determine movement profiles should be tailored according to the individual physiological capacity of the player (Abt and Lovell, 2009). Nevertheless, all previous analyses of physical performance highlight that exercise performed over the course of competition varies greatly in intensity and that the activity profile is intermittent in nature.

In general, activities at lower levels of intensity tend to dominate performance profiles at all levels of soccer, emphasising the predominantly aerobic nature of the game. The ratio of low- to high-intensity exercise in terms of distance covered is about 5:2, or about 7:1 when based on time (Reilly, 2007). In a group of professional Italian players, Mohr, Krustrup and Bangsbo (2003) observed that ~90% of total match time was spent in movement at low intensities. The relative distance covered in 5 movement intensities for a sample of 300 outfield players is presented in Figure 10.3. Approximately 8% of the total distance covered was performed at high running speeds (>19.1 km/h).

Sprint-type activities are widely considered to be a crucial element of performance, yet they contribute only a small proportion to the overall motion activity during competition, accounting for about 10% of the total distance covered over the course of matches (Carling et al., 2008). In addition, the majority of sprints are short in distance (10–20 m) and duration (2–3 s), suggesting that acceleration capabilities are more important than peak running speed (Spencer, Bishop, Dawson and Goodman, 2005). Although movement at high intensities makes up only a small part of the total distance covered, top-class soccer players must perform between 150 and 250 intense actions per game (Mohr, Krustrup, and Bangsbo, 2003). Research in the English Premier League showed that players perform a run at high intensities (>19.8 km/h) every 72 s (Bradley, Sheldon, Wooster, Olsen, Boanas et al., 2009).

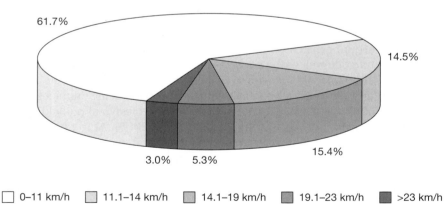

61.7%  14.5%  3.0%  5.3%  15.4%

☐ 0–11 km/h  ☐ 11.1–14 km/h  ☐ 14.1–19 km/h  ■ 19.1–23 km/h  ■ >23 km/h

**Figure 10.3** Analysis of the relative distances covered in 5 movement intensities in 300 outfield professional soccer players.

*Source*: Data adapted from Di Salvo, Baron, Tschan, Calderon Montero, Bachl et al. (2007).

184

Analyses of physical performance during selected short periods (e.g., 5-min intervals) demonstrate that players transiently perform substantially higher amounts of high-intensity running than the game average (Carling and Dupont, 2011). Consequently, very short recovery intervals between consecutive intense efforts can occur on several occasions throughout competition. The ability to reproduce and recover from these efforts (termed repeated sprint ability or RSA) is widely accepted as a critical component of high-intensity intermittent sports such as soccer. Gabbett and Mulvey (2008) found that international female players performed intense repeated-sprint bouts (defined as a minimum of 3 consecutive sprints, with recovery of less than 21 s between actions) almost 5 times per game and that recovery between sprints was generally active in nature (~93% of time). The role of the aerobic energy system is therefore paramount, as it provides energy during repeated high-intensity efforts and the active recovery between runs (Spencer et al., 2005). Information on repeated high-intensity exercise profiles and the intensity and duration of recovery periods that occur during competition has obvious implications for the design of conditioning elements in training programmes.

Another common feature of soccer at all levels is that only a small percentage (generally 1–3%) of the total distance covered by players is when in possession of the ball, although at elite standards the major part of this activity (~34%) is performed at high running speeds (>19.1km.h-1) (Carling, 2010). Circuits designed to train a player's capacity to run with the ball should therefore be based on movements carried out at high speeds to resemble the actual demands of the game. In addition, running with the ball increases physiological stress, as compared with normal running, leading to additional energy expenditure (Rupf, Thomas and Wells, 2007). Therefore, for a given speed of locomotion, the training stimulus will be higher when running with the ball. Nevertheless, the vast majority of running actions in field sports are 'off the ball'. These include supporting team-mates, tracking opposing players, executing decoy runs, countering runs by marking a player or challenging opponents for possession. These actions also require frequent changes in movement activities, such as accelerations and decelerations, changes of direction, turns, unorthodox movement patterns such as backwards and sideways running, as well as physical contact between players. On average, players in a professional soccer team were shown to perform about 40 very hard accelerations per game (Carling, unpublished data). In comparison to running at a constant pace, these intense locomotor actions are known to significantly increase metabolic demands (Osgnach, Poser, Bernardini, Rinaldo and di Prampero, 2010).

In general, there are marked differences in the total distance run and that covered in movement activities at different intensities across the various playing positions in soccer (Carling et al., 2008). Position-specific differences in physical activity profiles also occur at youth levels (Buchheit, Mendez-Villanueva, Simpson and Bourdon, 2010; Pereira Da Silva, Kirkendall and Leite De Barros, 2007) and in female soccer (Andersson, Randers, Heiner-Møller, Krustrup and Mohr, 2010). In an analysis of Premier League soccer, playing position was shown to have a significant influence on the time spent sprinting, running, shuffling, skipping and standing still (Bloomfield, Polman and O'Donoghue 2007). More detailed analyses of physical activity profiles shows that match-play data should be examined in relation to positional group (e.g., central and wide midfielders) rather than simply differentiating between defenders, midfielders and forwards, as each positional group has its own unique physical demands. Research has also shown that physical performance in players in the same position varies greatly according to the designated tactical role of players (Dellal, Chamari, Wong, Ahmaidi, Keller *et al.*, 2011).

In European club tournaments, significant differences in the amount of high-intensity exercise performed have been observed between full-backs and central defenders (Di Salvo, Baron, González-Haro, Gormasz, Pigozzi *et al.*, 2010). These authors also examined sprint activity patterns (runs >25.2 km/h) according to whether actions were 'explosive' (sprint characterised by a fast acceleration) or 'leading' (sprint characterised by a gradual acceleration) in nature. Substantial differences were observed across positional roles (Table 10.5). In addition, the intensity at which certain players recover following high-intensity actions can vary. Analysis of physical activity during recovery periods directly after high-intensity exercise bouts showed that central midfielders spent a greater amount of time at higher running intensities, as compared to other positions (Orendurff, Walker, Jovanovic, Tulchin, Levy *et al.*, 2010). As a whole, this research demonstrates a general need for a criterion model to enable the tailoring of training programmes to suit the specific needs of each positional role.

## Fatigue and variations in performance

Fatigue may be defined holistically as an exercise-induced impairment of performance (Knicker, Renshaw, Oldham and Cairns, 2011). Resistance to fatigue in soccer is a key factor in the effectiveness of a player's ability to continually perform efficient and precise movements (Stone and Oliver, 2009). Motion analyses of elite soccer match-play have comprehensively demonstrated both declines and variations in physical performance. In effect, players may experience impaired physical performance:

1   after short-term periods of intense activity;

2   at the beginning of the second-half;

3   overall in the second- versus the first-half;

4   in the final period towards the end of games;

5   during periods of fixture congestion.

Match-play activity profiles can also vary substantially across consecutive games, at different stages of the season and across seasons. A description of the nature of impairments and variations in performance occurring in competitive match-play is provided in Table 10.5.

Table 10.5 Total number of sprints and explosive and leading sprints performed according to positional role in European Champions League and UEFA Cup competition.

|  | Central defenders | Wide defenders | Central midfielders | Wide midfielders | Attackers |
|---|---|---|---|---|---|
| Total sprints | 17.3+8.7 | 29.5+11.7 | 23.5+12.2 | 35.8+13.4 | 30.0+12.0 |
| Explosive sprints | 4.5+4.2 | 7.2+5.5 | 6.3+5.8 | 8.4+6.3 | 7.2+5.7 |
| Leading sprints | 12.8+6.0 | 22.4+8.5 | 17.3+8.2 | 27.4+9.5 | 22.8+8.8 |

*Source*: Di Salvo *et al.* (2010).

186

**C. Carling and M. Court**

## First- versus second-half performance

There is conflicting evidence on differences in running performance across halves and decrements do not necessarily always occur in all players. A 14% slower overall speed in the second half of the game when compared with the first half has been reported in elite Australian soccer players (Burgess, Naughton and Norton, 2006). This result was attributed to fewer observations of the low-intensity movements (approximately 9% less walking and 12% less jogging) and more stationary periods. Engagement in game events such as kicking and passing was also 11% less frequent in the second versus first half of games. Information on differences in the total distance run per half in contemporary professional matches is reported in Table 10.6. Di Salvo et al. (2007) showed no significant difference across halves in high-intensity running performance for players in professional Spanish football and other top players participating in Champions League games, while the inverse was observed in English Premier League matches (Di Salvo et al., 2009).

## Performance towards the end of games

While the occurrence of fatigue can be indicated by differences in the physical performance overall across the first and second halves of matches, it may be more closely identified if activities during the game are broken up into smaller intervals (e.g., 15-min or 5-min segments). In elite players, Mohr, Krustrup and Bangsbo (2003) demonstrated a drop (35–45%) in the amount of high-intensity running in the last, as compared to the first, 15 min of play. However, the distance run at high intensities can remain constant throughout the second half, due to 'pacing' strategies (Carling and Bloomfield, 2010a). Players may perform fewer actions at low or moderate intensity in order to 'spare' their efforts for the final few crucial actions as their energy levels begin to get low.

## Transient fatigue

Research in elite soccer has shown that after the 5-min period during which the high-intensity running distance peaked, performance was significantly reduced in the following 5 min, as

**Table 10.6** Comparison of the total distance covered (metres) by contemporary elite soccer players during the first and second halves of competitive match-play.

| Study | Country | Total Distance | 1st Half | 2nd Half | Difference |
|---|---|---|---|---|---|
| Barros et al. (2007) | Brazil | 10012 | 5173 | 4808 | −365 |
| Burgess et al. (2006) | Australia | 10100 | 5300 | 4800 | −500 |
| Carling & Dupont (2010) | France | 11126 | 5694 | 5432 | −262 |
| Di Salvo et al. (2007) | Europe | 11393 | 5709 | 5684 | −25 |
| Mohr et al. (2003) | Italy | 10860 | 5510 | 5350 | −160 |
| | Denmark | 10330 | 5200 | 5130 | −70 |
| Rampinini et al. (2009) | Italy | 11828 | 5966 | 5862 | −104 |
| Rienzi et al. (2000) | South America/ England | 9020 | 4605 | 4415 | −190 |
| Zubiglia et al. (2007) | England | 10549 | 5297 | 5252 | −45 |
| | Spain | 10339 | 5121 | 5218 | +97 |

compared with the game average (Mohr et al., 2003; Carling and Dupont, 2011). In Premier League players, a 50% drop, as compared to levels below the game mean, was notably observed after the most intense 5-min period of activity suggesting, that players experienced a high degree of transient fatigue in match-play (Bradley et al., 2009). The physiological explanations for the causes of temporary fatigue development during match-play are still relatively unclear (Krustrup, Mohr, Steensberg, Bencke, Kjaer et al., 2006). However, while sprint-type performance often depends on the requirements of game situations, and particularly the recovery allowed by the natural ebb and flow of play (Reilly, 2007), increasing the ability of players to repeatedly perform and recover from sprint-type activities is essential.

## Performance at the beginning of the second-half

A significant fall in physical activity at the beginning of the second-half notably in comparison to the opening 15-mins of the first-half, has been reported (Mohr, Krustrup, Nybo, Nielsen and Bangsbo, 2004). Impaired performance was linked to players' resting during the half-time break leading to a drop in muscle temperature, and the lack of a warm-up session as performed prior to kick-off.

## Fixture congestion

Contemporary professional teams can play over 60 games per season and frequently participate in several games within a short timeframe. There is potential for residual fatigue and incomplete recovery, which may affect the activity profiles of players during subsequent games. Studies conducted in leagues in England (Odetoyinbo, Wooster and Lane, 2007), France (Carling and Dupont, 2011), Scotland (Dupont, Nedelec, McCall, McCormack, Berthoin et al., 2010) and Spain (Rey, Lago-Penas, Lago-Ballesteros and Dellal, 2010) generally do not report any statistical differences in athletic performance across successive matches played in over a short time interval although, in general, distances covered progressively dropped. Notably, measures of skill-related performance in the French League were also unaffected (Table 10.7). A recent case study also examined changes in performance in eight successive matches played over a 26-day period (Carling, Le Gall and Dupont, 2012). While the total distances run varied, high-intensity running performance was generally unaffected. The lack of decline in physical efforts may be linked to squad rotation and post-match recovery strategies.

## Intra- and inter-seasonal variations

Performance may vary substantially between successive matches and different phases of the season. In top-class soccer, the coefficient of variation in high-intensity running has been shown to be 9.2% between successive matches, whereas it was 24.8% between different stages of the season (Mohr, Krustrup and Bangsbo, 2003). Match-to-match variability in high-intensity performance was generally higher for centrally positioned players (midfielders and defenders) and lower for wide midfielders and attackers in the Premier League (Gregson, Drust, Atkinson and Salvo, 2010). Reasonable explanations for these variations in performance

C. Carling and M. Court

**Table 10.7** Comparison of physical and skill-related performance in professional midfield soccer players when competing in 3 successive matches within a timeframe of ≤7 days.

| Performance across matches | Consecutive matches | | |
|---|---|---|---|
| | 1 | 2 | 3 |
| **Physical Performance** | | | |
| Total distance (m) | 10494 ± 514 | 10949 ± 853 | 10795 ± 618 |
| High-speed distance (m) | 2667 ± 200 | 2629 ± 398 | 2414 ± 145 |
| Distance with ball (m) | 153 ± 41 | 210 ± 95 | 203 ± 68 |
| **Technical Peformance** | | | |
| Shots | 2.0 ± 1.8 | 1.3 ± 1.2 | 2.5 ± 2.2 |
| Shots on target | 66.1 ± 30.3 | 23.5 ± 20.8 | 25.2 ± 21.3 |
| Passes | 41.7 ± 11.0 | 50.8 ± 22.4 | 52.3 ± 23.9 |
| Successful passes (%) | 69.1 ± 14.0 | 77.5 ± 13.4 | 73.4 ± 16.5 |
| Possessions | 47.3 ± 10.1 | 52.5 ± 26.2 | 56 ± 15.1 |
| Possessions gained | 9.7 ± 3.4 | 9.0 ± 5.3 | 10.8 ± 5.6 |
| Possession lost | 13.7 ± 4.0 | 12.7 ± 6.9 | 13.8 ± 9.2 |
| Touches per possession | 2.1 ± 0.3 | 2.2 ± 0.3 | 2.0 ± 0.3 |
| Duels | 6.7 ± 2.9 | 5.7 ± 3.1 | 8.2 ± 3.8 |
| Duels won (%) | 46.5 ± 26.7 | 31.8 ± 23.6 | 52.8 ± 22.0 |

*Source*: Carling and Dupont (2011).

include: players do not always fully utilise their physical capacity; self-regulation of physiological stress by the players themselves; changes in their tactical role or simply a general decline in performance. Physical performance may also fluctuate across different stages of the season, in conjunction with the amount of training that is performed and changes in the physical condition of players (Drust, Atkinson and Reilly, 2007).

Information on physical performance can aid in examining the evolution of performance over several seasons to determine whether physical requirements are the same. The validity of current conditioning programmes and fitness tests can then be examined. Professional soccer players in the Premier League tend to cover greater distances in match-play than those in the old 1st Division, which has had obvious consequences for fitness training programmes. While contemporary outfield players across all playing positions are running further distances, the distance run relative to playing positions has remained consistent across the last three decades (Reilly, 2007).

## Factors influencing physical performance

Simple figures on distance covered and movement speeds observed in match-play may not always be a fair reflection of how a player performs, since many factors, both extrinsic and intrinsic, can substantially affect physical activity profiles. Motion analyses have been used over recent years to investigate a myriad of variables that shape and affect the physical performance profile of players in competition. While individual playing position is probably the most determining factor in the analysis, factors such as playing formation, opposition quality and standard of play all have a role and should be taken into account in the interpretation of data. Factors that can influence match performance profiles are therefore covered below.

## Playing formation

In a French League 1 team, players covered greater total distances against a 4-2-3-1, as compared with a 4-4-2 formation with more distance run in low/moderate movement intensities (Carling, 2011). Similarly, distances run in total high-intensity running out of possession were higher against a 4-2-3-1 and 4-3-3 formation, as compared with a 4-4-2 formation, suggesting that the reference team players had to work harder defensively to win back possession. In contrast, performance demands were generally unaffected across individual playing positions and declines in high-intensity running performance were not influenced by opposition formation. In a related study, Bradley, Carling, Archer, Roberts, Dodds et al. (2011) directly compared performance in players performing in three formations commonly used in the Premier League: 4-4-2, 4-3-3 and 4-5-1. No differences were observed across formations for the team as a whole in the total distance run or that in high-intensity, suggesting that team formation did not impact on the physical demands of play. However, high-intensity demands varied according to ball possession, as more distance was covered by players when their team had possession in a 4-4-2 and 4-3-3, as compared to a 4-5-1 formation. Conversely, more distance run at high intensities without possession was observed in players in a 4-5-1 versus 4-4-2 and 4-3-3 formations. These variations in performance may reflect the attacking and defensive characteristics inherent to the three common team formations. In both studies, some technical and tactical aspects of play were influenced by team formation.

## Regional differences

Comparative data have shown that substantial differences exist in movement demands across professional leagues. Data obtained using the same computerised match analysis system showed that Premier League players performed substantially greater total distances in high-intensity running than players in the La Liga, with differences occurring across the majority of playing positions (Dellal et al., 2011). Similarly, the overall distance (determined using the same manual motion analysis methodology) covered by professional players in South American was about 1000 m less than by peers in the Premier League (Rienzi, Drust, Reilly, Carter, and Martin, 2000). These results tended to uphold the common belief that matches in the Premier League are played at a faster pace than in other leagues, probably due to a more direct style of play. These findings also have important implications for fitness, as players moving between countries may need time to adapt physically (as well as tactically) to the particular styles of other leagues.

## Scoreline

There is limited information on the phenomenon of scoreline status in relation to physical performance in soccer. O'Donoghue and Tenga (2001) reported that players performed significantly more exercise when they were ahead, although this only relates to the 10-min period directly after a goal has been scored and is not sustained (Bloomfield, Polman and O'Donoghue, 2004). A more recent study (Lago, Casais, Dominguez and Sampaio, 2010) showed that elite soccer players generally performed less high-intensity activity when winning, as compared to losing, with drops in performance associated with changes in team tactics (notably keeping possession and slowing the game).

## Standard of play and team quality

Mohr, Krustrup and Bangsbo (2003) reported a 28% difference in high-intensity running distance in a top soccer team in Europe (competing in the Italian league and in the UEFA Champions League) versus professional players in the top league in Denmark. Top-class international female players also performed 28% more distance in high-intensity running than elite players at a lower level (Mohr et al., 2008). In addition, elite female soccer players performed more high-intensity running when playing in international games, as compared to for their clubs in domestic league games (Andersson et al., 2010). In contrast, high-intensity activity profiles and fatigue patterns were similar between international and professional domestic male players (Bradley, Di Mascio, Peart, Olsen and Sheldon, 2010).

There is contrasting evidence on the effects of the quality of opposition on physical performance. Rampinini, Coutts, Castagna, Sassi and Impellizzeri (2007) reported that the physical demands in a reference team were significantly influenced by the activity profile of opponents deemed to be either high or low in quality. Overall, demands and those in high-intensity running were greater against high-quality opposition (Champions League opponents and teams finishing in the highest eight places in the National League). In contrast, high-ranked teams in the Premier League (Di Salvo et al., 2009) and Serie A (Rampinini, Impellizzeri, Castagna, Coutts and Wisløff, 2009) were shown to perform less high-intensity running than low-ranked peers from the same league. Future work to investigate the relationship between tactical and technical performance indicators (e.g., percentage of ball possession, time the ball is in play, technical action completion rates) and physical performance in games against teams of different standards is warranted.

## Environmental conditions

Soccer training and competition often take place in unfavourable environments. These include high altitude, heat and humidity, cold and poor pitch conditions. During the 2010 World Cup, the total distance covered and that run at high intensities by teams, respectively, dropped by 4% and 11.5% in games at altitude, as compared to sea-level (Tucker and Dugas, 2010). A large decrease in high-intensity running has been observed toward the end of a friendly game played by professional soccer players in Spain in a hot environment (~31°C): -54% in the final, as compared to the first, 15-min period (Mohr, Mujika, Santisteban, Randers, Bischoff et al., 2010). In extremely cold conditions (≤5°C), high-intensity running distance reported in midfielders during the first 15-min interval of games was substantially affected when compared to performance in warmer temperatures, suggesting a need for improved pre-match warm-up strategies (Carling, Dupont and Le Gall, 2011).

191

## Practical implications of motion analysis data

In general, data from motion analyses can be used to determine the ratios of exercise to rest and low- to high-intensity exercise in match-play. This information can aid subsequently in the design and prescription of objective physical conditioning programmes to respond to the specific challenges of competition. Identification of these physical demands can also aid in developing individualised physical preparation regimes according to positional role. For example, wide-midfielders might benefit from additional repeated sprint activities to develop their ability to maintain performance and improve recovery during short repeated bouts of high-intensity running. In contrast, muscular power training might aid sprint performance in forwards, especially when accelerating past markers. Players who are aerobically well trained generally have better possibilities to maintain physical efforts towards the end of the game and recover following high-intensity efforts (Reilly, 2007). Aerobic-interval training using small-sided games during which intensity was controlled by heart-rate monitoring showed significant gains (14% and 18%, respectively) in the time spent in low- and high-intensity activities in match-play (Impellizzeri, Marcora, Castagna, Reilly, Sassi et al., 2006).

The use of results from physiological testing of anaerobic and aerobic capacity may be associated to match data to allow early identification of players who are more likely to suffer from a decline in performance. Rampinini, Bishop, Marcora, Ferrari Bravo, Sassi, et al. (2007) examined the validity of selected field tests as indicators of match-related physical performance in elite soccer. The results from a 'repeated sprint ability' test were highly correlated with the total distance covered in competition when sprinting. Krustrup, Mohr, Ellingsgaard and Bangsbo (2005) observed a strong relationship between an intermittent recovery test and match sprint performance in top female soccer players.

If a susceptibility to fatigue or a drop in performance is identified, the reasons for its occurrence should be explored and interventions should be implemented in training and preparation. Reduced performance at the end of games could be due to inadequate nutritional strategies, leading to insufficient glycogen levels in individual muscle fibres at the start of games (Krustrup et al., 2006). Monitoring training intensity using heart-rate telemetry may avoid players training too hard before matches. When physical performance might be impaired as a consequence of insufficient recovery time between matches, evidence-based post-competition recovery interventions can benefit future performance. Hydrotherapy and cryotherapy techniques (e.g., sauna, cold water immersion, jacuzzi) are effective in maintaining running performance in consecutive soccer games played within a short period of time (Buchheit, Horobeanu, Mendez-Villanueva, Simpson and Bourdon, 2011).

Substituting players before the onset of fatigue can restore imbalances in physical performance across teams. Mohr, Krustrup and Bangsbo (2003) and Carling and Bloomfield (2010b) reported that substitutes covered more distance than players who remained on the pitch. The latter study also demonstrated that substitutes ran more than the player they replaced. Mobile tracking systems (see www.sport-universal.com) are now providing coaches with real-time data upon which they can make objective decisions when attempting to identify players who are tiring and may need to be replaced over the course of games.

Physical performance at the beginning of games played in cold weather may be enhanced by increasing the duration and intensity of the pre-match warm-up, while adequate hydration and/or cooling vests may help to offset fatigue towards the end of games in hot and humid

C. Carling and M. Court

conditions. Changing conventional half-time practices by undertaking a few minutes of low-to moderate-intensity exercise may lead to improvements in physical and technical performance immediately after the pause.

Along similar lines, medical staff may attempt to anticipate injury by examining changes in physical performance. A general decline in performance over several matches (e.g., total distance run, frequency of high-intensity efforts) may suggest that a player is in need of a rest and could be susceptible to 'overtraining'. Similarly, players returning after medium- and long-term injuries could have their game profile scrutinised to see how they recovered from intense periods of play or their performance compared against benchmark data obtained from preceding matches.

Finally, motion analysis data can be employed to help design laboratory- or field-based protocols to simulate soccer-specific intermittent exercise. Tests can subsequently be used to examine the development of fatigue as well as the impact of training interventions, nutritional strategies and equipment on physical performance.

## SUMMARY

Match and motion analysis aims to provide the basis for objective, pertinent and meaningful feedback on physical, technical and tactical performance in competition. Manual and/or computerised techniques are used to record events underpinning match performance. Practitioners can subsequently evaluate, interpret and eventually transform the information into relevant practice sessions. At elite levels, match analysis has grown in popularity over recent years, due to a greater recognition by practitioners of its role in the coaching process. This recognition is partly due to major advances in computer and video technology, providing more efficient ways of obtaining and analysing data during match-play and training. It may also be due to acknowledgment of the key part that sports science plays in general in the daily functioning of contemporary professional soccer clubs. In addition, the plethora of scientific investigations highlighted in this chapter is providing practitioners at all standards of play with comprehensive sources of data and essential information on the specific performance demands in soccer. Real-time analysis as the match unfolds is now a reality and there are possibilities to access specific information on performance at any time during or immediately after competition. The miniaturisation and better durability of devices, their ability to generate and transmit vast amounts of information over considerable distances, combined with the development of algorithms for fast and/or accurate data processing, are ever improving. Work within professional soccer is currently moving towards the development of more intelligent systems to aid in the predictive modelling of performance using the intelligence gathered from indexes and ratings of key indicators of performance.

## REFERENCES

Abt, G. and Lovell, R. (2009). The use of individualized speed and intensity thresholds for determining the distance run at high-intensity in professional soccer. *Journal of Sports Sciences* 27, 893–898.

Alcock, A. (2010). Analysis of direct free kicks in the women's football World Cup 2007. *European Journal of Sport Science* 10, 279–284.

Andersson, H.A., Randers, M.B., Heiner-Møller, A., Krustrup, P. and Mohr, M. (2010). Elite female soccer players perform more high-intensity running when playing in international games compared with domestic league games. *Journal of Strength and Conditioning Research* 24, 912–919.

Bangsbo, J., Nørregaard, L. and Thorsøe, F. (1991). Activity profile of competition soccer. *Canadian Journal of Sports Science* 16, 110–116.

Barris, S. and Button, C. (2008). A review of vision-based motion analysis in sport. *Sports Medicine* 38, 1025–1043.

Bell-Walker, J., McRobert, A., Ford, P. and Williams, M.A. (2007). Quantitative analysis of successful teams at the 2006 World Cup finals. *Insight – The FA Coaches Association Journal* 4, 37–43.

Bloomfield, J.R., Polman, R.C.J. and O'Donoghue, P.G. (2004). Effects of score-line on work-rate in midfield and forward players in FA Premier League soccer. *Journal of Sports Sciences* 23, 191–192.

Bloomfield, J., Polman, R.C.J. and O'Donoghue, P.G. (2007). Physical demands of different positions in FA Premier League soccer. *Journal of Sports Science and Medicine* 6, 63–70.

Bradley, P.S., Carling, C., Archer, D., Roberts, J., Dodds, A., Di Mascio, M. *et al.* (2011). The effect of playing formation on high-intensity running and technical profiles in English FA Premier League soccer matches. *Journal of Sports Sciences* 19, 1–10.

Bradley, P.S., Di Mascio, M., Peart, D., Olsen, P. and Sheldon, B. (2010). High-intensity activity profiles of elite soccer players at different performance levels. *Journal of Strength and Conditioning Research* 24, 2343–2351.

Bradley, P.S., Sheldon, W., Wooster, B., Olsen, P., Boanas, P. and Krustrup, P. (2009). High-intensity running in English FA Premier League soccer matches. *Journal of Sports Sciences* 15, 159–168.

Breen, A., Iga, J., Ford, P. and Williams, M. (2007). World Cup 2006 – Germany. A quantitative analysis of goals scored. *Insight – The FA Coaches Association Journal* 6, 45–53.

Buchheit, M., Mendez-Villanueva, A., Simpson, B.M. and Bourdon, P.C. (2010). Match running performance and fitness in youth soccer. *International Journal of Sports Medicine* 31, 818–825.

Buchheit, M., Horobeanu, C., Mendez-Villanueva, A., Simpson, B.M. and Bourdon, P.C. (2011). Effects of age and spa treatment on match running performance over two consecutive games in highly trained young soccer players. *Journal of Sports Sciences* 17, 1–8.

Burgess, D.J., Naughton, G. and Norton, K.I. (2006). Profile of movement demands of national football players in Australia. *Journal of Science and Medicine in Sport* 9, 334–341.

Carling, C. (2010). Analysis of physical activity profiles when running with the ball in a professional soccer team. *Journal of Sports Sciences* 28, 319–326.

Carling C. (2011). Influence of opposition team formation on physical and skill-related performance in a professional soccer team. *European Journal of Sports Sciences* 11, 155–164.

Carling, C. and Bloomfield, J. (2010a). The effect of an early dismissal on player work-rate in a professional soccer match. *Journal of Science and Medicine in Sport* 13, 126–128.

Carling, C. and Bloomfield, J. (2010b). Work-rate of substitutes in elite soccer: a preliminary study. *Journal of Science and Medicine in Sport* 13, 253–255.

Carling, C. and Dupont, G. (2011). Are declines in physical performance associated with a reduction in skill-related performance during professional soccer match-play? *Journal of Sports Sciences* 29, 63–71.

Carling, C. and Williams, A.M. (2008). Match analysis and elite soccer performance: integrating science and practice. In T. Reilly (ed.), *Science and Soccer* (pp. 32–47). Maastricht, Netherlands: Shaker Publishing.

Carling, C., Dupont, G. and Le Gall, F. (2011). The effect of a cold environment on physical activity profiles in elite soccer match-play. *International Journal of Sports Medicine* 32, 1–4.

Carling, C., Le Gall, F. and Dupont, G. (2012). Are physical performance and injury risk in a professional soccer team in match-play affected over a prolonged period of fixture congestion? *International Journal of Sports Medicine* 33, 36–42.

Carling, C., Reilly, T. and Williams, A.M. (2009). *Performance Assessment for Field Sports*. London: Taylor and Francis.

Carling, C., Williams, A.M. and Reilly, T. (2005). *The Handbook of Soccer Match Analysis*. London: Routledge.

Carling, C., Bloomfield, J., Nelsen, L., and Reilly, T. (2008). The role of motion analysis in elite soccer: contemporary performance measurement techniques and work-rate data. *Sports Medicine* 38, 839–862.

Castagna, C., D'Ottavio, S. and Abt, G. (2003). Activity profile of young soccer players during actual match play. *Journal of Strength and Conditioning Research* 17, 775–780.

Coutts, A.J. and Duffield, R. (2010). Validity and reliability of GPS devices for measuring movement demands of team sports. *Journal of Science and Medicine in Sport* 13, 133–135.

Dellal, A., Chamari, K., Wong, D.P., Ahmaidi, S., Keller, D., Barros, R. *et al.* (2011). Comparison of physical and technical performance in European soccer match-play: FA Premier League and La Liga. *European Journal of Sport Science* 11, 51–59.

Di Salvo, V., Gregson, W., Atkinson, G., Tordoff, P. and Drust, B. (2009). Analysis of high intensity activity in Premier League soccer. *International Journal of Sports Medicine* 30, 205–212.

Di Salvo, V., Baron, R., González-Haro, C., Gormasz, C., Pigozzi, F. and Bachl, N. (2010). Sprinting analysis of elite soccer players during European Champions League and UEFA Cup matches. *Journal of Sports Sciences* 28, 1489–1494.

Di Salvo, V., Baron, R., Tschan, H., Calderon Montero, F.J., Bachl, N. and Pigozzi, F. (2007). Performance characteristics according to playing position in elite soccer. *International Journal of Sports Medicine* 28, 222–227.

Drust, B., Atkinson, G. and Reilly, T. (2007). Future perspectives in the evaluation of the physiological demands of soccer, *Sports Medicine* 37, 783–805.

Dupont, G., Nedelec, M., McCall, A., McCormack, D., Berthoin, S. and Wisløff, U. (2010). Effect of 2 soccer matches in a week on physical performance and injury rate. *American Journal of Sports Medicine* 38, 1752–1758.

Ensum, J., Taylor, S. and Williams, M. (2002). World Cup 2002 – Korea/Japan. A quantitative analysis of attacking set plays. *Insight – The FA Coaches Association Journal* 4, 68–72.

Ensum, J., Williams, M., and Grant, A. (2000). Analysis of the attacking set plays in Euro 2000. *Insight – The FA Coaches Association Journal* 4, 36–39.

Frencken, W.G., Lemmink, K.A. and Delleman, N.J. (2010). Soccer-specific accuracy and validity of the local position measurement (LPM) system. *Journal of Science and Medicine in Sport* 13, 641–645.

Gabbett, T.J. and Mulvey, M.J. (2008). Time-motion analysis of small-sided training games and competition in elite women soccer players. *Journal of Strength and Conditioning Research* 22, 543–552.

Gregson, W., Drust, B., Atkinson, G. and Salvo, V.D. (2010). Match-to-match variability of high-speed activities in Premier League soccer. *International Journal of Sports Medicine* 31, 237–242.

Franks, I.M. (2004). The need for feedback. In M.D. Hughes and I.M. Franks (eds), *Notational Analysis of Sport: Systems for Better Coaching and Performance* (pp. 8–16). London: E. and F.N. Spon.

Hughes, M.D. and Bartlett, R.M. (2002) The use of performance indicators in performance analysis. *Journal of Sports Sciences* 20, 739–754.

Impellizzeri, F.M., Marcora, S.M., Castagna, C., Reilly, T., Sassi, A., Iaia, F.M. *et al.* (2006). Physiological and performance effects of generic versus specific aerobic training in soccer players. *International Journal of Sports Medicine* 27, 483–92.

James, N. (2006). The role of notational analysis in soccer coaching. *International Journal of Sports Science and Coaching* 1, 185–198.

Jennings, D., Cormack, S., Coutts, A.J., Boyd, L. and Aughey, R.J. (2010). The validity and reliability of GPS units for measuring distance in team sport specific running patterns. *International Journal of Sports Physiology and Performance* 5, 328–341.

Knicker, A.J., Renshaw, I., Oldham, A.R. and Cairns, S.P. (2011). Interactive processes link the multiple symptoms of fatigue in sport competition. *Sports Medicine* 41, 307–328.

Krustrup, P., Mohr, M., Ellingsgaard, H. and Bangsbo, J. (2005). Physical demands during an elite female soccer game: importance of training status. *Medicine and Science in Sports and Exercise* 37, 1242–1248.

Krustrup, P., Mohr, M., Steensberg, A., Bencke, J., Kjaer, M. and Bangsbo, J. (2006). Muscle and blood metabolites during a soccer game: implications for sprint performance. *Medicine and Science in Sports and Exercise* 38, 1165–1174.

Lago, C. (2009). The influence of match location, quality of opposition, and match status on possession strategies in professional association football. *Journal of Sports Sciences* 27, 1463–1469.

Lago, C., Casais, L., Dominguez, E. and Sampaio, J. (2010). The effects of situational variables on distance covered at various speeds in elite soccer. *European Journal of Sport Science* 10, 103–109.

Lago-Peñas, C., Lago-Ballesteros, J. and Rey, E. (2011). Differences in performance indicators between winning and losing teams in the UEFA Champions League. *Journal of Human Kinetics* 27, 135–146.

Lago-Peñas C., Lago-Ballesteros, J., Dellal, A. and Gómez, M. (2010). Game-related statistics that discriminated winning, drawing and losing teams from the Spanish soccer league. *Journal of Sports Science and Medicine* 9, 288–293.

Mohr, M., Krustrup, P. and Bangsbo, J. (2003). Match performance of high-standard soccer players with special reference to development of fatigue. *Journal of Sports Sciences* 21, 519–528.

196

Mohr, M., Krustrup, P., Andersson, H., Kirkendal, D. and Bangsbo, J. (2008). Match activities of elite women soccer players at different performance levels. *Journal of Strength and Conditioning Research* 22, 341–349.

Mohr, M., Krustrup, P., Nybo, L., Nielsen, J.J. and Bangsbo, J. (2004). Muscle temperature and sprint performance during soccer matches – beneficial effect of re-warm-up at half-time. *Scandinavian Journal of Medicine and Science in Sports* 14, 156–162.

Mohr, M., Mujika, I., Santisteban, J., Randers, M.B., Bischoff, R., Sloan, R. *et al.* (2010). Examination of fatigue development in elite soccer in a hot environment: a multi-experimental approach. *Scandinavian Journal of Medicine and Science in Sports* 20 (Suppl 3), 125–132.

O'Donoghue, P.G. and Tenga, A. (2001). The effect of score-line on work rate in elite soccer. *Journal of Sports Sciences* 19, 25–26.

Oberstone, J. (2009). Differentiating the top English Premier League football clubs from the rest of the pack: identifying the keys to success. *Journal of Quantitative Analysis in Sports* 5, Article 10.

Odetoyinbo, K., Wooster, B. and Lane, A. (2007).The effect of a succession of matches on the activity profiles of professional soccer players. In F. Korkusuz and E. Ergen (eds), *VIth World Congress on Science and Football, Abstracts*, 16–20 January. *Journal of Science and Medicine in Sport* 6 (suppl. 10), 16.

Orendurff, M.S., Walker, J.D., Jovanovic, M., Tulchin, K.L., Levy, M. *et al.* (2010). Intensity and duration of intermittent exercise and recovery during a soccer match. *Journal of Strength and Conditioning Research* 24, 2683–2692.

Osgnach, C., Poser, S., Bernardini, R., Rinaldo, R. and di Prampero, P.E. (2010). Energy cost and metabolic power in elite soccer: a new match analysis approach. *Medicine and Science in Sports and Exercise* 42, 170–178.

Pereira Da Silva, N., Kirkendall, D.T. and Leite De Barros Neto, T. (2007). Movement patterns in elite Brazilian youth soccer. *Journal of Sports Medicine and Physical Fitness* 47, 270–275.

Rampinini, E., Coutts, A.J., Castagna, C., Sassi, R. and Impellizzeri, F.M. (2007). Variation in top level soccer match performance. *International Journal of Sports Medicine* 28, 1018–1024.

Rampinini, E., Impellizzeri, F.M, Castagna, C., Coutts, A.J. and Wisløff, U. (2009). Technical performance during soccer matches of the Italian Serie A league: effect of fatigue and competitive level. *Journal of Science and Medicine in Sport* 12, 227–233.

Rampinini, E., Bishop, D., Marcora, S.M., Ferrari Bravo, D., Sassi, R. and Impellizzeri, F.M. (2007). Validity of simple field tests as indicators of match-related physical performance in top-level professional soccer players. *International Journal of Sports Medicine* 28, 228–235.

Reep, C. and Benjamin, B. (1968). Skill and chance in association football. *Journal of the Royal Statistical Society* 131, 581–585.

Reilly, T. (2003). Motion analysis and physiological demands. In T. Reilly and A.M. Williams (eds), *Science and Soccer*, 2nd edn (pp. 59–72). London: Routledge.

Reilly, T. (2007). *Science of Training: Soccer*. London: Routledge.

Reilly, T. and Thomas, V. (1976). A motion analysis of work-rate in different positional roles in professional football match-play. *Journal of Human Movement Studies* 2, 87–97.

Rey, E., Lago-Peñas, C., Lago-Ballesteros, C.L. and Dellal, A. (2010). The effects of a congested fixture period on the activity of elite soccer players. *Biology of Sport* 27, 181–185.

Rienzi, E., Drust, B., Reilly, T., Carter, J.E. and Martin, A. (2000) Investigation of anthropometric and work-rate profiles of elite South American international soccer players. *Journal of Sports Medicine and Physical Fitness* 40(2), 162–169.

Rupf, R., Thomas, S. and Wells, G. (2007). Quantifying energy expenditure of dribbling a soccer ball in a field test. In *VIth World Congress of Science and Football, Book of Abstracts* (p. 132), Antalya, Turkey.

Spencer, M., Bishop, D., Dawson, B. and Goodman, C. (2005). Physiological and metabolic responses of repeated-sprint activities: specific to field-based team sports. *Sports Medicine* 35, 1025–1044.

Stone, K.J. and Oliver, J.L. (2009). The effect of 45 minutes of soccer-specific exercise on the performance of soccer skills. *International Journal of Sports Physiology and Performance* 4, 163–175.

Strudwick, T. and Reilly, T. (2001). Work-rate profiles of elite Premier League Football players. *Insight – The FA Coaches Association Journal* 4, 55–59.

Taylor, J.B., Mellalieu, S.D., James, N. and Shearer, D.A. (2008). The influence of match location, quality of opposition, and match status on technical performance in professional association football. *Journal of Sports Sciences* 26, 885–895.

Taylor, S. and Williams, A.M. (2002). World Cup 2002– Korea/Japan: a quantitative analysis of Brazil's performances. *Insight – The FA Coaches Association Journal* 4, 29–32.

Tenga, A., Ronglan, L.T. and Bahr, R. (2010). Measuring the effectiveness of offensive match play in professional soccer. *European Journal of Sport Science* 10, 269–277.

Tucker, R. and Dugas, J. (2010). The effect of altitude on the 2010 World Cup. http://www.sportsscientists.com/2010/07/football-analysis-altitude-and-goal.html. July 5.

Yates, I., North, J., Ford, P. and Williams, M. (2007). A quantitative analysis of Italy's World Cup performances. A comparison of World Cup winners. *Insight – The FA Coaches Association Journal* 5, 55–59.

# CHAPTER 11

## COACHING AND COACH EDUCATION

C. Cushion

### INTRODUCTION

In their review of coaching science research, Gilbert and Trudel (2004) identified in excess of 1,000 coaching-related publications. An examination of this research revealed a bewildering range of theoretical and empirical perspectives and insights into coaching. However, despite the apparent depth of empirical work that recognises the 'coaching process', an in-depth understanding of coaching and a conceptual underpinning to inform practice remain lacking (Cushion, Armour and Jones, 2006; Cushion, 2007a). We seem as far removed from consensus or clarity about the nature of coaching as ever and have no clear conceptual framework to inform practice or the development of practice (Cushion and Lyle, 2010; Cushion, 2007a).

In soccer, the difficulty is that coaches work without any reference to an established coaching process model and, in reality, base their coaching largely on feelings, intuitions, events and previous experience (Cushion et al., 2006; Ford, Yates and Williams, 2010; Williams and Hodges, 2005). Furthermore, although some research findings have impacted on practice (e.g., Smith and Smoll, 2007), there is no evidence for the systematic application of these, or any other findings, in the development of coaching or coach education (Abraham and Collins, 1998; Abraham, Collins and Martindale, 2006), in terms of either methodology or results (Cushion, 2007b). As both Gilbert (2007) and Cushion (2007b) remark, they have yet to meet a coach that referenced a research-based coaching model when describing what they do, nor have they seen such a model explicitly underpinning coach education.

These criticisms notwithstanding, there is a growing body of literature which recognises that coaching does not imply a set of behaviours to be mimicked, nor solely a cognitive enterprise, but a social activity built on a web of complex, context-dependent and interdependent activities that come together to form a holistic process (Jones, Armour, and Potrac, 2004; Lyle, 2002; Cushion et al., 2006). It is a remarkably complex, intricate, yet coherent process incorporating a myriad of individual variations that each coach, player and environment add to the blend. Perhaps it is this very complexity that has resulted in a dearth of research exploring the conceptual development of the coaching process (Lyle, 1999), possibly because it is too complex to research neatly or to draw straightforward conclusions about (Cushion et al., 2006).

With increased research attention devoted to coaching, and yet little apparent impact on coaching practice or coach education, this chapter attempts to give an overview and critical evaluation of 'what we currently know' about coaching and coach education. It is of course beyond the scope of this chapter to 'review' coaching research in its entirety, but drilling into key issues and linking these arguments with others provides a critical examination of the state of the field and provides a framework for understanding and bridging the 'theory–practice' gap (Abraham and Collins, 1998).

## CONCEPTUAL DEVELOPMENT: UNDERSTANDING THE NATURE OF COACHING PRACTICE

The conceptual features of the coaching process are wide ranging and multifaceted, and there remains a need to clarify this process so that effective coaching methods can be established (Cushion et al., 2006; Lyle, 2002). A number of researchers have argued that without studies directed toward describing the complexity inherent in specific contexts, understanding of coaching will remain imprecise and speculative (Saury and Durand, 1998; Jones et al., 2004; Cushion et al., 2006). However, it could be argued that thus far researchers have taken an overly simplistic approach to coaching, resulting in a dearth of useful research into its conceptual development (Cushion, et al., 2006; Jones, Armour and Potrac, 2003). As Lyle (1999, 2002) points out, a fragmented or episodic approach to coaching knowledge tends to underestimate the complexity of the process, and because coaching can be represented as 'episodes' and therefore parts of it can be described in individual terms, it is easy to overlook the degree in which the interrelatedness and interconnectedness of coaching sustains the process (Cushion et al., 2006; Cushion, 2007a; Jones, 2007). Consequently, it becomes (and has become) easy to take an asocial, linear view of coaching (e.g., 'plan-do-review'). This tendency, in turn, leads to an immature or limited understanding that hides meaning but gives the illusion of a more complete understanding. As Jones and Wallace (2005) suggest, we do not have a sufficiently in-depth understanding of the phenomenon of coaching, as a precursor to saying what should or should not be done in coaching. As a result, its complexity has not been acknowledged, nor sufficiently understood, before attempting to produce models; consequently, 'oversimplification of the phenomenon and over-precision of prescriptions is the unfortunate price paid' (Jones and Wallace, 2005: 123). The outcome has been an overly simplistic approach that fails to fully encompass coaching practice (Lyle, 2002; Cushion et al., 2006).

While the conceptual development and understanding of the coaching process has been limited, a promising and growing body of work has begun to emerge that explores coaching practice. This line of enquiry has been worthwhile in recognising more readily the complexity inherent in coaching and demonstrating that it is not something that is merely delivered but is a dynamic social activity that vigorously engages coach and athlete (Cushion et al., 2006; Jones, 2007). Coaching is a practical, social activity that has as its characteristics 'multi-dimensionality, simultaneity, uncertainty, publicity and historicity' (Côté et al., 1995: 255). Saury and Durand (1998) argue that coaching can be characterised as complex, uncertain, dynamic, singular and with conflicting values. These authors suggest that the 'actions of coaches were full of context based, opportunist improvisations and extensive management of uncertainty and contradictions' (p. 268). Increasingly, researchers have suggested that each coaching situation is unique, thus practice is characterised in terms of 'structured improvisation' that is neither entirely reason based nor planned, and is far from systematic but highly problematic and individual: a set of reciprocal relations between athlete, coach and context

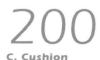

C. Cushion

(Saury and Durand, 1998; Sève and Durand, 1999; d'Arrippe-Longueville *et al.*, 1998; Cushion 2001; Poczwardowski *et al.*, 2002; Jones *et al.*, 2003, 2004).

While accounts of coaching practice such as these tend to be sport specific, this research knowledge has been gathered from a range of sports, including soccer, albeit within elite/ performance contexts. Therefore, the degree to which the cumulative findings of this work can be generalised to all soccer coaching contexts is a matter for debate. Yet, there is, arguably, enough in the findings to challenge more 'traditional' conceptions (Cushion and Lyle, 2010). The utility of the work for soccer perhaps lies in its more sophisticated and rich view of coaching practice. It is able to identify in coaching what Wenger (1998) identifies as the explicit language, roles, tools, documents and the implicit relationships, tacit conventions, subtle cues, untold rules of thumb, recognisable intuitions, specific perceptions, well-tuned sensitivities, embodied understandings, underlying assumptions and shared world-views. While most of these can never be articulated, they are unmistakable signs of coaching practice and make up part of a distinct culture, and understanding this is, arguably, crucial to coaching effectiveness (Cushion and Lyle, 2010; Cushion, 2007a).

An immersion in, and engagement with, the detail of coaching practice reveals much about its construction and complexity (Cushion, 2007a). There seems to be a beginning of some clearer and coherent concepts around understanding ambiguity and inconsistencies in practice. Structured improvisation, or the interaction of structure and agent, suggests that continuity in coaching comes not from stability but from adaptability (Cushion, 2007a). The ever-changing nature of coaching practice means we must focus on the totality of that practice and the practitioner in the soccer environment, and not simply on 'episodes' that occur in the process.

An understanding of coaching practice remains the cornerstone of conceptual development (Cushion, 2007b). For example, how coaching impacts on the subjectivities of those involved and how it is experienced as both a social space and a social structure offers fertile ground for conceptualising coaching (Cushion, 2007b). Any consideration of interaction and discourse within the coaching process, and of the coaching process itself, without a consideration of context, is both flawed and limited. Therefore, to develop coaching in soccer contexts, thinking should not be about producing definitive definitions or simplistic models, but instead about thinking with greater depth and detail so as to increase our understanding of practice. One of the simplest ways of beginning this thinking is to examine what coaches actually do in context, and the underpinning rationales for this practice.

## COACH BEHAVIOUR

The coach is commonly responsible for team performance and outcomes. Coaches therefore occupy a position of centrality and influence in efforts to improve performance (Cushion *et al.*, 2006; Smith and Smoll, 2007), with what they say and do impacting on players' achievement and well-being. As a result, understanding which behaviours translate into positive experiences and functioning on the part of the athletes is critical for researchers and practitioners alike (Amorose, 2007) and is a route into understanding coaching practice and the assumptions informing that practice. Coach behaviour research, utilising systematic observation, has emerged as a significant research activity (Nash and Collins, 2006) and one of the largest single categories within the general body of coaching knowledge (Gilbert and

Trudel, 2004). Of course the complex nature of coaching and the coaching process means that the different elements of coach behaviour are in fact interrelated and interdependent (Cushion, 2010; Cushion *et al.*, 2006), and coaches will engage with and deploy a range of discrete behaviours. Moreover, in reality, behaviours overlap and do not occur in neat, ordered ways, and whilst they are described as such here, these behaviours should not be thought of as separate or isolated.

### Instruction

Effective soccer coaching and player learning are linked to the quality of the coach's instructional behaviour (e.g., Carreira Da Costa and Pieron, 1992; DeMarco *et al.*, 1996; Gallimore and Tharp, 2004; Hodges and Franks, 2004). While there are principles that underlie the provision of effective instruction (Hodges and Franks, 2004), these principles alone are unable to account for the dominance of this behavioural approach within and across coaching, and over time these behavioural strategies are not solely based upon their efficacy for player learning. With this in mind, instruction has been consistently reported as the most frequently used 'active' coaching behaviour in soccer, regardless of performance level; see Table 11.1 (e.g., Cushion and Jones, 2001; Ford *et al.*, 2010). Moreover, behaviours that relate to task accomplishment (e.g., training, instruction and positive feedback) are, generally speaking, the most preferred by players (Reimer, 2007; Chelladurai and Reimer, 1998). This factor is reinforced by prior socialisation (as a player and a coach), along with well-established beliefs and traditions within soccer that validate and acknowledge certain behaviour as 'effective' (Cushion and Jones, 2006; Potrac *et al.*, 2007). Therefore, high levels of instruction reflect beliefs about effective and appropriate coaching behaviour that derive from previous playing and coaching experiences, and reproduce and reinforce an 'instructional' and directive approach (Cushion, 2010; Potrac *et al.*, 2007). This emphasis on instructional behaviour can be seen in terms of fulfilling the requirements of the role of a soccer coach, particularly when they are strongly associated with performance success.

The pressure to succeed in soccer and the accountability for and kudos of such success (real or perceived) sees the coach attempting to control as many variables as possible through high levels of instructional behaviour (Coakley, 2004; Bloom *et al.*, 1999; Potrac *et al.*, 2007). Coaches perhaps perceive the need to have the capacity to have an impact on their players' performances, thus achieving the desired outcomes (Jones *et al.*, 2004; Potrac *et al.*, 2002, 2007). This means not being viewed as weak, indecisive or lacking in knowledge or expertise (i.e., asking players for solutions). Coach education reinforces this perception and encourages coaches to use tried and tested (and safer) traditional methods that prove their knowledge and expertise, namely, instruction (Coakley, 2004; Jones *et al.*, 2004; Potrac *et al.*, 2002, 2007). 'The consequence of such action is that players are, in turn, increasingly socialised into expecting instructional behaviours from coaches, and thus resist other coaching methods' (Potrac *et al.*, 2007: 40), as these behaviours are deemed consciously or subconsciously to be associated with performance accomplishment.

**Table 11.1** Key coach behaviour findings from recent soccer studies.

| Author | Cushion and Jones (2001) | Smith and Cushion (2006) (in-game) | Potrac, et al. (2002) | Potrac et al. (2007) | Ford et al. (2010) | Partington and Cushion (2011) |
|---|---|---|---|---|---|---|
| Sample | 4 Premier League, 4 Championship (practice) | 4 Premier League, 2 Championship (practice) | 1 Premier League (Case study- practice) | 4 English Professional (practice) | 25 coaches – 3 Premier league, 9 Championship 7 semi-pro/amateur (differentiated practice) | 11 Premier League (differentiated practice) |
| Instruction | 63% | 27% | 57.53% | 59.84% | 30% | 42.65% |
| Questioning | 3.1% | 2.29% | 2.97% | 2.38% | † | 7.39% |
| Silence | 10.45% | 30.28% | 13.19% | 14.54% | 16%* | 4.4–8.8%** |

*Notes:*
† Questioning reported combined with instruction.
* Mean silence score for the range of practice activities.
** Range of silence scores across practice activities.

## Silence

Silence has been identified as a significant behaviour within coaching practice and can account for up to 40% of total behaviours in both training and competition (Smith and Cushion, 2006). This finding seems logical, as clearly coaches cannot constantly be engaged in 'active' coaching behaviours (Miller, 1992). However, coaches whose observation has been interpreted as 'passive' have been described as 'off-task' (Claxton, 1988). This suggestion has been superseded, with silence becoming increasingly understood as a deliberate coaching strategy, being used as a tool for promoting learning (Ford *et al.*, 2010; Partington and Cushion, 2011; Potrac *et al.*, 2007; Smith and Cushion, 2006).

Researchers describe a pattern of coaching behaviours in which periods of silence are punctuated with verbal cues, short reminders and specific commands or correction (Cushion and Jones, 2001; Partington and Cushion, 2011; Potrac *et al.*, 2007; Smith and Cushion 2006). When the coaches were not 'actively' providing feedback, they were in fact 'on-task', intently watching the action in silence. Therefore, the research evidence would indicate that the coaches' silence was an intentional behavioural strategy. Interestingly, coaches have expressed concern that too much verbal intervention would deny players not only opportunities to learn but also the opportunity to demonstrate what has already been learnt (Smith and Cushion, 2006; Partington and Cushion, 2011). Clearly, during moments of silence, coaches are involved in a number of cognitive processes. These can include observing and analysing the players' performance, allowing opportunities for them to learn for themselves and checking learning and athletes' decision making.

## Positive reinforcement: praise and scold

A positive working climate is a vital part of delivering quality soccer coaching. Smith and Smoll (2002) identified a positive approach to coaching where 'effective' coaching behaviours include: high frequencies of reinforcement for effort and performance; encouragement following errors; mistake-contingent and general instruction; and minimising punitive behaviours and non-responses. This approach is also advocated by Amorose and Horn (2000), who champion behaviour that contains a high frequency of positive and informational feedback, and low frequencies of punishment-oriented feedback. Soccer coaches frequently provide liberal support and encouragement to their performers. This is evidenced by behavioural research that reports praise as a substantial element in coaching practice, often being the second or third-largest category of behaviour overall (e.g., Cushion and Jones, 2001; Lacy and Darst, 1985; Miller, 1992; Potrac *et al.*, 2007; Bloom *et al.*, 1999). Potrac *et al.* (2002) contend that soccer coaches understand the significance of establishing a positive learning environment, recognising that athletes are more responsive to a positive coach and that positive behaviour can have an impact on motivation and self-efficacy in players. More subtly than this, coaches could use this behaviour to reinforce desired athlete behaviour, as Benfarri *et al.* (1986) note the method and style of transmission is critical in forming the recipients' perceptions.

Too much praise, however, can be seen as losing its value and thus becoming meaningless to athletes. The overuse of praise, especially general praise, can be interpreted as non-specific

C. Cushion

feedback that dilutes its effects (Schmidt, 1991). Alongside high levels of praise and contributing to a notion of a 'positive' coaching environment is a low level of scold behaviour, with some recorded praise-to-scold ratios as high as 33:1 (Potrac et al., 2002). The ability to punish another can be regarded as 'dysfunctional because it alienates people and builds up resentment' (Slack, 1997: 181). Some coaches' restricted use of scold behaviour is perhaps evidence of recognition of the unproductive nature of such behaviour and the potential damage that can be caused to coach–athlete relationships (Jowett, 2007). That said, researchers have also reported coaching behaviour in the professional domain as harsh, abusive and negative (e.g., Cushion and Jones, 2006), illustrating something of the context dependency of coaching behaviour.

## Expectancy effects

An important factor influencing behaviour in soccer is coaches' expectations or judgements of their players that, in turn, can have an impact on performance and behaviour (Cushion, 2010; Horn and Lox, 1993). This issue is important because it illustrates the bi-directional or dialectic nature of coach behaviour (LaVoi, 2007). Coaches often assume that players are passive recipients, that their behaviour is successfully received and that neither coach nor player is affected by the interaction. However, coach behaviour is not benign and there is a dialectic relationship with both coach and player, influenced by their interaction.

Given the competitive and evaluative nature of soccer, coaches form expectations of players (e.g., Wilson et al., 2006; Solomon, 1998). These are judgements or assessments about the physical competence or sporting potential of each player and are based on certain information available to the coach. A coach's expectations develop from a variety of factors but generally fall into two categories: person cues and performance information (Horn and Lox, 1993). Person cues include, for example, the player's age, social background, ethnicity and physical attributes. These cues are not used exclusively, but are combined with performance information about the player that could include past performance, physical test scores, ability and comments from other coaches (Horn and Lox, 1993; Solomon et al., 1996). Coaches also use impressions of players in practice situations informed by, for example, observation of behaviours related to the player's motivation, enthusiasm, pleasantness, response to criticism and interaction with staff and team-mates (Horn and Lox, 1993). In soccer, this is often defined in terms of players having a 'good attitude' or not. In addition, it is common for two coaches to form different sets of expectations for a player, based on which aspects of the available information they value most. The outcome of this process is that these expectations can be expressed to players through verbal and non-verbal behaviours (Cushion and Jones, 2006; Wilson et al., 2006). The link between coach behaviour and expectations has found differential feedback between high- and low-expectancy players. Cushion and Jones (2006) and Wilson et al. (2006) identified significant differences in the nature of coach behaviour based on an athlete's position in the group, with clear 'favourites' and 'rejects' suffering differential treatment within the coaching process. Some coaches appear to be 'pygmalion' (Horn and Lox, 1993) with clear differences between the quality and frequency of athlete–coach interaction. Expectancy theory assumes that a coach's feedback patterns will differ because players are perceived as high or low expectancy (Solomon et al., 1996). However, this assumption is worth considering: put simply, expectation effects are responsible for some differences in coach behaviour, but not all.

Perception of ability may not be the only basis for differential treatment and behaviour patterns. In accordance with the principles of behaviour modification and reinforcement theory, coaches ordinarily use performance feedback to cultivate and shape desired player behaviours (Sinclair and Vealey, 1989). Markland and Martinek (1988) noted that players working with more successful coaches (defined by win/loss record) received more feedback than from their less successful peers. This finding was mirrored by Solomon et al. (1996), who, while investigating expectancy effects, found that head coaches and assistants differed in the amount of feedback given. Head coaches gave feedback based on mistakes, whereas assistant coaches delivered more general positive feedback. Moreover, Claxton (1988) found that expert coaches used more questioning behaviours and would give less instruction than their non-expert colleagues. This research demonstrates other possible reasons for differential feedback, namely the coach's 'success' or level of expertise. Differential feedback and differences in coach behaviour have been attributed to numerous factors related to the coach. These include, but are not limited to, for example, job expectation, interaction opportunities, differentiation of roles, the philosophy of the programme and the goals of the sessions (Solomon, 1998).

## Coach behaviour – concluding thoughts

Coach behaviour is complex, involving the interplay of the individual's perceptions of self, other and the relationship (LaVoi, 2007). The functional significance of any interaction/ behaviour does not lie solely with 'what' the coach says or does, but depends on how the player(s) perceives, interprets and evaluates a coach's behaviour (Horn, 2002). Soccer players are remarkably perceptive in detecting differences in treatment or reactions from coaches, differences that coaches themselves would either be unaware of or at times deny (Solomon, 1998; Wilson et al., 2006; Cushion and Jones, 2006). As Tudge and Rogoff (1989) suggest, social interaction does not carry 'blanket benefits' and the circumstances in which coach behaviour facilitates development and learning need to be carefully planned and considered. Therefore, coaches need 'relational expertise', a capacity to observe patterns of connection and disconnection, including an awareness of self, other and relationship (Jordan, 1995; LaVoi, 2007).

Despite the seemingly 'muddy water', researchers have confirmed that coaching behaviour remains 'very situation specific and dependent on the interaction of a myriad of influencing variables' (Jones, 1997: 30), only some of which are beginning to be studied. It remains logical to conclude that there is 'no stereotypic coaching personality or set of behaviours which leads to success in coaching' (Markland and Martinek, 1988: 299). As has been argued, the coach's behaviour will often reflect more deep-seated values, and coaching practice, an essentially social practice, does not occur in a vacuum and therefore cannot be value free. Values are always represented in and through coach behaviour, although coaches may or may not be conscious of them or accurately identify their actual behaviour (Partington and Cushion, 2011). All coaches will have developed a personal set of views on coaching, on issues regarding soccer and about interpersonal relationships (Cushion, 2010). These views will have evolved over time and will be derived from experience and other kinds of education (Cushion *et al.*, 2003; Gilbert and Trudel, 2001; Cushion, 2006). Therefore, coaches need to reflect critically on why they behave as they do, in order to be able to make coaching judgements that are meaningful within their particular situation and challenge, rather than reinforce, certain beliefs or practices.

Coach behaviour should vary across athletes and situations; thus, providing specific recommendations on how to behave becomes difficult. However, it is important to see beyond coaching style and the directive/non-directive debate, and to position the needs of the player as paramount. Arguably, effective coaches are able to focus on the needs of individual players, and behaviour should be shaped around individual players' progress and responses, as well as the context at any given moment. The intent should always be to connect coach behaviour to player learning. Therefore, the quality of the support and behaviour provided by the coach is the key. There is not a 'one size fits all' approach and the optimal behaviour will depend on the characteristics of the situation and the player. Regardless of the 'style' of coach behaviour, directive or non-directive, if this is perceived by the player as imposing the coach's way of thinking, feeling or acting and is not aligned with the player's needs, then it will be seen as controlling and will not be positively received. In this sense, the coach needs to be an authority rather than in authority (Drewe, 2000; Jones and Standage, 2006), while being active rather than passive in the coaching process.

## COACH EDUCATION AND LEARNING

The coaching environment has traditionally been viewed as a place where players learn. More recently, however, this context has begun to be recognised as a place in which coaches' learning and development takes place (Cushion *et al.*, 2003; Cushion, 2006). Learning is an important term, as it places the emphasis on the person in whom change is expected to occur or has occurred and is therefore described as an 'act or process by which behavioural change, knowledge, skills, and attitudes are acquired' (Jarvis, 2004: 100–101). Learning can happen through a number of means, for example, through experience, reflection, study or instruction. In this sense, learning can embrace all of the mechanisms through which coaches acquire the knowledge that informs their practice. Learning occurs not only inside but also outside of educational settings (Cushion *et al.*, 2010). Consequently, while the coach-learner is the essential element in the learning process, the coach-educator is not, as learning often occurs without teaching.

### Informal learning

Soccer coaches' learning takes place in a wide variety of contexts, predominantly in informal situations beyond dedicated formal learning environments (Cushion *et al.*, 2003; Merriam and Caffarella, 1999). Learning in informal situations has become a well-established pathway for soccer coaches, with its implications for knowledge development and professional socialisation being recognised in the literature (Cassidy *et al.*, 2009; Cushion *et al.*, 2003). This 'imbalance may be as much a commentary on the efficacy of other learning provision than on the effectiveness of learning in informal situations' (Cushion et al., 2010). The dominance of informal and self-directed learning is due largely to the limitations and low impact of current formal provision (Cushion et al., 2003, 2010). Moreover, coach education has traditionally lacked any coherent or overarching structure, which has meant that coaches have been left to 'go it alone', resulting in an often ad hoc, negotiated and individual learning curriculum (Cushion et al., 2010; Cushion 2010, 2011; Nelson et al., 2006). Therefore, learning in informal situations, such as through day-to-day practice in clubs, occurs without a prescribed curriculum and is usually facilitated by an 'other'. This can ignore power relations where the 'other' dominates the learning process and where particular ideological interpretations of high-status knowledge are enforced (Cushion et al., 2010). Without a form of reflective process, coaches uncritically accrue experience by informal means (Cushion et al., 2010; Kidman, 1997; Gilbert and Trudel, 2001) and are more likely to 'non-reflectively' accept and be socialised into the knowledge, values, beliefs and expectations of the sporting culture in which they work (Jarvis, 2006).

## Reflection

The theory of reflection appears to offer a great deal for understanding how soccer coaches learn experientially (e.g., Cushion et al., 2003; Cushion, 2006; Cassidy et al., 2009). However, reflection can be undertaken in a superficial way, which in fact might be little different from simply recounting events in a form of descriptive writing (Cushion et al., 2010; Cushion, 2011). Several authors have commented on the inadequacy of much activity performed in the name of reflection because it is in fact largely non-critical and non-reflective (e.g., Kim, 1999; Moon, 2004), suggesting, thus, that reflection has a range of application, with a continuum from shallow description at the one end to deep critical reflection at the other (Cushion et al., 2010; Cushion, 2011). As Cushion (2011) argues, the key to this process is learning the skill of reflection and allowing enough time for the skill to be developed and supported. Knowles et al. (2001) suggest that the 'development of reflective skills is not a simplistic process even with structured support. Coach educators cannot therefore assume that development of reflective skills will be a naturally occurring phenomena [sic] that runs parallel to increasing coaching experience' (p. 204). Reflective strategies can be used in learning, but these approaches require time and commitment and need to be built into coach education programmes beyond the completion of coaching 'log-books' (Gilbert and Trudel, 2006).

## Mentoring

Mentoring in coaching is the most visible example of a practice where formal and informal learning meet (Colley et al., 2003a). Influencing the experiences and interactions of coaches by a mentor is suggested by a number of authors (e.g. Cushion et al., 2003; Werthner and Trudel, 2006; Trudel and Gilbert, 2006) and it is this process that goes some way to reproducing traditional practice in soccer coaching. As part of a formal coach education programme, mentoring is conceived as bringing increasing formalisation of a practice that is inherently informal (Colley et al., 2003a).

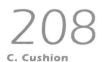
C. Cushion

The success of learning will be dependent upon the quality of the relationship between mentor and protégé (Dymock, 1999; Cushion, 2006). There are common issues identified that negatively impact on mentoring, including the lack of time and training, personal or professional compatibility, undesirable attitudes or behaviours, and workloads that went unnoticed (Cushion et al., 2010; Cushion, 2011). Mentees have reported a lack of mentor interest and training, as well as problematic behaviours (overly critical, defensive, controlling) (Cushion et al., 2010). Ehrich et al. (2004) state that 'mentoring is a highly complex dynamic and interpersonal relationship that requires at the very least, time, interest and commitment of mentors and mentees and strong support from educational or organisational leaders responsible for overseeing programmes' (p. 533).

## Formal learning

Activities conforming to this definition of coach learning include large-scale coach certification programmes developed by the national governing bodies and higher education courses relating to coaching and sport science (Nelson et al., 2006). Formal coach education has under-standably attracted considerable attention, with numerous scholars having researched and specifically written about this topic, including in relation to soccer (e.g., Abraham and Collins, 1998; Cassidy et al., 2009; Cushion et al., 2003; Lyle, 2002, 2007; Trudel and Gilbert, 2006). Closer inspection reveals that, to date, few researchers have attempted to directly investigate and evaluate coach education programmes in soccer or other sports (Cushion et al., 2010; McCullick et al., 2009). As a result, there remains no evidence to link coach education certification with coaching competency or developments in practice, despite many courses being competency based (Cushion et al., 2010).

Coaches have tended to attach much less importance to formal coach education for the acquisition of knowledge (Gould et al., 1990; Irwin et al., 2004; Schempp et al., 1998). When asked to comment on their experiences, coaches have suggested that: (1) courses often give little more than a basic understanding but offer a starting-point (Abraham et al., 2006; Jones et al., 2004); (2) they often arrive already knowing about, and putting into practice, much of what is covered, meaning that little new knowledge is gained (Gilbert and Trudel, 1999; Irwin et al., 2004); (3) some of the theoretical material covered is considered too abstract from everyday practice to be considered worthwhile (Lemyre et al., 2007); (4) courses can be guilty of trying to cram too much information into a relatively short period of time (Lemyre et al., 2007); and (5) they have come to question much of the information acquired during courses later in their careers (Irwin et al., 2004). As a result of such experiences, some coaches have admitted to attending later awards because of their compulsory requirement only (Wright et al., 2007). The element of compulsion and the need for certification mean that coaches are unlikely to directly contest the programme or coach educator (Cushion et al, 2003; Chesterfield et al., 2010). Specifically, in soccer, Chesterfield et al. (2010) found that coaches purposely gave an outward appearance of acceptance, while sometimes harbouring and restricting their disagreement with, and rejection of, the official coaching orientation.

Some provision in formal situations could perhaps even be described as 'indoctrination', which can be defined as 'activities that set out to convince us that there is a 'right' way of thinking and feeling and behaving' (Rogers, 2002: 53; Nelson et al., 2006; Cushion et al.,

and coach education

2010; Cushion, 2011). Chesterfield *et al.* (2010) provided evidence supporting the claim that coach education in soccer can be considered indoctrination in certain instances, with the course delivering and assessing against a 'right way' to coach. In this respect, indoctrination denies the learner choice, instead exposing them to a single set of expected values and attitudes; this might include a prescribed method of delivery, feedback sequence, coaching philosophy, or tactical and technical approach (Jones *et al.*, 2003; Nelson *et al.*, 2006; Cushion *et al.*, 2010; Cushion, 2011). Currently, formal coach learning in soccer defines what knowledge is necessary for coaches to practise and how that knowledge can 'best' be transmitted, and certification requires coaches to structure sessions, deliver information to players and provide feedback in a prescribed manner in order to be deemed competent (Nelson *et al.*, 2006; Cushion *et al.*, 2010; Cushion, 2011). With this in mind, coach education that delivers this discourse might be better described as training, or even indoctrination in certain instances (Cushion *et al.*, 2010).

## DEVELOPING COACH EDUCATION

To develop coach learning for soccer, coach education ought to ensure that it is meeting the needs of coaches and players. Linked to this is understanding of how coach educators can ensure that learning leads to enhanced coach and player development. Any current prescriptions for coach learning are 'substantively and strategically' incomplete because they are missing data and evidence (McLaughlin and Zarrow, 2001; Armour, 2010). As a result, it seems crucial to determine the complex ways in which coaches learn and, in turn, how coach and player learning are linked. However, learning is complex, not linear, and, as a result, is difficult to quantify. There are a myriad of variables that impact on learning that can make 'measuring' in experimental or causal studies problematic. There has been scant systematic research on the effects of coach learning on improvements in coaching practice or on player outcomes. Coach learning needs effective longitudinal evaluation, without which it is impossible to determine what works, why and for whom.

Currently, for soccer coaches, learning most frequently occurs outside educational settings, and often in environments where the primary purpose is not coach learning (Cushion *et al.*, 2010). This situation arises due to the limitations of current formal provision, the lack of an overarching structure, and issues around volunteerism, which combine to allow a negotiated and individual learning curriculum. However, this curriculum is not unproblematic; it can ignore underlying power relations and promote and reinforce certain ideological inter-pretations of knowledge and practice. Gilbert and Trudel (2006) suggest that, as experience and interaction with others are inevitable phenomena in coaching, this type of learning deals with knowing, not knowledge (Sfard, 1998), and control of the learning content is therefore impossible. To develop coach learning and ensure an even developmental experience, coach education must find ways to control and facilitate these experiences (Cushion, *et al.*, 2003; Cushion, 2006; Werthner and Trudel, 2006). Reflection appears particularly important in framing coaches' learning from experience. However, reflection is a skill that needs to be developed and supported.

Formal mediated modes of learning are crucial to coach learning and the evolution of coaching, yet the evidence concerning formal coach learning is largely critical. Clearly,

210

evidence of the impact of formal learning is urgently required so as to enable the development of worthwhile coach education. Those developing coach education programmes should be mindful to incorporate more rigorous monitoring and evaluation processes. A key issue raised by Trudel and Gilbert (2006) that limits the potential of any new approach is that coaching courses tend to be condensed, and soccer coach education is no exception. The limited amount of time that coaches have to invest in their preparation has been noted (Abraham and Collins, 1998), and the appropriateness of 'weekend education programmes' is questionable if we want to facilitate coach learning and development by taking experience into account (Trudel and Gilbert, 2006). These reservations notwithstanding, any learning method needs clear tutor/facilitator training and support, and needs a well-planned curriculum with clear learning objectives (Cushion et al., 2010).

Overall, while much material exists about informal and formal learning, it is difficult, if not impossible, to be prescriptive about a specific, optimal mix. However, an important observation is that coach learning should be a mix. Colley et al. (2003) point out that it is often the blending of learning types that is significant, not their separation. Therefore, matching a varied blend of learning appropriately with the developmental stage of the coach is required. It would be unrealistic to think that coaches would, could or should switch off their ability to learn when operating in a given situation, be it formal, non-formal, or informal. It seems important that the field should assist coaches with developing the necessary abilities to fully engage in all situations so that they can maximise their on-going learning and development.

## SUMMARY

While sections of this chapter may seem disconnected, they, like coaching more broadly, can be perceived as key interactive and interdependent operational variables that structure a broad coaching process. The assumptions one has about the nature of coaching will direct coaching practice and coach behaviour and will inform the necessary knowledge and structures underpinning coach education. For example, an instrumental perspective to coaching that is reduced to the application of a generic set of rules and involves the application of a known set of predictable sequences will produce a certain type of coaching behaviour and training for coaches. This approach will be in contrast to a view of coaching as a dynamic and fluid endeavour that is inextricably linked to the constraints and opportunities of human interaction, thus precluding the simple application of any 'painting-by-numbers' approach to behaviour and coach education.

Coaching and perspectives on it, therefore, will often reflect deep-seated values. Values are always represented in and through coach behaviour, although coaches may or may not be conscious of them. All coaches will have developed a personal set of views on coaching, on issues regarding their sport, and about interpersonal relationships. These views will have evolved over time and will be derived from experience and the coaches' coaching and broader education. Therefore, coaches need to reflect critically on why they behave as they do in order to be able to make coaching judgements that are meaningful within their particular situation and that challenge, rather than reinforce, certain beliefs or practices.

# REFERENCES

Abraham, A., and Collins, D. (1998). Examining and extending research in coach development, *Quest* 50, 59–79.

Abraham, A., Collins, D., and Martindale, R. (2006). The coaching schematic: validation through expert coach consensus, *Journal of Sports Sciences* 24(6), 549–564.

Amorose, A. J. (2007). Coaching effectiveness: exploring the relationship between coaching behaviour and self-determined motivation. In M. S. Hagger, and N. L. D. Chatzisarantis (eds), *Intrinsic Motivation and Self-determination in Exercise and Sport* (pp. 209–227). Champaign, IL: Human Kinetics.

Amorose, A. J., and Horn, T. S. (2000). Intrinsic motivation: relationships with collegiate athletes' gender, scholarship status, and perceptions of their coaches' behaviour. *Journal of Sport and Exercise Psychology* 22, 63–84.

Armour, K. M. (2010). The learning coach, the learning approach: professional development for sports coach professionals. In J. Lyle, and C. Cushion (eds), *Sports Coaching: Professionalisation and Practice* (pp. 153–164). London: Elsevier.

Benfarri, R., Wilkinson, H., and Orth, C. (1986). The effective use of power, *Business Horizons* 29, 12–16.

Bloom, G. A., Crumpton, R., and Anderson, J. E. (1999). A systematic observation study of the teaching behaviours of an expert basketball coach. *The Sport Psychologist* 13, 157–170.

Carreira Da Costa, F., and Pieron, M. (1992). Teaching effectiveness: comparison of more and less effective teachers in an experimental teaching unit. In T. Williams, L. Almond, and A. Sparkes (eds), *Sport and Physical Activity: Moving towards Excellence* (pp. 169–176). London: E and FN Spon.

Cassidy, T., Jones, R., and Potrac, P. (2009). *Understanding Sports Coaching: The Social, Cultural and Pedagogical Foundations of Coaching Practice*. Abingdon: Routledge.

Chelladurai, P., and Reimer, H. A. (1998). Measurement of leadership in sport. In J. Duda (ed.), *Advances in Sport and Exercise Psychology Measurement*. Morgantown, WV: Fitness Information Technology.

Chesterfield, G., Potrac, P., and Jones, R. L. (2010). 'Studentship' and 'impression management': COACHES' experiences of an advanced soccer coach education award. *Sport, Education and Society* 15(3), 299–314.

Coakley, J. (2004). *Sports in Society: Issues and Controversies*, 8th edn. New York: McGraw-Hill.

Colley, H., Hodkinson, P., and Malcolm, J. (2003) *Informality and Formality in Learning: A Report for the Learning and Skills Research Centre* (London: Learning and Skills Research Centre).

Côté, J., Salmela, J., Trudel, P., Baria, A., and Russell, S. (1995). The coaching model: a grounded assessment of expert gymnastic coaches' knowledge, *Journal of Sport and Exercise Psychology* 17(1), 1–17.

Claxton, D. (1988). A systematic observation of more and less successful high school tennis coaches. *Journal of Teaching in Physical Education* 7, 302–310.

Cushion, C. J. (2001). 'The coaching process in professional youth football: an ethnography of practice'. Unpublished PhD thesis. Brunel University, UK.

Cushion, C. J. (2006). Mentoring: harnessing the power of experience. In R. Jones (ed.), *The Sports Coach as Educator: Reconceptualising Sports Coaching* (pp.128–144). London: Routledge.

Cushion, C. J. (2007a). Modelling the complexity of the coaching process. *International Journal of Sport Science and Coaching* 2(4), 395–401.

Cushion, C. J. (2007b). Modelling the complexity of the coaching process: A response to commentaries. *International Journal of Sport Science and Coaching* 2(4), 427–433.

Cushion, C. J. (2010). Coach and athlete learning: A social approach. In R. Jones, P. Potrac, C. Cushion, and L. T. Ranglan (eds), *The Sociology of Sports Coaching* (pp. 166–178). London: Routledge.

Cushion, C. J. (2011). Coaches' learning and development. In R. Bailey, and I. Stafford (eds), *Coaching Children in Sport* (pp. 57–68). London: Routledge.

Cushion, C. J., and Jones, R. L. (2001). A systematic observation of professional top-level youth soccer coaches. *Journal of Sport Behaviour* 24, 1–23.

Cushion, C. J., and Jones, R. L. (2006). Power, discourse and symbolic violence in professional youth soccer: the case of Albion FC. *Sociology of Sport Journal* 23, 142–161.

Cushion, C. J., and Lyle, J. (2010). Conceptual development in sports coaching. In J. Lyle, and C. Cushion, *Sports Coaching: Professionalisation and Practice* (pp. 43–62). London: Elsevier.

Cushion, C. J., Armour, K. M., and Jones, R. L. (2003). Coach education and continuing professional development: experience and learning to coach. *Quest* 55, 215–230.

Cushion, C. J., Armour, K. M., and Jones, R. L. (2006). Locating the coaching process in practice: models 'for' and 'of' coaching. *Physical Education and Sport Pedagogy* 11(1), 83–99.

Cushion, C. J., Nelson, L., Armour, K., Lyle, J., Jones, R. L., Sandford, R., and O'Callaghan, C. (2010). *Coach Learning and Development: A Review of Literature*. Leeds: Sports Coach UK.

d'Arrippe-Longueville, F., Fournier, J. F., and Dubois, A. (1998). The perceived effectiveness of interactions between expert French judo coaches and elite female athletes. *The Sport Psychologist* 12, 317–332.

DeMarco, G., Mancini, V., and Wuest, D. (1996). Reflections on change: a qualitative and quantitative analysis of a baseball coach's behaviour. *Journal of Sport Behaviour* 20(2), 135–163.

Drewe, S. (2000). An examination of the relationship between coaching and teaching. *Quest* 52, 79–88.

Dymock, D. (1999). Blind date: a case study of mentoring as workplace learning. *The Journal of Workplace Learning* 11(8), 312–317.

Ehrich, L., Hansford, B., and Tennent, L. (2004). Formal mentoring programs in education and other professions: a review of the literature. *Educational Administration Quarterly* 40(4), 518–540.

Ford, P. R., Yates, I., and Williams, M. A. (2010). An analysis of practice activities and instructional behaviours used by youth soccer coaches during practice: exploring the link between science and application. *Journal of Sports Sciences* 28, 483–495.

Gallimore, R., and Tharp, R. (2004). What a coach can teach a teacher, 1975–2004: reflections and reanalysis of John Wooden's teaching practices. *The Sport Psychologist* 18, 119–137.

Gilbert, W. (2007). Modelling the complexity of the coaching process: a commentary. *International Journal of Sport Science and Coaching* 2(4), 427–433.

Gilbert, W., and Trudel, P. (1999). Framing the construction of coaching knowledge in experiential learning. *Sociology of Sport Online* 2(1), http://physed.otago.ac.nz/sosol/v2i1/v2i1s2.htm.

Gilbert, W., and Trudel, P. (2001). Learning to coach through experience: reflection in model youth sport coaches. *Journal of Teaching in Physical Education* 21, 16–34.

Gilbert, W., and Trudel, P. (2004). Analysis of coaching science research published from 1970–2001. *Research Quarterly for Exercise and Sport* 75, 388–399.

Gilbert, W., and Trudel, P. (2006). The coach as a reflective practitioner. In R. L. Jones (ed.) *The Sports Coach as Educator: Reconceptualising Sports Coaching* (pp. 114–127). London: Routledge.

Gould, D., Giannini, J., Krane, K., and Hodge, K. (1990). Educational needs of elite US national team, Pan American and Olympic coaches. *Journal of Teaching Physical Education* 9, 332–334.

Hodges, N. J., and Franks, I. M. (2004). Instructions, demonstrations and the learning process: creating and constraining movement options. In A. M. Williams, and N. J. Hodges (eds), *Skill Acquisition in Sport: Research, Theory and Practice* (pp. 145–174). London: Routledge.

Horn, T. S. (2002). Coaching effectiveness in the sport domain. In T. S. Horn (ed.), *Advances in Sport Psychology* (pp. 309–354). Champaign, IL: Human Kinetics.

Horn, T. S., and Lox, C. (1993). The self-fulfilling prophecy theory: when coaches' expectations become reality. In J. M. Williams (ed.), *Applied Sport Psychology; Personal Growth to Peak Performance*. Mountain View, CA: Mayfield Publishing Company.

Irwin, G., Hanton, S., and Kerwin, D. G. (2004). Reflective practice and the origins of elite coaching knowledge. *Reflective Practice* 5(3), 425–442.

Jarvis, P. (2004). *Adult Education and Lifelong Learning: Theory and Practice*, 3rd edn. London: Routledge.

Jarvis, P. (2006). *Towards a Comprehensive Theory of Human Learning*. London: Routledge.

Jones, R. L. (1997). 'Effective' instructional coaching behaviour: a review of literature. *International Journal of Physical Education* 24(1), 27–32.

Jones, R. L. (2007). Coaching redefined: an everyday pedagogical endeavour. *Sport Education and Society* 12(2), 159–174.

Jones R. L., and Standage, M. (2006). First among equals: shared leadership in the coaching context. In R. L. Jones (ed.), *The Sports Coach as Educator: Reconceptualising Sports Coaching* (pp. 65–76). London: Routledge.

Jones, R. L., and Wallace, M. (2005). Another bad day at the training ground: coping with ambiguity in the coaching context. *Sport, Education and Society* 10, 119–134.

Jones, R. L., Armour, K. M., and Potrac, P. (2003). Constructing expert knowledge: a case study of a top-level professional soccer coach. *Sport, Education and Society* 8(2), 213–229.

Jones, R. L., Armour, K. M., and Potrac, P. (2004). *Sports Coaching Cultures: From Practice to Theory*. London: Routledge.

Jordan, J. V. (1995). *Transforming Disconnection*. Working paper No. 75, Wellesly MA: Stone Center.

Jowett, S. (2007). Interdependence analysis and the 3 + 1 C's in the coach–athlete relationship. In S. Jowett, and D. Lavallee (eds), *Social Psychology in Sport* (pp. 15–29). Champaign, IL: Human Kinetics.

214

Kidman, L. (1997). A self-reflective analysis process for coach education. *Pedagogy in Practice* 3(1), 18–36.

Kim, H. S. (1999). Critical reflective inquiry for knowledge development in nursing practice. *Journal of Advanced Nursing* 29(5), 1205–1212.

Knowles, Z., Gilbourne, D., Borrie, A., and Nevill, A. (2001). Developing the reflective sports coach: a study exploring the processes of reflective practice within a higher education coaching programme. *Reflective Practice* 2(2), 185–207.

Lacy, A. C., and Darst, P. W. (1985). Systematic observation of behaviours of winning high school head football coaches. *Journal of Teaching in Physical Education* 4, 256–270.

LaVoi, N. M. (2007). Interpersonal communication and conflict in the coach–athlete relationship. In S. Jowett and D. Lavallee (eds), *Social Psychology in Sport* (pp. 75–90). Champaign, IL: Human Kinetics.

Lemyre, F., Trudel, P., and Durand-Bush, N. (2007). How youth-sport coaches learn to coach. *The Sport Psychologist* 21, 191–209.

Lyle, J. (1999). Coaching philosophy and coaching behaviour. In N. Cross and J. Lyle (eds), *The Coaching Process: Principles and Practice for Sport* (pp. 25–46). Oxford: Butterworth-Heinemann.

Lyle, J. (2002). *Sports Coaching Concepts: A Framework for Coaches' Behaviour.* London: Routledge.

Lyle, J. (2007). A review of the research evidence for the impact of coach education. *International Journal of Coaching Science* 1(1), 17–34.

Markland, R., and Martinek, T. J. (1988). Descriptive analysis of coach augmented feedback given to high school varsity female volleyball players. *Journal of Teaching in Physical Education* 7, 289–301.

McCullick, B., Schempp, P., Mason, I., Foo, C., Vickers, B., and Connolly, G. (2009). A scrutiny of the coaching education program scholarship since 1995. *Quest* 61(3), 322–335.

McLaughlin, M. W., and Zarrow, J. (2001). Teachers engaged in evidence based reform: trajectories of teacher's inquiry, analysis and action. In L. Leiberman, and L. Miller (eds), *Teachers Caught in the Action: Professional Development that Matters* (pp. 79–101). New York: Teacher's College.

Merriam, S. B., and Caffarella, R. S. (1999). *Learning in Adulthood*, 2nd edn. San Francisco, CA: Jossey-Bass.

Miller, A. W. (1992). Systematic observation behavior similarities of various youth sport soccer coaches. *Physical Educator* 49(3), 136–143.

Moon, J. A. (2004). *A Handbook of Reflection and Experiential Learning: Theory and Practice.* London: Kogan Page.

Nash, C., and Collins, D. (2006). Tacit knowledge in expert coaching: science or art? *Quest* 58(4), 465–477.

Nelson, L. J., Cushion, C. J., and Potrac, P. (2006). Formal, nonformal and informal coach learning: a holistic conceptualisation. *International Journal of Sports Science and Coaching* 1(3), 247–259.

Partington, M., and Cushion, C. J. (2011). An investigation of the practice activities and coaching behaviours of professional top-level youth soccer coaches. *Scandinavian Journal of Medicine and Science in Sport.* DOI: 10.1111/j.1600-0838.2011.01383.x.

Poczwardowski, A., Barott, J. E., and Henschen, K. P. (2002). The athlete and coach: their relationship and its meaning. Results of an interpretive study. *International Journal of Sport Psychology* 33, 116–140.

Potrac, P., Jones, R. L., and Armour, K. (2002). 'It's all about getting respect': the coaching behaviours of an expert English soccer coach. *Sport Education and Society* 7, 183–202.

Potrac, P., Jones, R. L., and Cushion, C. J. (2007). Understanding power and the coach's role in professional English soccer: a preliminary investigation of coach behaviour. *Soccer and Society* 8, 33–49.

Reimer, H. A. (2007). Multi-dimensional model of coach leadership. In S. Jowett, and D. Lavallee (eds), *Social Psychology in Sport* (pp. 57–73). Champaign IL: Human Kinetics.

Rogers, A. (2002). *Teaching Adults*, 3rd edn. Buckingham: Open University Press.

Saury, J., and Durand, M. (1998). Practical knowledge in expert coaches: on site study of coaching in sailing. *Research Quarterly for Exercise and Sport* 69(3), 254–266.

Schempp, P., Manross, D., and Tan, S. (1998). Subject expertise and teachers' knowledge. *Journal of Teaching in Physical Education* 17, 342–356.

Schmidt, R. A. (1991). *Motor Control and Performance: From Principles to Practice*. Champaign, IL: Human Kinetics.

Sève, C., and Durand, M. (1999). The action of a table tennis coach as situated action. *Avante* 5, 69–86.

Sfard, A. (1998). On two metaphors for learning and the dangers of choosing just one. *Educational Researcher* 27, 4–13.

Sinclair, D. A., and Vealey, R. S. (1989). Effects of coaches' expectations and feedback on the self-perceptions of athletes. *Journal of Sport Behaviour* 12, 77–91.

Slack, T. (1997). *Understanding Sport Organisations: The Application of Organisation Theory*. Champaign, IL: Human Kinetics.

Smith, M., and Cushion, C. J. (2006). An investigation of the in-game behaviours of professional, top-level youth soccer coaches. *Journal of Sport Sciences* 24(4), 355–366.

Smith, R. E., and Smoll, F. L. (2002). *Way To Go Coach! A Scientifically Proven Approach to Coaching Effectiveness*, 2nd edn. Portolla Valley, CA: Warde.

Smith, R. E., and Smoll, F. L. (2007). Social-cognitive approaches to coach behaviour. In S. Jowett, and D. Lavallee (eds) *Social Psychology in Sport* (pp. 75–90). Champaign, IL: Human Kinetics.

Solomon, G. B. (1998). Coach expectations and differential feedback: perceptual flexibility revisited. *Journal of Sport Behaviour* 21(3), 298–310.

Solomon, G. B., Striegel, D. A., Eliot, J. F., Heon, S. N., Maas, J. L., and Wayda, V. (1996). The self-fulfilling prophecy in college basketball: implications for effective coaching. *Journal of Applied Sport Psychology* 8, 44–59.

Trudel, P., and Gilbert, W. (2006). Coaching and coach education. In D. Kirk, D. Macdonald and M. O'Sullivan (eds), *The Handbook of Physical Education* (pp. 516–539). London: Sage Publications.

Tudge, J. R. H., and Rogoff, B. (1989). Peer influences on cognitive development: Piagetian and Vygotskyian perspectives. In M. H. Bornstein, and J. S. Bruner (eds), *Interaction in Human Development*. Hillsdale, NJ: Lawrence Erlbaum.

Wenger, E. (1998). *Communities of Practice: Learning, Meaning and Identity*. Cambridge: Cambridge University Press.

Werthner, P., and Trudel, P. (2006). A new theoretical perspective for understanding how coaches learn to coach. *The Sport Psychologist* 20, 198–212.

Williams, A. M., and Hodges, N. (2005). Practice, instruction and skill acquisition in soccer: challenging tradition. *Journal of Sports Sciences* 23(6), 637–650.

Wilson, M., Cushion, C. J., and Stephens, D. (2006). 'Put me in coach . . . I'm better than you think!' Coaches' perceptions of their expectations in youth sport. *International Journal of Sport Science and Coaching* 1(2), 149–162.

Wright, T., Trudel, P., and Culver, D. (2007). Learning how to coach: the different learning situations reported by youth ice hockey coaches. *Physical Education and Sport Pedagogy* 12(2), 127–144.

# CHAPTER 12

## BIOMECHANICS APPLIED TO SOCCER SKILLS

A. Lees

## INTRODUCTION

Biomechanics offers methods by which the very fast actions which occur in sport can be recorded and analysed in detail. There are various reasons for undertaking such analyses. One is to understand the general mechanical effectiveness of the movement, another is the detailed description of the skill, yet another is an analysis of the factors underlying successful performance. An important application of biomechanics within any sport, and soccer in particular, is the definition and understanding of skills. Information presented in this chapter can help in the coaching process and, as a result, enhance the learning and performance of those skills.

There is a wide range of skills which form the foundation of performance in soccer. Those which have been the subject of biomechanical analysis are the more technical ones which are concerned directly with scoring. For example, in soccer, shooting at goal is an aspect of kicking and is the means by which goals are scored. Similarly, heading the ball and throwing-in can be important elements of attacking play, while goal-keeping skills are important in preventing the scoring of goals.

Other skills are important in the game, but have received much less attention in terms of biomechanical analysis. For example, kicking actions such as passing and trapping the ball, tackling, falling behaviour, jumping, running, sprinting, starting, stopping and changing direction are all important skills in soccer, but have received little detailed attention. The skills in other codes of football have similarly received little attention in terms of biomechanical analysis. This chapter is concerned with those skills in which biomechanics has been successfully applied in order to gain an insight into their mechanical characteristics.

## KICKING

Kicking is without doubt the most widely studied skill in soccer. Although there are many variations of this skill, due to ball type, speed and position, nature and intent of kick, the variant which has been most widely reported in the literature is the maximum velocity instep kick of a stationary ball, a skill which essentially corresponds to the penalty kick in soccer.

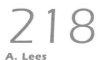

The mature form of the kicking skill has been described by Wickstrom (1975). It is characterised by an approach from a short distance, placement of the supporting leg at the side and slightly behind the stationary ball. The kicking leg is first taken backwards and the leg flexes at the knee. The forward motion of the kicking leg is initiated by rotating the hip about the supporting leg and by bringing the thigh of the kicking leg forwards. The leg is still flexing at the knee at this stage. Once this initial action has taken place, the thigh begins to decelerate until it is essentially motionless at ball contact. During this deceleration, the shank vigorously extends to give the knee almost full extension at ball contact. The leg remains straight through ball contact and begins to flex during the long follow-through. The foot will often reach above the level of the hip during the follow-through. A series of kinetograms of the kicking action are given in Figure 12.1.

The approach made by skilled players when performing an instep kick is made from an angle to the direction of ball flight, at a distance of a few steps and using a curved run. An angled approach is favoured by players, and self-selected approach angles of around 43° have been reported by Egan, Vwerheul and Savelsbergh (2007), supporting previous research where it was reported that an approach angle of around 45° generated maximum ball speed (Isokawa and Lees, 1988). Players also prefer to use an approach distance which requires them to take a small number (2–4) of steps. An approach of this type generates a modest approach speed of around 3–4 m.s$^{-1}$ (Kellis and Katis, 2007). Thus, the nature of the approach rather than the speed appears to be important for performance. The length of the last step is important in maximal kicking. Lees and Nolan (2002) reported a larger last step length for two professional players performing a maximal instep kick (0.72 and 0.81 m), as compared to a sub-maximal kick (0.53 and 0.55 m). These authors associated the longer length of the last step with a greater degree of pelvic retraction, which in turn allowed an increased range for pelvic protraction (i.e, forward rotation of the kicking side). The approach path made by skilled players is curved and, as a consequence, the body is inclined towards the centre of rotation. It is likely that the purpose of the curved run is to ensure the body produces and maintains a lateral inclination as the kick is performed. The inclined kicking leg foot is more able to get under the ball to make better contact (Plagenhoef, 1971). Moreover, a more inclined lower body would allow an extended kicking leg knee at impact, generating higher foot velocity. Finally, a curved approach provides a stable position for executing the kick, thus contributing to the accuracy and consistency of kick performance.

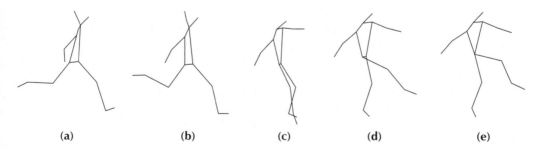

(a)      (b)      (c)      (d)      (e)

**Figure 12.1** Kinetograms of the key positions during a soccer kick showing: (a) maximum hip retraction; (b) forward movement of the thigh and continued knee flexion; (c) ball contact; (d) post-impact follow-through; and (e) knee flexion as follow-through proceeds.

As the support foot contacts the ground a force is generated. The ground reaction forces have been reported for a maximal instep kick as 15–20, 4–6 and 5–6 N.kg⁻¹ in the vertical, posterior (braking) and lateral (towards the non-kicking side) directions respectively (Kellis, Katis and Gissis, 2004; Lees, Steward, Rahnama and Barton, 2009). In particular, the horizontal forces are directed solely in the posterior and lateral (to non-kicking side) directions. These forces, together with the reduced velocity of the hip after support foot contact, suggest that the motion of the body is slowed during the kicking action. This slowing may have benefits for stabilising the action, enabling greater muscle forces to be produced, or to influence the kicking leg action. The support leg knee is flexed to 26° at foot contact and remains flexed throughout the duration of the kick, being flexed to 42° at ball contact (Lees et al., 2009). The flexion of the knee continues for longer than necessary, in order to absorb the impact of landing, and is a cause of the slowing forward motion. It begins to extend just before ball contact, stabilising the action, as the slow contraction velocity of muscles around the support leg knee enables these muscles to generate their highest levels of force.

A notable feature of kicking skill is the inclination of the body at ball contact. The body is inclined backwards to the vertical and laterally to the non-kicking side at ball contact. With regard to the trunk, Parassas, Terauds and Nathan (1990) reported a backward lean of 13° and 17° in skilled players performing a low- and high-trajectory kick, respectively. Lees and Nolan (2002) reported a backward lean of 12° and 0°, and lateral inclinations to the non-kicking side of 10° and 16° at ball contact for two professional players performing a maximal instep kick. In collegiate-level players, Orloff et al. (2008) reported trunk backward lean of 3° and 13° and a lateral lean of 3° and -8° in males and females, respectively, the negative sign indicating a lean to the kicking side.

The pelvis is retracted before support foot contact and protracts through a significant range of motion to ball contact. Mean rotation for pelvic retraction to protraction at ball contact in skilled players have been reported as 30° and 36°, respectively (Levanon and Dapena, 1998; Lees and Nolan, 2002; Lees et al., 2009). Although none of these studies established maximal ranges of motion at the joints, it is likely, given the good agreement in these data, that skilled kickers use a maximal or close to maximal pelvic range of motion.

The kicking leg has been studied widely, and recent reviews (Lees and Nolan, 1998; Kellis and Katis, 2007; Lees, Asai, Bull-Anderson, Nunome and Sterzing, 2010) have provided a good account of the kinematic and kinetic data associated with this limb. The definition of the mature skill above suggests that there are four phases to kicking leg motion. The period from kicking foot take-off to maximum hip extension is termed the *back swing phase*; the period from maximum hip extension to maximum knee flexion is termed the *leg cocking phase*; the period from maximum knee flexion to ball contact is termed the *leg acceleration phase* (Nunome, Asai, Ikegami, and Sakurai, 2002); finally, after ball contact is the *follow through phase*. The two intermediate phases are the most important from a performance point of view. The interaction between the thigh and shank can be seen in Figure 12.2, which shows their angular velocities throughout the movement. On this graph, each phase is marked, and it can be seen that during the leg cocking phase the thigh rotates forwards while the shank rotates backwards. In the leg acceleration phase both the shank and the thigh increase in angular velocity. The muscular energy for this increase must come from the muscles around

A. Lees

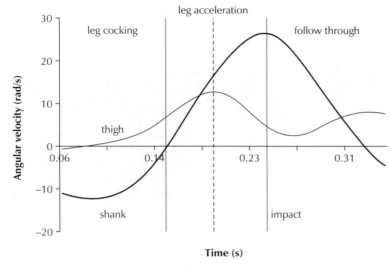

**Figure 12.2** Angular velocity of the upper leg and shank during a soccer kick. Three phases of the kick are marked, with impact being at the end of the leg acceleration phase.

the hip and thigh. In the latter part of the leg acceleration phase, just before impact, there is an increase in shank angular velocity, and at the same time a decrease in the thigh angular velocity. There appears to be an interaction between the two segments. A high angular velocity of the shank means a high foot velocity, and this is important in the production of a well-hit kick. It can be seen that, in order to achieve high foot velocity, energy must be built up in the early phases of the movement. Therefore, the range of movement that the hips and leg move through, and the muscular strength applied during these stages, will determine the maximal speed of the foot at impact.

The upper body demonstrates some important characteristics. The non-kicking-side arm is abducted and horizontally extended before support foot contact and then adducts and horizontally flexes to ball contact (Shan and Westerhoff, 2005). In addition, the shoulders are rotated such that they move out of phase with the rotation of the pelvis. This adjustment leads to a trunk twist during the preparation phase of the kick and untwist during the execution phase. Shan and Westerhoff (2005) reported that the non-kicking-side shoulder went through a range of horizontal extension of 158° and a range of abduction of 36°, as compared to 63° and 20°, respectively, during the previous running strides. The greater range of motion suggests that the non-kicking-side arm has a role to play in the kick. The horizontal elevation of the arm is frequently attributed to the maintenance of balance, but this is more likely to reflect a 'tension arc' which goes across the body from the kicking leg as it is withdrawn to the non-kicking-side arm as it is extended and abducted (Figure 12.3). The forward motion of both limbs yields a release of this tension arc (a shorten arc) and is an expression of the stretch–shorten cycle. Shan and Westerhoff (2005) also reported greater ranges of motion in the hip, knee and ankle for skilled players, as compared to novice players, suggesting a more prominent use of this stretch–shorten cycle.

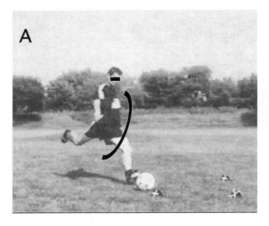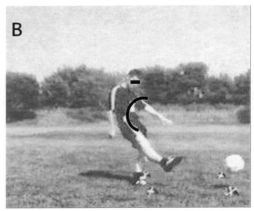

Figure 12.3  An illustration of (A) the tension arc and (B) the shorten arc.

The retraction of the kicking leg and non-kicking-side arm lead to a twist in the torso which is described by the 'hip–shoulder' separation angle. This movement is measured by the difference in orientation angles of a line representing the hip joints and a line representing the shoulder joints projected onto the transverse plane. This variable may also be considered to represent the 'tension arc'. Lees and Nolan (2002) reported that range of motion for hip–shoulder separation reached 38° and 42° for maximal instep kicks in two professional players, but was lower in sub-maximal kicks by 6° and 12° respectively. The higher values for the maximal kick suggest that hip–shoulder separation is an important performance variable.

Kicking, like many of the skills in soccer, is developmental in nature and it has been shown that it develops from an early age. Bloomfield, Elliott and Davies (1979) analysed the kicking action of young boys from the age of 2 to 12 years. They looked at various indicators of performance and were able to characterise six levels of development. These ranged from level 1 (average age 3.9 years), where the children often hit the ball with their knee or leg, to level 6 (average age 11.2 years), where the mature kicking pattern as described above had been achieved by 80% of the children. The intermediate ages for levels 2 to 5 were 4.11, 4.8, 6.11 and 8.2 years, respectively. Although chronological age was not found to be a good predictor of the level of skill development, the age ranges suggest that the skill develops rapidly between the ages of 4 and 6 years. This finding has implications for skill development in children of a very young age and is an illustration of the role biomechanics can play in this area.

Muscle strength is represented by joint moments, and these have been widely reported for kicking (for a review, see Kellis and Katis, 2007). Nunome *et al.* (2002) were the first to report full three-dimensional joint moments (i.e., for the ab/adduction and int/extension axes) for the kicking leg. Furthermore, three-dimensional joint moment data for the kicking leg have been reported by Kawamoto, Miyagi, Ohashi and Fukashiro (2007), who attributed the better performance of experienced players to the greater hip joint moments (hip flexion, adduction and external rotation were 168, 100 and 41 Nm, respectively), as compared to inexperienced players (94, 115 and 26 Nm, respectively).

It would be expected that there is a relationship between muscle strength and performance, due to the fact that the muscles are directly responsible for increasing foot velocity. Such a relationship has been reported by several researchers. Cabri et al. (1988) reported that there was a high correlation between knee flexor and extensor strength, as measured by an isokinetic muscle function dynamometer and kick distance. There was also a significant relationship between hip flexor and extensor strength, but this was weaker than that for the knee. If muscle strength is related to performance, it would be expected that training should show positive effects on ball speed or distance. De Proft et al. (1988) reported that over a season of training specific leg muscle strength, muscle strength increased and so too did kick performance as measured by distance. The correlations between leg strength and distance increased from the beginning to the end of the season.

Although the evidence reviewed above suggests that there is a good relationship between muscle strength and performance, there are other factors which contribute to successful kicks. These factors can be appreciated from a consideration of the relationship between foot and ball velocity before and after contact. By considering the mechanics of collision between the foot and ball (following the treatment of Plagenhoef, 1971), the velocity of the ball can be stated as:

$$V_{(ball)} = \frac{V_{(foot)} \cdot [M] \cdot [1 + e]}{[M + m]} \qquad (1)$$

where V = velocity of ball and foot respectively; M = effective striking mass of the leg; m = mass of the ball; and e = coefficient of restitution. The effective striking mass is the mass equivalent of the striking object (in this case the foot and leg) and relates to the rigidity of the limb.

The term $M / [M + m]$ gives an indication of the rigidity of impact and relates to the muscles involved in the kick and their strength at impact. Therefore, one would expect that the best correlations with performance would be with eccentric muscle strength, and the data from Cabri et al. (1988) suggest that this is the case.

The term $[1 + e]$ relates to the firmness of the foot at impact. Because the ball is on the ground, the foot contacts the ball on the dorsal aspect of the phalanges and lower metatarsals. The large force of impact serves to plantar-flex the foot forcefully and it will do so until the bones at the ankle joint reach their extreme range of motion. At this stage, the foot will deform at the metatarsal-phalangeal joint. There is little to prevent considerable deformation here and this will affect the firmness of impact and the value of 'e', the coefficient of restitution. If contact between the foot and ball is made closer to the ankle joint, then the impact will be firmer. In punts or drop kicks it is possible to achieve this point of contact.

The term $M / [M + m]$ would be expected to have a value of about 0.8 based on realistic data for the masses of the foot and the ball. The term $[1 + e]$ would be expected to have a value of about 1.5. Therefore, the product of the two suggests that the ball should travel at about 1.2 times the velocity of the foot; in other words, the ball leaves the foot faster than the foot is travelling. The relationship now becomes

$$V_{(ball)} = 1.2 * V_{(foot)} \qquad (2)$$

223

This ratio of ball to foot velocity is an indicator of a successful kick. Foot velocities for competent soccer players are between about 16 and 22 m.s$^{-1}$ and ball velocities are in the range of 24 to 30 m.s$^{-1}$ (Lees and Nolan, 1998), which always give a ball:foot velocity ratio greater than 1.

For submaximal kicking, there still appears to be a relationship between foot and ball velocity. Zernicke and Roberts (1978) report a regression equation between the two variables of foot and ball velocity over a ball speed range of 16 to 27 m.s$^{-1}$.

$$V_{(ball)} = 1.23 * V_{(foot)} + 2.72 \qquad (3)$$

This value is reassuringly close to the relationship for maximal kicking (equation 2) suggested above on the basis of theoretical data.

Other types of kick have also been studied. The side-foot kick is often used to make a pass. In order to make a side-foot kick, the foot has to be angled outwards. This alignment prevents the leg from flexing in the same way as it would for an instep kick. Therefore, the foot velocity during a side-foot kick is lower than during the instep kick. As contact with the ball is made on the firm bones of the shank and ankle, the foot provides a much better surface for the impact. The resultant ball velocity is much higher in the side-foot kick than it would be with the same foot velocity for an instep kick. A further advantage is that the flatter side of the foot allows a more accurate placement of the ball. Levanon and Dapena (1998) compared the instep with side-foot kicks and reported that during the side-foot kick for a right-footed player, the player orientates the pelvis, the right leg and foot more towards the right. Although the velocity of the foot at impact in the side-foot kick is lower than in the instep kick, most of the speed of the foot in both cases is generated by knee extension. Other analyses have investigated the volley (Gómez-Píriz et al., 2009), the outstep kick (Katis and Kellis, 2010) and the punt kick (McCrudden and Reilly, 1993).

## SOCCER THROW-IN

The throw-in is both a method of restarting the game and a tactical skill. Consequently, throwing-in the ball to achieve a long distance is an important soccer skill. The long-range throw-in can be performed from a stationary position or with a run-up; with feet together or feet staggered. The throw-in is initiated by bending the knees and taking the ball backwards with both hands behind the head. As the ball is travelling backwards with respect to the body, there is an upward extension of the knee joint and a marked pushing of the hips both forward and upward. These actions serve to prime the upper body for the recoil which will propel the ball forwards (Figure 12.4). As the upper body starts to come forwards there is a sequential unfolding, starting with the hips, then followed by the shoulders, elbows and finally the wrists and hands until ball release. This sequential series of rotations about the medio-lateral axis serves to build up initial rotational velocity using the large muscles of the legs and trunk first, and then to transfer this energy out towards the distal segments in order to gain high end-speed velocity as seen in Figure 12.5. This mechanism is identical in principle to that used to attain high foot velocity in the kick.

The range of a throw-in is determined by the height, angle and speed of release. As height of release is fixed for a given player, most researchers simply report the angle and speed of

224

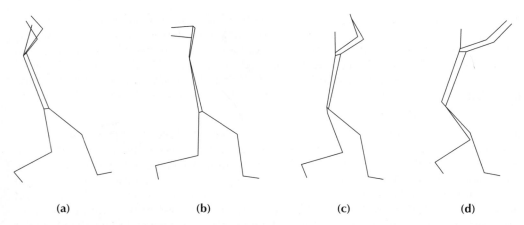

**(a)**          **(b)**          **(c)**          **(d)**

**Figure 12.4** A kinetogram of a player performing a run-up throw-in (the ball is omitted from this illustration). The different positions highlighted include: (a) retraction of ball behind the head; (b) maximum ball retraction; (c) trunk and shoulder forward flexion to bring the ball forward; and (d) elbow extension to ball release.

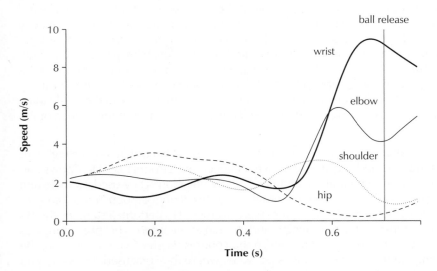

**Figure 12.5** The joint velocities for a run-up throw-in. These graphs illustrate the rapid increase in velocity achieved by the wrist and ball during the last phase of the motion.

release. Chang (1979) investigated one player performing four types of throw-in including: (a) standing square, with feet side by side; (b) standing staggered, with one foot in front of the other; (c) using a run-up and (d) handspring. Disregarding the handspring throw-in, which is not commonly used in contemporary soccer, the release velocities ranged from 14.6 to 15.2 m.s$^{-1}$ and release angles from 21 to 45° to the ground. Levendusky *et al.* (1985) investigated the staggered standing throw-in and reported a mean ball release speed of

18.3 m.s$^{-1}$ and release angle of 29°. They also identified that the throw-in followed a proximal-to-distal sequence of segment rotations from the trunk to the lower arm. Messier and Brody (1986) presented a more detailed comparison of two types of throw-in (standing staggered and handspring). The staggered throw-in produced a mean ball release velocity of 18.1 m.s$^{-1}$ and release angle of 28° to the ground. Finally, Kollath and Schwirtz (1988) reported that the mean ball release velocity was 14.2 and 15.3 m.s$^{-1}$ and release angle 33° and 32° for the standing and run-up throw-ins, respectively.

It is generally agreed that the run-up throw-in is the better technique for players to use. The potential advantage of the run-up throw-in is that the ball has an initial forward speed. However, it is not this speed which enhances the performance of the running throw-in. Lees, Kemp and Moura (2005) investigated the standing and run-up throw-ins (both using a staggered stance) in skilled players. Using three-dimensional motion analysis, they reported significantly greater release velocity, and hence range of throw, for the run-up throw-in, confirming previous findings. They attributed this greater performance to an enhanced joint torque at the shoulder. The joint torque profiles are given in Figures 12.6a and 6b. These show that the accelerating torque about the shoulders dominates with a small proximal-to-distal sequence evident for the shoulder and elbow joints. For the run-up throw-in a significant relationship was found between the negative shoulder retraction torque and the positive propulsion torque (r= -0.539), but for the standing throw-in this was non-significant. The explanation was that during the forward motion of the trunk segment there is a backward motion of the upper limb segments so a run-up produces a greater *difference* in velocity between the trunk and upper limb segments and thus a greater torque. The significantly greater retraction torque at the shoulder is strongly correlated with the following propulsive torque. It is likely that a 'stretch–shorten' cycle is occurring, where the muscles of the shoulders are forcibly stretched (due to the greater velocity difference between segments in the run-up throw) and then allowed to shorten rapidly. This action leads to an increase in the pre-loading of muscle and, as a result, more work is done, explaining the enhanced performance of the run-up throw-in.

Strength and practice affect the performance of most skills, so it is likely that training regimens based on strength training and practice will have an effect on performance. De Carnys and Lees (2009) reported a strength training and practice investigation. They used 13 male and 10 female skilled players who were divided into three groups (control group N = 7; strength group N = 9; practice group N = 7). Participants were instructed to perform 5 standing throws and 5 throws with a run-up of 5 m in length and the range recorded. This procedure was repeated once a week for 6 weeks, during which the controls received no intervention, the practice group completed 3 practice sessions per week where they practised throw-ins, and the strength group attended a twice-weekly session during which a set muscle strength training routine was followed. There was an improvement in performance for the intervention groups between weeks 1 and 6. For the run-up throw-in, both strength training (from 17.05 m to 18.27 m) and practice (from 16.40 m to 17.81 m) were found to significantly increase performance. The increase in range was due to the increase in speed of release. It was suggested that a combination of the two practice regimens might be the most effective.

Other forms of the throw-in skill have appeared in order to take advantage of its attacking capability. One such variant is the 'handspring' throw-in, which first appeared in US collegiate football during the 1980s (Messier and Brody, 1986). The player runs up with the ball in both

# 226

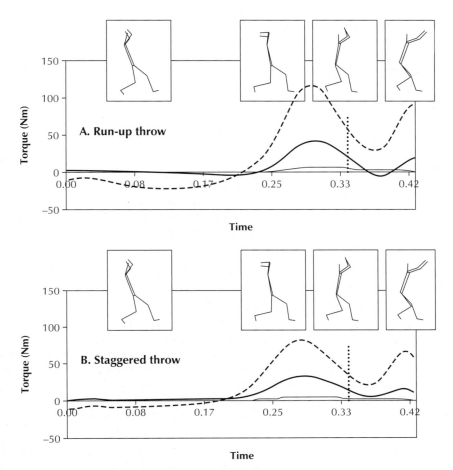

**Figure 12.6** Joint torque at the shoulder (thick line), elbow (medium line) and wrist (thin line) for (a) the run-up throw-in and (b) the staggered throw-in. Note the greater (negative) retraction torque during the earlier stages of the run-up throw. The dashed line indicates release.

hands. The ball is placed on the ground and the player rotates over it as in a handspring. After the feet hit the ground the body is rotating forwards with the arms and ball over the head. During the recovery from the handspring the ball is released. The rules state that for a throw-in to be legal the player must face the field of play, have both feet in contact with the ground, be on or outside the touchline at release and deliver the ball from behind and over the head using both hands equally. The handspring throw-in is a novel approach to the throw-in which does not contravene the rule. The advantage of this type of throw is that it has a greater velocity of release and, consequently, a greater range. Data for the two groups at ball release are shown in Table 12.1 and show that the handspring throw-in achieves considerably greater range with a lower angle of projection than the conventional throw-in. The handspring throw-in would therefore be more suitable for playing strategies requiring a fast long-range delivery.

**Table 12.1** Mechanical data for the conventional and handspring throw-in at release.

|  | Conventional | Handspring |
|---|---|---|
| Ball velocity (m.s$^{-1}$) | 18.1 | 23.0 |
| Angle of release (deg) | 28.0 | 23.0 |
| Distance (m) | 29.3 | 44.0 |

## GOAL-KEEPING

Goal-keeping skills are important in preventing opponents from scoring. The goal-keeper has to anticipate attacks on goal and be positioned accordingly. There are a number of movement skills that the goal-keeper needs to master, but very few of them have been subjected to biomechanical analysis.

With regard to positioning, Figure 12.7 shows the position that the goalkeeper adopts to reduce the angle of shot from the opponent.

The diving motion made by goal-keepers in saving a set (penalty) shot was reported by Suzuki *et al.* (1988). They analysed two skilled and two less skilled goalkeepers in terms of their ability to dive and save. They found that the more skilled keepers dived faster (4 m.s$^{-1}$ as opposed to 3 m.s$^{-1}$) and more directly at the ball. In this case the skilled keeper was able to perform a counter-movement jump and launch himself into the air and then turn to meet the ball. The less skilled keeper failed to perform a counter-movement, thereby restricting take-off velocity and failing to turn the body effectively to meet the ball. In this analysis, both quantitative and qualitative methods were used to clarify the differences in performance between the two groups.

Spratford, Mellifont and Burkett (2009) quantified the movement patterns of six elite goalkeepers making diving saves to their preferred and non-preferred side at three different dive heights. Synchronised three-dimensional kinematic and kinetic biomechanical data

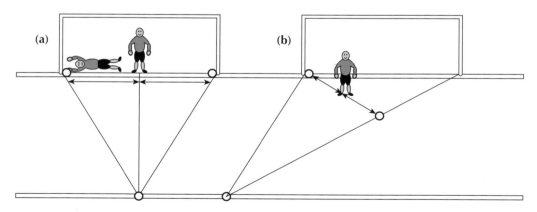

**Figure 12.7** Diagram to show how the goal-keeper's diving range changes with ball position.

A. Lees

analysis found the diving direction to significantly influence the movement patterns of the diving save. The non-preferred side displayed greater lateral rotation of the pelvis and thorax at the initiation event. At take-off the thorax displayed no significant difference in rotation, although a difference still remained for the pelvis. These over-rotations were subsequently linked to greater peak knee joint moments, lower peak ankle joint moments, less hip extension at take-off, and the centre of mass to travelling more slowly and less directly to the ball. Thus, there would appear to be an advantage in having prior knowledge of limb preference in an opposing goal-keeper, who will be less effective diving to the non-preferred side.

In an analysis of goal-keeping dive actions, Graham-Smith, Lees and Richardson (1999) conducted an investigation whereby a ball was projected into several areas of the goalmouth (A–L in Figure 12.8). Seven basic goal-keeping actions were identified, as indicated in the shaded areas of Figure 12.8 and in Table 12.2. These actions were characterised by the use of a cross-over and side-steps when reaching for the ball.

The penalty kick in soccer is a major set piece which offers the opportunity to score goals and, with penalty shoot-outs common in major tournaments, to win games. Two types of strategy used by goal-keepers have been suggested by Khun (1988). These are an 'early strategy' and 'late strategy'. In the former, the goal-keeper dives before the ball is hit while in the latter the goalkeeper dives at contact or after the ball was hit. In European club matches, Khun (1988) reported that 77% of dives were early, while only 23% were late. However, the late-strategy dives were more successful, with a 60% chance of success, as compared to only 8% success for the early strategy. A trend for the preferred use of the late strategy was suggested by Morya, Bigatão, Lees and Ranvaud (2005), based on evidence from club matches and from the 2002 World Cup, where around 40% of the dives were late. Although the success rate of these dives was less (around 36%) than that reported by Khun (1988), they were more successful than the early dives, which still had a low success rate of around 11%. Thus, the late strategy would seem to be a beneficial strategy for goalkeepers to use. When using a late strategy, the goal-keeper must look for visual cues from the kicker's actions before ball contact in order to help his/her decision making.

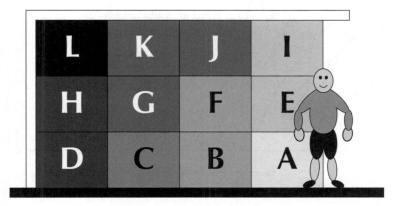

**Figure 12.8** Diagram to show the 12 goal-keeping areas and their relationship to the 7 diving actions.

**Table 12.2** Goal-keeping action types used to save in each of the 12 goal areas of Figure 12.8.

| Goal-keeping action | Cross-over step | Side step |
|---|---|---|
| Type 1 area A<br>Collapse both legs and drop to ground | 0 | 0 |
| Type 2 area E and I<br>Single or 2 legged jump to get in line with ball | 0 | 0 |
| Type 3 area B and F<br>Right leg comes under body and dive off left leg | 0 | 1 |
| Type 4 area C<br>Small step to right followed by low dive driving off left leg | 0 | 1 |
| Type 5 area G, J and K<br>Small step followed by drive upwards off right leg | 0 | 1 |
| Type 6 area D and H<br>Crossover step before diving off left leg | 1 | 0 |
| Type 7 area L<br>2 cross over steps and dive off right leg | 2 | 0 |

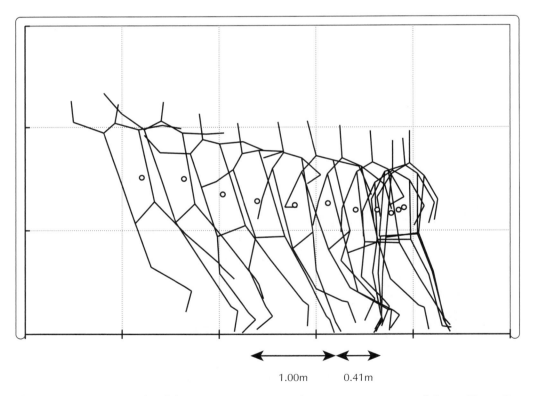

1.00m     0.41m

**Figure 12.9** An example of diving action Type 7 with two cross-over steps followed by a dive from the right leg.

When taking a penalty two types of kick are commonly used, depending on the desired outcome of the kick. The instep kick is used when a faster ball speed is required, while the side-foot kick is used where more precision is required. In a typical penalty kick, the player may decide to kick the ball powerfully or kick the ball more accurately. Sixteen out of the 17 penalty kicks in the 2006 World Cup tournament were taken using the side-foot technique, indicating the importance of accurate placement over ball speed. Generally, for a side-foot kick, which is kicked straight ahead, players tended to orientate the pelvis towards the kicking leg side and to externally rotate the kicking leg and foot in order to orientate the side of the foot to the intended direction of ball travel. These changes in the orientation of segments as the kick unfolds could provide postural cues for the goal-keeper to decide on the likely direction the ball will take.

The ability of goal-keepers to use postural cues is important in sports where the ball velocity dictates the decisions that must be made in advance of the action. If the goal-keeper could employ an anticipatory method for where the ball is likely to be kicked, there would be a greater chance that the penalty kick could be saved. Using notational analysis methods, Franks and Harvey (1997) studied all penalty kicks in World Cup competitions from 1982 to 1994 and concluded that the placement of the support foot 200–250 ms before ball contact was the earliest reliable predictor of where the shot was likely to result. Lees and Owens (2011) investigated this and other possible cues and found that at kicking foot take-off (about 200 ms before contact) differences were evident in the progression angle of the support. For goal-keepers to use a 'late strategy' where they move at or after ball contact they must use visual cues and make a decision on which way to dive as early as during the period of support of the kicking foot prior to ball contact. Of the cues investigated, the best one seemed to be the orientation of the support foot as it is brought through and before it is planted on the ground. In general terms, the orientation of the support foot indicates the direction of the ball, so a foot orientated to the kicker's left indicates a ball travelling to the kicker's left, while a more forward orientation indicates a ball travelling straight ahead. Other cues are available, such as the rotation of the pelvis and extension of the hip, but these are more ambiguous with regard to interpretation, and others are available but occur too late for the goal-keeper to use.

## SUMMARY

This overview has illustrated the way in which biomechanics can be applied to gain an insight into the performance of skills in soccer. Many skills in the game are amenable to biomechanical analysis and several of them have now been analysed in depth. The most frequently analysed skill is kicking and we now know much about different forms of the kick, including the instep, side-foot, outside foot, volley and punt kicks. The kick is often described in temporal phases, and biomechanical analyses have described the main kinematic and kinetic features of each. Attempts have been made to explain the importance of the sequence of actions which unfold as the kick progresses and biomechanical analysis has helped us to understand the factors that affect performance. These factors relate to the influence of the upper body, biological mechanisms (such as the stretch–shorten cycle and proximal-to-distal sequencing) and foot–ball interaction. Physical factors such as muscle strength have also been shown to play a role in the performance of the kick. The developmental nature of the kick has also been of interest to researchers.

The throw-in and goal-keeping have been other skills analysed biomechanically. The benefits of one style of performance over another have been established and the underlying explanations for their success given. There are various ways to perform these skills but good performances are characterised by sound technique, utilisation of biological mechanism of performance and muscle strength. It is necessary to develop these aspects through practice and training and it would be particularly important to include a formal programme of skill development based on biomechanical analysis in a practical setting.

It is evident that there are other soccer skills not addressed in this chapter. They are important to the game but have received little attention at this time. It is likely, with the development of analytical methods and a widening of interest in the analysis of soccer skills, that these shortfalls will be addressed. There are still many opportunities for biomechanists to apply their analytical methods to soccer skills and to contribute to the development of soccer science.

## REFERENCES

Bloomfield, J., Elliott, B. C. and Davies, C. M. (1979). Development of the punt kick: a cinematographical analysis. *Journal of Human Movement Studies* 6, 142–150.

Cabri, J., De Proft, E., Dufour, W. and Clarys, J. P. (1988). The relation between muscular strength and kick performance. In T. Reilly, A. Lees, K. Davids and W. J. Murphy (eds), *Science and Football* (pp.186–193). London: E. and F. N. Spon.

Chang, J. (1979). The biomechanical analysis of selected soccer throw-in techniques. *Asian Journal of Physical Education* 2, 254–260.

De Carnys, G. and Lees, A. (2009). The effect of strength training and practice on soccer throw-in performance. In T. Reilly and F. Korkusuz (eds), *Science and Football VI* (pp. 302–307). Oxford: Routledge.

De Proft, E., Cabri, J., Dufour, W. and Clarys, J. P. (1988). Strength training and kick performance in soccer. In T. Reilly, A. Lees, K. Davids and W. J. Murphy (eds), *Science and Football* (pp.108–113). London: E. and F. N. Spon.

Egan, C. D., Vwerheul, M. H. G. and Savelsbergh, G. J. P. (2007). Effects of experience on the coordination of internally and externally timed soccer kicks. *Journal of Motor Behaviour* 39, 423–432.

Franks, I. M. and Harvey, T. (1997) Cues for goalkeepers: high-tech methods used to measure penalty shot response. *Soccer Journal* 42, 30–38

Gómez Píriz, P. T., Gutiérrez Dávila, M., Cabello Manrique, D., and Lees, A. (2009) Biomechanics of the volley kick by the soccer goalkeeper. In B. Drust, T. Reilly, and A. M. Williams (eds), *International Research in Science and Soccer* (pp. 47–53). London: Routledge.

Graham-Smith, P., Lees, A. and Richardson, D. (1999) Analysis of technique of goalkeepers during the penalty kick. *Journal of Sports Sciences* 19, 916.

Isokawa, M. and Lees, A. (1988). A biomechanical analysis of the instep kick motion in soccer. In T. Reilly, A. Lees, K. Davids and W. J. Murphy (eds), *Science and Football* (pp. 449–455). London: E. and F. N. Spon.

Katis, A. and Kellis, E. (2010). Three-dimensional kinematics and ground reaction forces during the instep and outstep soccer kicks in pubertal players. *Journal of Sports Sciences* 28, 1233–1241.

Kawamoto, R., Miyagi, O., Ohashi, J. and Fukashiro, S. (2007). Kinetic comparison of a side foot soccer kick between experienced and inexperienced players. *Sports Biomechanics* 6, 187–198

Kellis, E. and Katis, A. (2007). Biomechanical characteristics and determinants of instep soccer kick. *Journal of Sports Science and Medicine* 6, 154–165.

Kellis, E., Katis, A., and Gissis, I. (2004). Knee biomechanics of the support leg in soccer kicks from three angles of approach. *Medicine and Science in Sports and Exercise* 36, 1017–1028.

Khun, W. (1988). Penalty-kick strategies for shooters and goalkeepers. In T. Reilly, A. Lees, K. Davids and W. J. Murphy (eds), *Science and Football* (pp. 489–492). London: E. and F. N. Spon.

Kollath, E. and Schwirtz, A. (1988). Biomechanical of the soccer throw-in. In T. Reilly, A. Lees, K. Davids and W. J. Murphy (eds), *Science and Football* (pp 460–467). London: E. and F. N. Spon.

Lees, A. and Nolan, L. (1998) Biomechanics of soccer – a review. *Journal of Sports Sciences* 16, 211–234.

Lees, A. and Nolan, L. (2002). Three dimensional kinematic analysis of the instep kick under speed and accuracy conditions. In W. Spinks, T. Reilly and A. Murphy (eds), *Science and Football IV* (pp. 16–21). London: E. and F. N. Spon.

Lees, A. and Owens, L. (2011). Early visual cues associated with a directional place kick in soccer. *Sports Biomechanics* 10, 126–135.

Lees, A., Kemp, M. and Moura, F. (2005). A biomechanical analysis of the soccer throw-in with a particular focus on the upper limb motion. In T. Reilly, J. Cabri and D. Araujo (eds), *Science and Football V* (pp. 89–94). London: Routledge.

Lees, A., Steward, I., Rahnama, N. and Barton, G. (2009). Understanding lower limb function in the performance of the maximal instep kick in soccer. In T. Reilly and G. Atkinson (eds), *Proceedings of the 6th International Conference on Sport, Leisure and Ergonomics* (pp. 149–160). London: Routledge.

Lees, A., Asai, T., Bull-Anderson, T., Nunome, H. and Sterzing, T. (2010). The biomechanics of kicking: A review. *Journal of Sports Sciences* 28, 805–817.

Levanon, J. and Dapena, J. (1998) Comparison of the kinematics of the full-instep and pass kicks in soccer. *Medicine and Science in Sports and Exercise* 30, 917–927.

Levendusky, T. A., Clinger, C. D., Miller, R. E. and Armstrong, C. W. (1985) Soccer throw-in kinematics. In J. Terauds and J. N. Barham (eds), *Biomechanics in Sports II* (pp. 258–268). California: Del Mar.

McCrudden, M. and Reilly, T. (1993). A comparison of the punt and the drop-kick. In T. Reilly, J. Clarys and A. Stibbe (eds), *Science and Football II* (pp. 362–368). London: E. and F. N. Spon.

Messier, S. P. and Brody, M. A. (1986). Mechanics of translation and rotation during conventional and handspring soccer throw-ins. *International Journal of Sport Biomechanics* 2, 301–315.

Morya, E., Bigatão, H., Lees, A. and Ranvaud, R. (2005). Evolving penalty kick strategies: world cup and club matches 2000–2002. In T. Reilly, J. Cabri and D. Araujo (eds), *Science and Football V* (pp. 236–242). London: Routledge.

233

Nunome, H., Asai, T., Ikegami, Y. and Sakurai, S. (2002). Three dimensional kinetic analysis of side-foot and instep kicks. *Medicine and Science in Sports and Exercise* 34, 2028–2036.

Orloff, H., Sumida, B., Chow, J., Habibi, L., Fujino, A. and Kramer, B. (2008). Ground reaction forces and kinematics of plant leg position during instep kicking in male and female collegiate soccer players. *Sports Biomechanics* 7, 238–247.

Parassas, S. G., Terauds, J. and Nathan, T. (1990). Three dimensional kinematic analysis of high and low trajectory kicks in soccer. In N. Nosek, D. Sojka, W. Morrison and P. Susanka (eds), *Proceedings of the VIIIth Symposium of the International Society of Biomechanics in Sports* (pp. 145–149). Prague: Conex.

Plagenhoef, S. (1971). *The Patterns of Human Motion*. New Jersey: Prentice-Hall.

Shan, G. and Westerhoff, W. (2005). Full-body kinematic characteristics of the maximal instep kick by male soccer players and parameters related to kick quality. *Sports Biomechanics* 4, 59–72.

Spratford, W., Mellifont, R., and Burkett, B. (2009). The influence of dive direction on the movement characteristics for elite football goalkeepers. *Sports Biomechanics* 8, 235–244.

Suzuki, S., Togari, H., Isokawa, M., Ohashi, J. and Ohgushi, T. (1988). Analysis of the goalkeeper's diving motion. In T. Reilly, A. Lees, K. Davids and W. J. Murphy (eds), *Science and Football* (pp. 468–475). London: E. and F. N. Spon.

Wickstrom, R. L. (1975). Developmental kinesiology. *Exercise and Sports Science Reviews* 3, 163–192.

Zernicke, R. and Roberts, E. M. (1978). Lower extremity forces and torques during systematic variation of non-weight bearing motion. *Medicine and Science in Sports* 10, 21–26.

A. Lees

# PART IV
# DIFFERENT POPULATIONS

# CHAPTER 13

## WOMEN'S SOCCER

D. Scott and H. Andersson

## INTRODUCTION

Women's soccer has over 29 million participants around the world and in 2010 it was reported that 512 international matches were played by 141 countries (Fédération Internationale de Football Association [FIFA], 2011). Germany and the United States of America (USA), two of the leading countries in the development of women's soccer, each have over 1 million registered female players (Deutscher Fussball-Bund, 2011). The women's game gained more credibility in 2007 during the Fifth World Cup Finals in China, since FIFA allocated prize money for the qualifying teams and for the teams that advanced from the group stages, thereby indicating a growing interest in, and recognition of, the women's game on the world stage. In the 2011 World Cup finals in Germany, 73,000 spectators attended the opening game in Berlin and 14.1 million viewers watched it on TV in Germany (20% of the German population), showing the increasing public popularity of female soccer. Furthermore, the career opportunities for female players are growing and players are now able to train and compete full time. Several countries, such as Germany, Sweden, England, France, the USA and Russia have full- and part-time professional players competing in their leagues, including overseas international players. Consequently, along with the growing professional environment for female players the work profile and the physical demands for elite players are also increasing, meaning that players need to plan and prepare more optimally for match-play.

The majority of the scientific research on soccer is based on male players. Recently, however, researchers have attempted to address gaps in the scientific literature on female players by focusing on the unique aspects of the women's game in regard to nutrition (Martin, Lambeth, and Scott, 2005), physical characteristics (Vescovi, Rupf, Brown, and Marques, 2011), performance testing (Castagna, Impellizzeri, Manzi, and Ditroilo, 2010), fatigue and recovery (Andersson et al., 2008; Sjökvist et al., 2011) and the physical demands during game play (Krustrup, Mohr, Ellingsgaard, and Bangsbo, 2005; Gabbett and Mulvey, 2008; Mohr, Krustrup, Andersson, Kirkendal, and Bangsbo, 2008; Krustrup, Zebis, Jensen, and Mohr, 2010; Andersson, Randers, Heiner-Møller, Krustrup, and Mohr, 2010). In this chapter, specific considerations for female players are addressed, and include recent scientific research and highlight the current status and physical standards of elite female players competing on the world stage.

## PHYSICAL CHARACTERISTICS

The physical characteristics of female players from varying levels of competition have been well described in the literature. The mean values for height (158–170 cm), weight (55–65 kg) and $\dot{V}O_{2max}$ (38.6 mL.kg$^{-1}$.min$^{-1}$ to 57.6 mL.kg$^{-1}$.min$^{-1}$) vary, depending on the position on the field and measuring methods employed (Davis and Brewer, 1993; Jensen and Larsson, 1992; Polman, Walsh, Bloomfield, and Nesti, 2004; Rhodes and Mosher, 1992; Siegler, Gaskill, and Ruby, 2003; Tamer, Gunay, Tiryaki, Cicioolu, and Erol, 1997; Tumilty and Darby, 1992). Recently, data on the specific physical characteristics of *elite* female players have been published (Andersson, Ekblom, and Krustrup, 2007; Krustrup et al., 2005; Krustrup et al., 2010; Gabbett and Mulvey, 2008; Sjökvist et al., 2011). A summary of the physical characteristics of elite female players is shown in Table 13.1. The mean values for height, weight, age, percentage of body fat, $\dot{V}O_{2max}$, YOYO IE-2 and YOYO IR-1 test (two soccer-specific endurance tests), maximal sprint time and countermovement jump (CMJ) from some of the most successful nations in women's soccer are presented. The table shows that the elite female player is on average 20–26 years old (range), 162–171 cm tall and weighs 58–65 kg. The performance measurements show an average maximal oxygen uptake ranges between 49–55 mL.kg$^{-1}$.min$^{-1}$, an average 10-m sprint time of 1.79–2.31 s, and that the average jump height is 29–35 cm. In the more football-specific endurance test the players run on average 1265–2182 m in the YOYO IE-2 test and 1097–1379 m in the YOYO IR-1 test. Nevertheless, top female players in the US and Swedish National leagues were reported to run > 2000 m in the YOYO IR-1 test and jump higher than 45 cm, in recent unpublished data.

## GAME LOAD

### Physical load during a game

Published reports dating back to the early 1990s indicate that female soccer players covered approximately 8.5 km in total distance during a game (Davis and Brewer, 1993). More recent reports show that the total distance covered during a game is approximately 10 km (Andersson et al., 2010; Mohr et al., 2008), which is similar to that reported in male players (Mohr, Krustrup, and Bangsbo, 2003). The running distance at high speeds (above 15 km/h) during a game is, however, reported to be lower for female players (~1.3–1.5 km) (Krustrup et al., 2005; Andersson et al., 2010), as compared to elite male players (~ 1.9–2.4 km) (Mohr et al., 2003). The different physiological characteristics of male and female players may account for these differences, with male players generally having a greater level of aerobic capacity and faster sprint speeds than female players. Nevertheless, when comparing high-level male players in a Nordic domestic league to top-class female players during international games the difference in high-speed distances is not great (~1.9 km vs. 1.7 km) (Mohr et al., 2008). This finding suggests that top international female players have the physical ability to run similar distances at high speeds as professional male players. Furthermore, the distances covered at high speeds seem to differ more depending on the competition level in both male and female players rather than gender differences (Mohr et al., 2003; Mohr et al., 2008). Similarly it was reported that top-class female players ran further at high speeds (1.68±0.09 km), compared to high-level female players at a lower competition level (1.33±0.10 km) (Mohr et al., 2008).

## 238

**Table 13.1** Physical characteristics and physical performance measurements of elite female players.

| Nationality/ author | Year | Competition level | n | Age (yrs) | Height (cm) | Weight (kg) | % body fat | $\dot{V}O_{2max}$ $(ml.kg^{-1}$ $.min^{-1})$ | YOYO IE-2 test (m) | YOYO IR-1 test (m) | 20-m sprint (s) | 30-m sprint (s) | CMJ (cm) |
|---|---|---|---|---|---|---|---|---|---|---|---|---|---|
| Australia/ Gabbett and Mulvey 2008 | 2008 | Highest div. | 13 | 21 ±2 | | | | 51.4 ±5.4 | | | | | |
| Denmark/ Krustrup et al. 2005 | 2005 | Highest div. | 14 | 24 | 167 | 58.5 | 14.6 [§] | 49.4 | | 1379 | | | |
| Denmark/ Krustrup et al. 2010 | 2010 | Highest div. | 23 | 23 | 169 | 60.1 | 18.5[§] | 52.3 ±1.3 | 1265 ±133 | | | | 35 ±1 |
| England/ unpublished data | 2004 | Highest div. | 22 | 24 ±2 | 162 ±1 | 61.7 ±6 | 22.1[§] | | | | | | |
| England/ unpublished data | 2009 | National team | 27 | 25 ±3 | 168 ±1 | 62.1 ±6 | 17.2[§] | | 2182 ±89 | | | | |
| Norway/ unpublished data* | 2008 | Highest div. | 9 | 21 ±2 | 167 ±2 | 62.0 ±1.6 | | 54.1 ±0.2 | | | 1.80 ±0.02 | 3.21 ±0.03 | 29.3 ±1.4 |
| Sweden / unpublished data | 2010 | National team | 17 | 26 | 171 ±1 | 64.2 ±1 | | | 1744 ±65 | | 1.79 ±0.01 | 3.16 ±0.02 | 31.4 ±1.0 |

Table 13.1 Continued

| Nationality/ author | Year | Competition level | n | Age (yrs) | Height (cm) | Weight (kg) | % body fat | $\dot{V}O_{2max}$ $(ml.kg^{-1}$ $.min^{-1})$ | YOYO IE-2 test (m) | YOYO IR-1 test (m) | 20-m sprint (s) | 30-m sprint (s) | CMJ (cm) |
|---|---|---|---|---|---|---|---|---|---|---|---|---|---|
| Sweden/ unpublished data* | 2008 | Highest div. | 9 | 23 ±4 | 168 ±2 | 64.5 ±2.2 | | 54.9 ±1.3 | | | 1.79 ±0.02 | 3.17 ±0.02 | 30.8 ±1.0 |
| USA/ unpublished data | 2008 | National team | 18 | 25 ±1 | 169 ±1 | 65.7 ±1 | | | 1824 ±87 | | | | |
| USA/McCurdy et al. 2010 | 2010 | Div. I (NCAA) | 15 | 20 ±1 | 165 ±2 | 61.7 ±7.7 | | | | | 2.31± 0.25 | | |
| USA/Sjökvist et al. 2011 | 2011 | Div. I (NCAA) | 14 | 20 ±2 | 168 ±4 | 61.9 ±6.5 | 20.9 ±3.4[†] | 53.9 ±5.7 | | 1097 ±100 | | 3.59 ±0.17 | |

Notes:
[†] Body fat measured with skin-fold calipers (three sites; Jackson et al., 1980).
[§] Skin-fold calipers (four sites, Durnin and Womersley, 1974).
* Unpublished data that originates from Anderson et al., 2008.

Also, the same female players were reported to cover further distances in high speeds during international games (1.53±0.1 km), as compared to domestic games (1.33±0.9 km), despite playing in the same position (Andersson *et al.*, 2010; Gabbett and Mulvey, 2008). Such findings further suggest that the distance at high speeds during a game relates to the level of competition.

In addition, unpublished research using more advanced technology (GPS units) has shown top-class players to cover 10.0±0.4 km in total distances and 1.86±0.26 km in high-intensity running, which is similar to the previous findings using traditional, video-based motion analysis methods. Since GPS is a more efficient tool for gathering data compared to video-based motion analysis, it is now more frequently used to assess the distance covered during training and match-play.

The relative aerobic load during a game is reported not to differ between female and male players showing average heart rate values of approximately 85–90% of heart rate maximum ($HR_{max}$), which corresponds to ~70% of $\dot{V}O_{2max}$ (Andersson *et al.*, 2010; Bangsbo, 1994). The aerobic load during a game is slightly different, depending on the field position. Figure 13.1 presents a typical heart rate profile during an international game for a central defender, central midfielder and forward. The heart rate was somewhat higher for the central midfielder compared to the defender and forward, more specifically the average HR for the defender was 85% of $HR_{max}$ in the first half and 82% of $HR_{max}$ in the second half, 89% and 87% of $HR_{max}$ for the midfielder, and 85% and 83% of $HR_{max}$ for the forward, respectively.

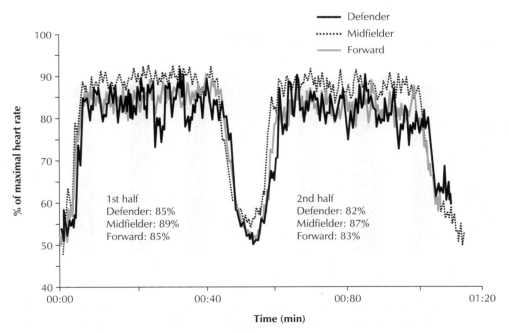

**Figure 13.1** The heart rate in % of $HR_{max}$ during an international game for a central defender, central midfielder, and forward.

The heart rate response throughout games, divided into 15-min periods, is depicted in Figure 13.2. The data are from international and domestic games (unpublished data) and show that the heart rate is high throughout the games. It also shows that the heart rate is somewhat higher in the international compared to the domestic game. Nevertheless, although the heart rate is high throughout the game, several studies have shown that the distance in high-intensity running (HIR) is lowered towards the end of the game, possibly suggesting development of fatigue (Andersson et al., 2010; Krustrup et al., 2005; Mohr et al., 2008). In Figure 13.3 the amount of HIR distance, divided into 15-min periods, during international and domestic games is displayed. The players covered less HIR during the last 15-min, as compared to any of the 15-min blocks during the first 60 min of the international game. Similarly, during the domestic games players covered less HIR distance in the last 15-min, as compared to any of the 15-min blocks during the first 45 min of games. These results indicate that although the aerobic load, measured as heart rate, is similar throughout the game, players perform less HIR running towards the end of games. Hence, heart rate measure alone may not be the most accurate way to estimate the total physical work performed by a player during match-play. Total physical work load should instead be evaluated more accurately by using a combination of methods such as heart rate and distances covered (GPS) during games.

Collectively, data on the physiological response in elite players during games have shown that the distance covered at high speeds, the occurrence of fatigue towards the end of games and high heart rate values indicate that the physical load is high during games for elite female players. It is therefore apparent that female players need to be optimally prepared physically to meet the physical demands required during match-play.

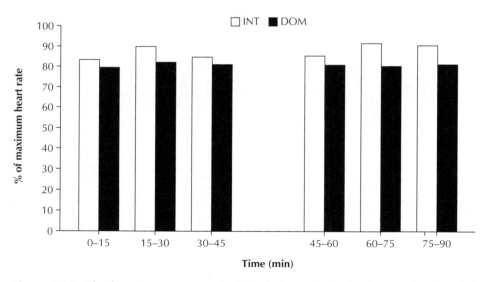

**Figure 13.2** The heart rate response in 15-min intervals during international and domestic games (English players – unpublished data). The heart rate is high throughout the game in both game types. The heart rate was slightly higher in the international compared to the domestic games.

D. Scott and H. Andersson

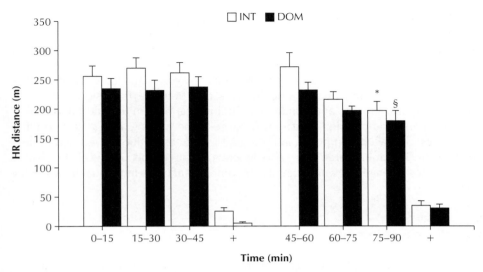

**Figure 13.3** The distance of high-intensity running performed during an international and domestic league game in 15-min intervals (Scandinavian players, Andersson *et al*. 2010).

*Note*: * indicates significantly (p<0.05) less HIR distance compared to the first 60 min of the international games and § significantly less HIR distance compared to the first 45 min of the domestic game.

*Source*: Figure reprinted with permission from the National Strength and Conditioning Association, World Headquarters, Bob Johnson Drive, Colorado Springs, CO, USA.

## Game frequency

The competitive season and thus the game frequency for many elite female players has increased greatly during the last decade, largely due to the introduction of more professional leagues. The competitive season can typically last for 7–8 months. In addition, there is a pre-season phase of training that can last for anywhere between 3 and 12 weeks, depending on the country and/or level of competition (Figure 13.4). The number of competitive games during a season depends on the level of competition of the individual player. Top elite female players will typically compete in 50–60 games during a major international tournament year, encompassing domestic league and cup games, club European games and national team games. Such game exposure is not too dissimilar to that of elite male players. The training and physical preparation of elite female players is therefore crucial to ensure optimisation of game performance, as well as maintenance of injury and health status throughout the demanding season.

## TRAINING LOAD

### Training frequency

The training frequency has also increased for elite female players in the last decade. In most countries that have a professional league, players can train 7–10 sessions per week (encompassing physical strength and conditioning training, and team technical and tactical training sessions) and compete in 1–2 games per week. The training and game frequency usually decreases for players competing in leagues at lower competition levels and in non-professional teams. The training frequency also depends on the competition level, the coach's strategy, the domestic league in which the player competes and the individual needs of the player.

### Training volume and intensity

In order to cope with the frequent and high load in match play, the training sessions of an elite female player must have sufficient volume and intensity to physically prepare in an optimal way. As mentioned above, training contains both physical conditioning and team tactical/technical training elements. The physical training consists of several different periods during a year, commonly known as macrocycles. An example of an annual plan for an elite female player is displayed in Figure 13.4. The season is structured in such a way that the players have to perform multiple games throughout a year, not just one major competition per year, as in many individual sports. A challenge for the support staff of the club and country is to integrate the competitive phase of both the domestic and international programmes, whilst at the same time optimising the physical development of each individual player. To ensure the training volume and intensity are sufficient to accrue the desired physical fitness levels at the optimal times, physical monitoring and tapering of the players becomes crucial. Monitoring players is also important to ensure correct recovery in preparation for games. Moreover, planning and preparation should include the challenges of travel (such as jet lag and travel fatigue), nutrition, hydration and training schedule at the new destination. All of these factors combined will have an effect on the training efficiency, potential health and injury risk of players, and, most importantly, performance and success during games.

### Strength training

Strength training is essential for female players to develop a good strength base, for injury prevention and subsequently to develop power and explosiveness. Strength training is typically included in the annual plan, consisting of a general preparation phase, a specific phase and a maintenance phase (Figure 13.4). In the general preparation phase (early in the pre-season), strength training may comprise two to three training sessions per week, and includes exercises to improve general strength and injury prevention (for example, core and knee-stability, and hamstring exercises). In the specific preparation phase (later in the pre-season), strength training is intended to develop power and explosiveness (for example, clean and jerk, snatch, and plyometric-type exercises). The competition period may include one to two strength sessions

244

**An Example of a Periodised Training Year for an International Player**

| | January | February | March | April | May | June | July | August | September | October | November | December |
|---|---|---|---|---|---|---|---|---|---|---|---|---|
| Domestic Phase | | | | | | Competition Period | | | | | | |
| International Competition | Training Camp / China Cup | Training Camp | Algarve Cup | Away Fixture | Home Fixture | World Cup Finals | | | Training Camp | Home Fixture | Home Fixture | Training Camp |
| Phase of Preparation | Gen-Specific Phase | Specific Preparation | | Maintenance of Fitness and Recovery for Game Play | | | | | Regeneration | Transition | General Preparation | |
| Type of Physical Training | Shift from aerobic/strength fitness sessions to explosive/power training | Shift to more speed and power physical focus, individual fitness requirements and more game play | | Maintenance of components of fitness developed during the preparation phases of training, increasing amount of technical training, more game play, more recovery sessions to recover following games and prepare for forthcoming games | | | | | Alternative sports, non-impact aerobic | Gradual increase in volume and intensity of training | Strength and aerobic development focus, with unloading and transition periods of training | |

**Figure 13.4**  An example of a training periodisation over a year for an elite female player.

per week, and the aim is mostly to maintain the strength developed during pre-season and for completion of pre-habilitation exercises for individual players.

As mentioned, strength training is central to injury prevention, especially during a relatively long competitive season. Some types of injuries are more common in female players than in male players. The incidence of anterior cruciate ligament injuries has, for example, been reported to be higher among female than male players, especially in youth players (Prodromos, Han, Rogowski, Joyce, and Shi, 2007). At present, there is a lack of scientific evidence explaining the exact cause for this higher incidence of ACL injuries in women, but high game frequency relative to age (Söderman, Pietilä, Alfredson, and Werner, 2002), as well as differences in anatomical and biomechanical factors between female and males have been suggested as contributing factors (Hewett, Myer, and Ford, 2006). Some researchers have shown that regular inclusion of specific knee injury prevention programmes in training may reduce the occurrence of ACL-injury risk in young female players (Mandelbaum et al., 2005; Gilchrist et al., 2008; Bien, 2011). These reports emphasise the importance of including regular strength and knee-stability training for female players, especially young players. Special attention should therefore be devoted to correct strength-training technique and optimal muscle strength in certain muscle groups such as the gluteus maximus (for example, lunges, single leg Romanian dead lifts (RDL)), hamstring-quadriceps strength ratio (for example, back squats, dead-lifts, good-mornings), as well as muscles involved in core strength and stability.

### Endurance training

The aerobic endurance capacity for soccer players is important, as it enables players to train at high volumes and increase their recovery potential. As shown in Table 13.1, the maximal oxygen uptake ($\dot{V}O_{2max}$) values for elite female players have been reported to be approximately 49–55 mL.kg$^{-1}$.min$^{-1}$ which is somewhat lower than values reported for male players (55–68 mL.kg$^{-1}$.min$^{-1}$; Hoff, 2005). The absolute maximal oxygen uptake among trained athletes is, however, known to be about 10–20% lower in females, as compared to males, and this variation is attributed to differences in body composition, body size and haemoglobin content (Åstrand and Rodahl, 1986). Importantly though, the ability to train and improve aerobic and anaerobic capacities does not, in general, differ between males and females. Although not reported in female players, high-intensity interval training has been shown to increase aerobic capacity in male players and may include exercises with and without the ball (Helgerud, Engen, Wisloff, and Hoff, 2001; Dupont, Akakpo, and Berthoin, 2004). Such exercises may consist of longer intervals with heart rate values above 85–90% of HR$_{max}$, comprised of small-sided games at 4 min work x 2 min rest or running intervals at 4 min work x 3 min rest (Helgerud et al., 2001).

Although aerobic capacity is of importance for soccer players, the ability to run at high speed is even more significant for match performance (Mohr et al., 2003). It has been shown that players with higher scores on a soccer-specific endurance test, aiming to test the ability to recover between high-speed runs (YOYO Intermittent Recovery Test, YOYO IR), ran longer distances at high speeds during the game for both male and female players (Krustrup et al.,

## 246

2005; Mohr et al., 2003). Thus, in addition to improving aerobic capacity, fitness training for elite female players should more specifically aim to improve the ability to work at high speeds, through speed endurance-type training. Training sessions aimed at improving speed endurance can be included in the specific preparation phase (late in the pre-season) and during the competitive period (Figure 13.4). There are two forms of speed endurance training: production and maintenance training. Although there are a limited number of published reports involving female players, studies on male players show that production training is a very effective way to elicit adaptations in several muscle variables, as well as to improve performance in repeated high-intensity exercises (Iaia and Bangsbo, 2010). Production training involves exercises lasting 10–40 s near maximal speed, separated by rest periods of 1–5 min (>5 times the exercise duration); for example, 30 s exercise and 3 min rest. Maintenance training has been shown to improve the ability to sustain intense exercise and involves exercises of 5–90 s with shorter resting period (>1–3 times the exercise duration); for example 30 s work and 30 s rest (Paton and Hopkins, 2005). The recommendations on how to improve fitness for players are similar for female and male players.

## Monitoring training and game load

Heart rate monitoring and analysis is a commonly used method for assessing the individual training and match load. An accurate $HR_{max}$ for each player must, however, be ascertained for this method to be valid. Figure 13.5 depicts a heart rate curve from a 90-min training session for a Swedish elite female player (unpublished data). In the middle section of the training, the players competed in a small-sided game for 2–3 min and rested for 3–4 min. During the small-sided game, the average heart rate was 89–94% of $HR_{max}$. The last section of the training included shorter intervals where the players worked for ~30 s and rested for

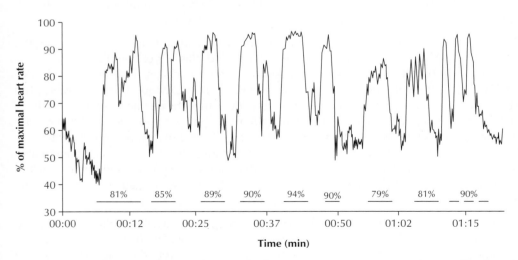

**Figure 13.5** A heart rate curve during a high-intensity training session for an elite female player (unpublished data).

~60 s and the average heart rate was 90% of $HR_{max}$. In total, the player spent 22.5 min above 85% of $HR_{max}$ during the training session and 17.5 min of this time above 90% of $HR_{max}$. Such training sessions can be classified as high intensity and, if completed often enough, will most likely improve the player's aerobic endurance capacity.

Since heart rate monitoring systems can be expensive, a relatively easy and inexpensive method for monitoring training loads has been developed by Foster et al. (2001). This monitoring technique uses the session-RPE method, a method which has demonstrated significant correlations with other published methods based on the heart rate response to exercise (Impellizzeri, Rampinini, Coutts, Sassi and Marcora, 2004). This method involves multiplying the player's own perceived exertion rating, using the category ratio scale (CR-10) (Foster et al., 2001), of each session by the training duration to determine the internal training load (TL). This product represents, in a single number, the magnitude of internal TL in arbitrary units (AU). The player's training load can be assessed for each individual session, as well as accumulated weekly TL. A typical weekly TL for the US Women's National Team (WNT) in the general preparation phase of training is shown in Figure 13.6a. The concurrent detail of each session type and the players' average heart rate data during each session are also displayed. During the training week, the players completed 11 training sessions and had one day off. The training sessions encompassed 1 recovery session, 2 strength training sessions, 3 technical sessions, 4 aerobic HI sessions and 1 aerobic MI session. Each player wore a heart rate monitor continuously during the training sessions, and rated each session with an average CR-10 score within 30 min of the completion of the training to ensure that the perceived effort was relevant to the complete session and not simply the most recent activity. The total training duration for this week was 530 min and the average TL was 3510 AU, which is a high TL, as expected during a general preparation training week. The players completed an average of 210 min working above 85% of $HR_{max}$, as shown in Figure 13.6a. As this training week was during the general preparation phase, the main aim was to focus on the development of strength and aerobic fitness. In summary, with the strength sessions employed and the amount of HI training completed, the goals of the training were achieved.

Figure 13.6b shows a similar model and data for an individual player training during the competition phase of the season. Over the 7-day period, this player completed 3 technical sessions, 1 aerobic HI session, 2 strength sessions, 1 recovery session, 1 game, and had 1 day off. The training time for the week was 470 min and the TL was 2850 AU for this player. The TL and training duration in this example are slightly lower than the demands during the general preparatory phase, since the main aim during this training phase is to prepare the player for the game, and then to enable the player to recover following that game, in preparation for the next game. However, what can be seen is that during this week of training the player completed more minutes above 90% of $HR_{max}$, than during the preparation phase, which is largely due to the game demands. During the competitive phase, the games are naturally the main focus for the players (Impellizzeri et al., 2004).

Figure 13.7 shows a comparison of the daily TL throughout a week for players during the general preparation (GP) and competition (C) phases of training. For the GP phase there is an increase in the TL from Monday to Wednesday, with a recovery day and day off on the Thursday, and then an increasing TL for the remaining 3 days of the training week. For the C period, the game is played on the Saturday, so the day prior to the game is tapered, with a

248

**(a) A Typical Pre-Season Training Week for US National Women's Team Players**

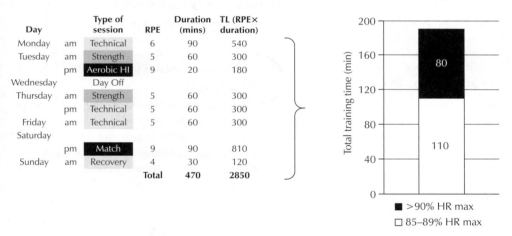

| Day | | Type of session | RPE | Duration (mins) | TL (RPE× duration) |
|---|---|---|---|---|---|
| Monday | am | Technical | 8 | 30 | 240 |
| Tuesday | am | Strength | 5 | 50 | 300 |
| | pm | Aerobic HI | 9 | 20 | 180 |
| Wednesday | am | Technical | 5 | 50 | 350 |
| | pm | Aerobic HI | 9 | 50 | 450 |
| Thursday | | Day Off | | | 0 |
| Friday | am | Strength | 5 | 90 | 450 |
| | pm | Aerobic HI | 9 | 20 | 180 |
| Saturday | am | Technical | 5 | 50 | 350 |
| | pm | Recovery | 4 | 30 | 120 |
| Sunday | am | Technical | 7 | 50 | 420 |
| | pm | Aerobic HI | 9 | 50 | 450 |
| | | **Total** | | **530** | **3510** |

- ■ >90% HR max
- □ 85–89% HR max

**(b) A Typical Training Week During the Competition Period for An Individual Player**

| Day | | Type of session | RPE | Duration (mins) | TL (RPE× duration) |
|---|---|---|---|---|---|
| Monday | am | Technical | 6 | 90 | 540 |
| Tuesday | am | Strength | 5 | 60 | 300 |
| | pm | Aerobic HI | 9 | 20 | 180 |
| Wednesday | | Day Off | | | |
| Thursday | am | Strength | 5 | 60 | 300 |
| | pm | Technical | 5 | 60 | 300 |
| Friday | am | Technical | 5 | 60 | 300 |
| Saturday | | | | | |
| | pm | Match | 9 | 90 | 810 |
| Sunday | am | Recovery | 4 | 30 | 120 |
| | | **Total** | | **470** | **2850** |

- ■ >90% HR max
- □ 85–89% HR max

**Figure 13.6a and b** The figures show an example of training load (training time x RPE-10), total time (min) spent above 85% of $HR_{max}$ during the sessions, and a detailed training content across seven days of training. (a) Data from the US national team during the general preparation phase. (b) Data from an individual player during 7 days of training in the competitive season.

lower TL, and similarly the day following this game is a period of recovery, with a day off. A usual low-intensive training week during the competitive phase can typically accrue a TL of 2000–2500 AU for individual players, and may consist of 1 game, 1 strength maintenance session, possibly 1 HI aerobic session, 2–3 moderate technical sessions, and the inclusion of 2 complete days off. Nevertheless, the training load is largely dependent on the playing time

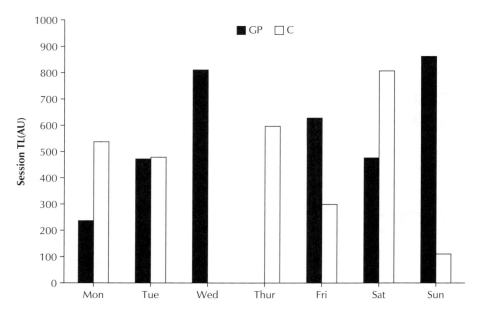

**Figure 13.7** A comparison of the daily TL through a training week during the general preparation (GP) and competition (C) phases of training. Sat in the competitive phase is a match.

of individual players, especially as the season progresses and players become more fatigued, as well as the fitness and injury status of each individual player.

At present, there is a limited amount of data available on the session-RPE method in soccer, and so, to accurately analyse and interpret TL and heart rate data, information should be continually collected over a number of sessions, so that baseline values can be determined for each individual player. Furthermore, by collecting data continuously, TL for each type of session (for example, strength training, tactical sessions, speed training) can be calibrated and training can be adapted accordingly. Altogether, this process enables coaches to plan the training more effectively and to monitor players more closely in each part of the training. This process will ultimately help the players to perform optimally during games.

## NUTRITION FOR FEMALE PLAYERS

The nutritional requirements for soccer training and games are not too dissimilar between elite male and female players. The biggest gender difference is that male players require a greater energy intake, due to their relatively larger body size and thus higher metabolism, and not necessarily due to lower training intensity and duration of female players, as has been suggested previously (Maughan and Shirreffs, 2007). As has already been discussed, at the elite level, the relative training and match load of female players are very similar to those of their male counterparts. Although some female players are full-time professional players, many females still have to combine full-time occupations and family commitments with full-time training

**D. Scott and H. Andersson**

schedules. This hectic lifestyle may lead to difficulties in obtaining an optimal nutritional intake and well-balanced diet. The key details of nutrition which players should focus on are the timing, quantity and type of carbohydrate and protein to be consumed in relation to training and games, as well as iron and calcium, which are commonly low in female players (Clark, Reed, Crouse, and Armstrong, 2003; Scott, Chisnall, and Todd, 2002).

Several researchers have reported female players to consume a low dietary intake of carbohydrate (CHO) (Clark et al., 2003; Mullinix, Jonnalagadda, Rosenbloom, Thompson, Kicklighter, 2003; Martin et al., 2005). Since carbohydrate is an essential fuel during training and games, a low intake of carbohydrate is likely to be inadequate to replace muscle and liver glycogen stores, which deplete rapidly during repeated bouts of high-intensity exercise performed during training and competition (Bangsbo, 1994). Ultimately, both the quality of training and game performance may be compromised on a regular basis, due to earlier onset of fatigue, with such nutritional deficiencies. Similarly, Martin et al. (2005) reported that England women's national team players on average consumed $1.2\pm0.3$ g.kg$^{-1}$.day$^{-1}$ of protein per day, which is at the lower end of the recommended range for elite and professional athletes (1.2–1.7 g.kg$^{-1}$.day$^{-1}$) (Maughan and Burke, 2002). A low intake of protein compromises the functional capacity, growth and repair of muscles and all other tissues in the body. This effect will clearly have an impact on the quality and intensity of training which players can complete, and will ultimately impact on the physical development and training adaptations of players. It is therefore vital that female players focus on their intake of CHO and protein, especially in relation to type of training and games, and develop good nutritional strategies to maximise recovery following sessions. This monitoring process will enable good training intensity in subsequent sessions and thus help to optimise performance and development in physical capacities. The recommendations to achieve optimal CHO and protein intake are similar for female and male players.

## Iron deficiency

Iron deficiency in female athletes appears to be common (Bean, 2003) and can be due to insufficient dietary intake, menstrual losses, iron losses in sweat, gastrointestinal and bladder blood loss, or haemaglobinuria from red blood cell damage in the plantar fascia during running (Tunstall-Pedoe, 1984). Furthermore, female athletes who train and compete at high levels are at a greater risk of iron depletion, which can lead to the development of anaemia. Iron depletion, with or without anaemia, may have a negative effect on physical and mental performance. Iron depletion affects the production of haemoglobin, and consequently, the oxygen transportation in the blood is reduced. This affects the ability to improve or sustain high aerobic endurance capacity. Iron deficiency and anaemia is characterised by symptoms such as excessive fatigue, weakness, dizziness, headaches and frequent infections/illness. Since iron deficiency tends to develop slowly, adaptation occurs and the disorder often goes unrecognised for some time. Iron levels should therefore be monitored regularly in female players. Landahl et al. (2005) found that 58% of the Swedish national squad players were iron deficient and 29% had iron deficiency anaemia six months prior to the FIFA Women's World Cup in 2003. Similarly, Scott, Bennett, and Hodson (2007) found that 42% of the England national squad had iron deficiency and 14% were characterised as having iron deficiency anaemia. In similar unpublished data (2010), 56% of the USA national squad were iron deficient, although none had symptoms of iron deficiency anaemia. Although caution should be exerted in comparing the degree of iron deficiency, dependant on the exact criteria used, it does seem that the prevalence of iron deficiency in female players is higher than for the general female population (Milman, Clausen, and Byg, 1998). This finding highlights the extra demands placed on elite female players to maintain adequate iron stores, as well as the potential for reduced aerobic capacity performance during training and games. Kang and Matsuo (2004) observed that 4 weeks of iron supplementation in elite female players significantly increased body iron stores and prevented training-induced decreases in haemoglobin concentration. Iron status is a result of the balance between the small amounts of dietary iron which are absorbed each day and the sum of the small iron losses as outlined above, and evaluation and management of iron status should be undertaken on an individual basis by a sports medicine expert. The use of iron supplementation may benefit performance (Fogelholm *et al.*, 1995) and regular monitoring should be employed to identify players at risk. Furthermore, since iron intake is, in general, lower than the recommended guidelines (Clark *et al.*, 2003; Martin *et al.*, 2005), the long-term management plan should include dietary advice to increase the intake of iron, and appropriate strategies to reduce any unwarranted iron loss. Such strategies should include:

- an increased intake of iron-rich foods – haem sources of iron are more easily absorbed by the body, and include foods such as red meat, liver, sardines, turkey;
- inclusion of fortified foods, non-haem sources of iron, such as breakfast cereals, cooked beans and lentils, baked potato with the skin;
- alongside the consumption of iron-rich foods, consuming iron absorption enhancers (mainly vitamin C sources), whilst limiting iron absorption inhibitors (mainly caffeine, fibre and tannin sources), as set out in Table 13.2.

Table 13.2 Nutrients that enhance and inhibit the iron absorption.

| Iron absorption enhancers | Iron absorption inhibitors |
|---|---|
| Meat, fish, poultry | Coffee and tea |
| Fruits: orange, orange juice, cantaloupe, strawberries, grapefruit | Vegetables: spinach, chard, beet greens, rhubarb and sweet potato |
| Vegetables: broccoli, brussels sprouts, tomato, tomato juice, potato, green and red peppers | Whole grains and bran Soy products |

### Calcium

The primary importance of calcium for women is its function in bone development. Young women (adolescents and young adults) need to make sure their diet includes sufficient calcium, as they can achieve their peak bone mass just after this age. Adequate amounts of calcium will help their bones to reach optimum density and can help to protect against the development of osteoporosis later in life. Mature women need calcium to prevent breakdown of

D. Scott and H. Andersson

bone, since, after the age of 40 years, bone mass in women is lost typically at a rate of about 0.5–1.0% per year (Cohn et al., 1976). Female players tend to have higher bone mineral density than sedentary women (Pettersson, Nordström, Alfredson, Henriksson-Larsén, and Lorentzon, 2000; Scott, et al., 2007), largely due to the weight-bearing nature of soccer training and games. Dairy products are the best source of calcium; however, these are commonly avoided by female athletes, due to their fat content. Consumption of reduced-fat versions of dairy products should therefore be encouraged in female players, with foods such as milk, yoghurt, frozen yoghurt, ice cream and cheese being regularly consumed.

## Dietary supplements

In general, players eating a healthy, well-balanced diet do not need dietary supplements in order to sustain an optimal performance. For example, it has been shown that elite female players seem to have a natural effective antioxidant system that is able to cope with increased oxygen free radicals occurring during a game (Andersson, Karlsen, Blomhoff, Raastad, and Kadi, 2009). As previously mentioned, however, due to the relatively hectic lifestyle of many female players, it is not always possible to consume a well-balanced diet sufficient in energy quality and quantity. In such cases it may be an option for some players to consume additional nutritional supplements during certain phases of training. Nevertheless, dietary supplements may contain some traces of doping-classified substances, and some may cause gastro-intestinal problems and other side-effects in individuals. The use of any supplements should be discussed with a sports medicine and/or sports dietician expert prior to consumption.

## Fluid balance

Fluid balance is also a key component of any player's nutritional strategy. The intensity and duration of a session/game, as well as the environmental conditions, can all affect sweat losses incurred by players. Maughan, Burke, and Coyle (2004) found that during a training session, sweat and drinking rates for female players were lower than for their male counterparts. This gender difference may largely be due to the smaller body size of female players, but the authors also suggest that the observed differences were due to lower metabolic heat production in the female players (Maughan et al., 2004). Nevertheless, for female players completing high-intensity training sessions and games, this may be less of an explanation for the gender differences observed. Shirreffs, Sawkab, and Stone (2006) conducted a sweat analysis of England women's senior and U21 players during training and games and found that while sweat rates were lower in female, as compared to male players, the sodium concentration of the sweat was similar, thereby highlighting the need to replace the observed sodium losses in rehydration fluids. The choice of fluid intake depends largely on the duration and intensity of the training session completed, as well as the environmental conditions. Such factors should be considered when developing individual fluid replacement strategies for players, especially in relation to the concentration and type of energy and electrolytes contained in the fluid.

Players, and appropriate support staff, should develop methods for monitoring the hydration status of players. This monitoring can involve simple methods such as weighing players pre and post training or games to indicate sweat volume lost, and also players individually monitoring the frequency, volume and colour of their urine. More expensive methods include the use of monitoring tools such as osmometers to measure the actual osmolality of the urine, thereby giving players immediate and more accurate feedback on their hydration status.

## PERFORMANCE AND MENSTRUAL CYCLE

Although there is scarce information on the menstrual phase-associated changes in performance for soccer players, training ability or performance in other sports does not seem to be largely affected by menstruation. There is, however, inconsistency in the reports of menstrual phase-associated changes to exercise performance. The inconsistent findings may be confounded by the high variability in the concentrations of ovarian hormones between and within participants from day to day (Oosthuyse and Bosch, 2010). The variation in performance level seems to be small during all the phases of the menstrual cycle. Some women experience pre-menstrual discomfort, others dysmenorrhoea or painful menses. Participation in exercise can attenuate menstrual discomfort and oral contraceptives are commonly used to regulate the menstrual cycle by some sportswomen. Additionally, women on high training loads may be prone to disruptions to the normal menstrual cycle. This may be indicated by a shortened luteal phase or by absence of menses, known as amenorrhea. Amenorrhea is seen as a disturbance of the hypothalamic-pituitary-gonadal axis that regulates the menstrual cycle. The cause of amenorrhea is complex and may be related to competitive and personal stress, insufficient nutrition intake and low body-fat. A consequence of low oestrogen levels associated with prolonged training-induced amenorrhea is a loss of minerals (notably calcium) from bone. The osteoporosis observed in women in some endurance sports is, however, rarely found in women soccer players.

## SUMMARY

Women's soccer is now being played in all different cultures and is one of the fastest-growing female sports throughout the world. Furthermore, it is becoming professional in an increasing number of countries. The physical load for elite female players is high and, consequently, players complete demanding training schedules in order to optimally prepare for games. Moreover, the ability to run at high speeds during a game is vital for the match performance of successful elite players, and hence training must reflect this demand. A higher incidence of ACL injuries has been shown for female than for male players, especially in younger age groups, and highlights the importance of strength training, with correct technique and knee-stability programmes in the early stages of development for female players. Additionally, female players are more prone to iron deficiency than are male players, and low iron status may affect a player's training response. It is important for female players to monitor their iron status regularly and to develop strategies to ensure an adequate intake of iron in the diet. The training response and injury incidents do not, in general, seem to be affected by the different phases of the menstrual cycle. Finally, while there is a plethora of research on elite male

D. Scott and H. Andersson

players, by comparison very few studies have been completed on female players. With the ever-increasing number of female players worldwide, and more demanding training and game loads for elite players, further research is warranted to investigate the match demands, as well as physical preparation and recovery strategies specific to female players at all levels of the game.

## REFERENCES

Andersson, H., Ekblom, B., and Krustrup, P. (2007). Elite football on artificial turf versus natural grass: movement patterns, technical standards, and player impressions. *Journal of Sports Science* 26, 113–122.

Andersson, H., Karlsen, A., Blomhoff, R., Raastad, T., and Kadi, F. (2009). Plasma antioxidant responses and oxidative stress following a soccer game in elite female players. *Scandinavian Journal of Medicine and Science in Sports* 20, 600–608.

Andersson, H., Randers, M.B., Heiner-Møller, A., Krustrup, P., and Mohr, M. (2010). Elite female soccer players perform more high-intensity running when playing in international games compared to domestic league games. *Journal of Strength and Conditioning Research* 24, 912–919.

Andersson, H., Raastad, T., Nilsson, J., Pausen, G., Garthe, I., and Kadi, F. (2008). Neuromuscular fatigue and recovery in elite female soccer: effects of active recovery. *Medicine and Science in Sports and Exercise* 40, 372–380.

Åstrand, P.O., and Rodahl, K. (1986). *Textbook of Work Physiology: Physiological Bases of Exercise*. New York: McGraw Hill.

Bangsbo, J. (1994). The physiology of soccer: with special reference to intense intermittent exercise. *Acta Physiologica Scandinavica* Suppl, 619, 1–155.

Bean, A. (2003). *The Complete Guide to Sports Nutrition*, 4th edn. London: A and C Black Publishers Ltd.

Bien, D.P. (2011). Rationale and implementation of anterior cruciate ligament injury prevention warm-up programs in female athletes. *Journal of Strength and Conditioning Research* 25, 271–285.

Castagna, C., Impellizzeri, F.M., Manzi, V., and Ditroilo, M. (2010). The assessment of maximal aerobic power with the multistage fitness test in young women soccer players. *Journal of Strength and Conditioning Research* 24, 1488–1494.

Clark, M., Reed, D.B., Crouse, S.F., and Armstrong, R.B. (2003). Pre- and post-season dietary intake, body composition, and performance indices of NCAA Division I female soccer players. *International Journal of Sport Nutrition and Exercise Metabolism* 13, 303–319.

Cohn, S.H., Vaswani, A., Zanzi, I., Aloia, J.F., Roginsky, M.S., Ellis, K.J. (1976). Changes in body chemical composition with age measured by total-body neutron activation. *Metabolism*, 25, 85–95.

Davis, J.A., and Brewer, J. (1993). Applied physiology of female soccer players. *Sports Medicine* 16, 180–189.

Deutscher Fussball-Bund (2011). Member Statistics. http://www.dfb.de/uploads/media/DFB-Mitglieder-Statistik-2011_01.pdf.

Dupont, G., Akakpo, K., and Berthoin, S. (2004). The effect of in-season, high-intensity interval training in soccer players. *Journal of Strength and Conditioning Research* 18, 584–589.

Durnin, J.V., and Womersley, J. (1974). Body fat assessed from total body density and its estimation from skinfold thickness: measurements on 481 men and women aged from 16 to 72 years. *British Journal of Nutrition* 32, 77–97.

FIFA (2011). Increase participation and competitions. 5th FIFA Women's Football Symposium, Frankfurt, 15–17 July. http://www.fifa.com/mm/document/footballdevelopment/women/ 01/51/51/64/presentation_increaseparticipation_e.pdf.

Fogelholm, C.M., Kukkonen-Harjula, T.K., Taipale, S.A., Sievänen, H.T., Oja, P., and Vuori, I.M. (1995). Resting metabolic rate and energy intake in female gymnasts, figure-skaters and soccer players. *International Journal of Sports Medicine* 16, 551, 556.

Foster, C., Florhaug, J.A., Gottschall, L., Hrovatin, L.A., Parker, S., Doleshal, P., and Dodge, C. (2001). A new approach to monitoring exercise training. *Journal of Strength and Conditioning Research* 15, 109–115.

Gabbett, T.J., and Mulvey, M.J. (2008). Time-motion analysis of small-sided training games and competition in elite women soccer players. *Journal of Strength and Conditioning Research* 22, 543–552.

Gilchrist, J., Mandelbaum, B.R., Melancon, H., Ryan, G.W., Silvers, H.J., Griffin, L.Y., Watanabe, D.S., Dick, R.W., and Dvorak, J. (2008). A randomized controlled trial to prevent noncontact anterior cruciate ligament injury in female collegiate soccer players. *American Journal of Sports Medicine* 36, 1476–1483.

Helgerud, J., Engen, L.C., Wisloff, U., and Hoff, J. (2001). Aerobic endurance training improves soccer performance. *Medicine and Science in Sports and Exercise* 33, 1925–1931.

Hewett, T.E., Myer, G.D., and Ford, K.R. (2006). Anterior cruciate ligament injuries in female athletes. *American Journal of Sports Medicine* 34, 299–311.

Hoff, J. (2005). Training and testing physical capacities for elite soccer players. *Journal of Sports Science* 23, 573–582.

Iaia, F.M., and Bangsbo, J. (2010). Speed endurance training is a powerful stimulus for physiological adaptations and performance improvements of athletes. *Scandinavian Journal of Medicine and Science in Sports* 20, 11–23.

Impellizzeri, F.M., Rampinini, E., Coutts, A.J., Sassi, A., and Marcora, M. (2004). Use of RPE-based training load in soccer. *Medicine and Science in Sports and Exercise* 34, 1042–1047.

Jackson, A.S., Pollock, M.L., and Ward, A. (1980). Generalized equations for predicting body density of women. *Medicine and Science in Sports and Exercise* 3, 175–181.

Jensen, K., and Larsson, B. (1992). Variations in physical capacity among the Danish national soccer team for women during a period of supplemental training. *Journal of Sports Science* 10, 144–145.

Kang, H.S, and Matsuo, T. (2004). Effects of 4 weeks iron supplementation on haematological and immunological status in elite female soccer players. *Asia Pacific Journal of Clinical Nutrition* 13, 353–358.

Krustrup, P., Mohr, M., Ellingsgaard, H., and Bangsbo, J. (2005). Physical demands during an elite female soccer game: importance of training status. *Medicine and Science in Sports and Exercise* 37, 1242–1248.

Krustrup, P., Zebis, M., Jensen, J.M., and Mohr, M. (2010). Game-induced fatigue patterns in elite female soccer. *Journal of Strength and Conditioning Research* 24, 437–441.

Landahl, G., Adolfsson, P., Börjesson, M., Mannheimer, C., and Rödjer, S. (2005). Iron deficiency and anemia: a common problem in female elite soccer players. *International Journal of Sport Nutrition and Exercise Metabolism* 15, 689–694.

Mandelbaum, B.R., Silvers, H.J., Watanabe, D.S., Knarr, J.F., Thomas, S.D., Griffin, L.Y. Kirkendall, D.T., and Garrett, W. (2005). Effectiveness of a neuromuscular and proprioceptive training program in preventing anterior cruciate ligament injuries in female athletes. *American Journal of Sports Medicine* 33, 1003–1010.

Martin, L., Lambeth, A., and Scott, D. (2005). Nutritional practices of national female soccer players: analysis and recommendations. *Journal of Sports Science and Medicine* 5, 130–137.

Maughan, R.J., and Burke, L.M. (eds) (2002). *Handbook of Sports Medicine and Science: Sports Nutrition*. Massachusetts: Blackwell Publishing Ltd.

Maughan, R.J., and Shirreffs, S.M. (2007). Nutrition and hydration concerns of the female football player. *British Journal of Sports Medicine* 41 (Supple. 1), i60–i63.

Maughan, R.J., Burke, L.M., and Coyle, E.F. (eds) (2004). *Food, Nutrition and Sports Performance II. The International Olympic Committee Consensus on Sports Nutrition.* New York: Routledge.

McCurdy, K.W., Walker, J.L., Langford, G.A., Krutz, M.R., Guerrero, J.M., and McMillan, J. (2010). The relationship between kinematic determinants of jump and sprint performance in Division I women soccer players. *Journal of Strength and Conditioning Research* 24, 3200–3208.

Milman, N., Clausen, J., and Byg, K.E. (1998). Iron status in 268 Danish women aged 18–30 years: influence of menstruation, contraceptive method, and iron supplementation. *Annals of Hematology* 77, 13–19.

Mohr, M., Krustrup, P., and Bangsbo, J. (2003). Match performance of high-standard soccer players with special reference to development of fatigue. *Journal of Sports Science* 21, 519–528.

Mohr, M., Krustrup, P., Andersson, H., Kirkendal, D., and Bangsbo, J. (2008). Match activites of elite women soccer players at different performace levels. *Journal of Strength and Conditioning Research* 22, 341–349.

Mullinix, M.C., Jonnalagadda, S.S., Rosenbloom, C.A., Thompson, W.R., and Kicklighter, J.R. (2003). Dietary intake of female U.S. soccer players. *Nutrition Research* 23, 585–593.

Oosthuyse, T., and Bosch, A.N. (2010). The effect of the menstrual cycle on exercise metabolism. *Sports Medicine* 40, 207–227.

Paton, C.D., and Hopkins, W.G. (2005). Combining explosive and high-resistance training improves performance in competitive cyclists. *Journal of Strength and Conditioning Research* 19, 826–830.

Pettersson, U., Nordström, P., Alfredson, H., Henriksson-Larsén, K., and Lorentzon, R. (2000). Effect of high impact activity on bone mass and size in adolescent females: a comparative study between two different types of sports. *Calcified Tissue International* 67, 207–214.

Polman, R., Walsh, D., Bloomfield, J., and Nesti, M. (2004). Effective conditioning of female soccer players. *Journal of Sports Science* 22, 191–203.

Prodromos, C.C., Han, Y., Rogowski, J., Joyce, B., and Shi, K. (2007). A meta-analysis of the incidence of anterior cruciate ligament tears as a function of gender, sport, and a knee injury-reduction regimen. *Arthroscopy: The Journal of Arthroscopic and Related Surgery: Official Publication of the Arthroscopy Association of North America and the International Arthroscopy Association* 23, 1320–1325.

Rhodes, E.C., and Mosher, R.E. (1992). Aerobic and anaerobic characteristics of elite female university players. *Journal of Sports Science* 10, 143–144.

Scott, D., Bennett, P., and Hodson, A. (2007). Iron status in elite female soccer players. *Journal of Sports Science and Medicine* 6, 185–186.

Scott, D., Chisnall, P.J., and Todd, M.K. (2002). Dietary analysis of English female soccer players. In T. Reilly and A. Murphy (eds), *Science and Football IV* (pp. 245–250). London: E and FN Spon.

Shirreffs, S.M., Sawkab, M.N., and Stone, M. (2006). Water and electrolyte needs for football training and match-play. *Journal of Sports Science* 24, 699–707.

Siegler, J., Gaskill, S., and Ruby, B. (2003). Changes evaluated in soccer-specific power endurance either with or without a 10-week, in-season, intermittent, high-intensity training. *Journal of Strength and Conditioning Research* 17, 379–387.

Sjökvist, J., Laurent, M.C., Richardson, M., Curtner-Smith, M., Holmberg, H.C., and Bishop, P.A. (2011). Recovery from high-intensity training sessions in female soccer players. *Journal of Strength and Conditioning Research* 25, 1726–1735.

Söderman, K., Pietilä, T., Alfredson, H., and Werner, S. (2002). Anterior cruciate ligament injuries in young females playing soccer at senior levels. *Scandinavian Journal of Medicine and Science in Sports* 12, 65–68.

Tamer, K., Gunay, G., Tiryaki, G., Cicioolu, I., and Erol, E. (1997). Physiological characteristics of Turkish female soccer players. In T. Reilly, J. Bangsbo and M. Hughes (eds), *Science and Football III* (pp. 37–39). London: E and FN Spon.

Tumilty, D., and Darby, S. (1992). Physiological characteristics of female soccer players. *Journal of Sports Science* 10, 144.

Tunstall-Pedoe, D. (1984). Marathon medicine and introduction. *British Journal of Sports Medicine* 18, 238–240.

Vescovi, J.D., Rupf, R., Brown, T.D., and Marques, M.C. (2011). Physical performance characteristics of high-level female soccer players 12–21 years of age. *Scandinavian Journal of Medicine and Science in Sports* 21, 670–678. (E-publication ahead of print).

**D. Scott and H. Andersson**

# CHAPTER 14

## DISABLED PLAYERS

C. Boyd and V. Goosey-Tolfrey

### INTRODUCTION

As a result of the successful integration of disability soccer into the infrastructure of the Football Association (FA), participation in disability soccer has increased in England by 28,000 players in just five years (The FA, 2010). Currently, the FA operates seven international disability squads, each with a specific impairment (amputation, blind, cerebral palsy, deaf and hearing impaired [male and female], learning disability and visual impairment [partially sighted]). It has been over 30 years since amputee soccer competitions were initially established, yet they are not currently part of the Paralympic programme. In terms of the history of the Paralympic Games, the 7-a-side game for athletes with cerebral palsy (CP) and the 5-a-side soccer which is open to athletes with a visual impairment (VI) have been part of the Paralympic programme since the New York/Stoke Mandeville Games in 1984 and Athens 2004, respectively. It is beyond the scope of this chapter to discuss all the six international disability soccer divisions. In this chapter we attempt to raise awareness of soccer for persons with a disability. We highlight the available literature on the topic of disability soccer and then focus on the 7-a-side cerebral palsy (CP) game and 5-a-side Futsal Blind (B1) game so as to enable the reader to understand how to apply their soccer knowledge to special populations with specific issues and needs.

### RESEARCH ON DISABILITY SOCCER

The scientific data on disability soccer is extremely limited and the translation of able-bodied training theory to soccer players with a disability is not well understood. In an injury audit of athletes with a disability that included ambulant Paralympic CP and VI sportsmen it was concluded that abrasions, strains, sprains and contusions were more common than fractures and dislocations (Ferrara and Peterson, 2000). An interest in the amputee soccer player soon followed this work, with a description of the UK sport science support programme (Wilson, 2002), and a description of the dietary and anthropometric profiles of the Brazilian players according to their positional roles (da Silva Gomes, Ribeiro and de Abreu Soares, 2006). Research with a CP focus has also been scarce, but case study data has been reported by Andrade, Fleury and de Silva (2005). They highlighted the leg strength characteristics and bilateral limb discrepancies of Brazilian national team players, underlining the impact that this disability may have on performance. More recently, researchers have also investigated the attentional processes that support the performance of the Dutch CP soccer team (Steenbergen and van der Kamp, 2008) and the restrictions of activity in grassroots players with VIs (Macbeth, 2009). These aforementioned studies are varied and lack a coherent research theme, which limits the scientific integrity and application to this specific population of soccer players. Building upon the work of Wilson (2002), we report an applied sport science support programme to prepare both the CP and VI Great Britain squads for the Beijing 2008 Paralympic Games and beyond. This longitudinal study is the only research that has documented detailed information on the training and preparation of disabled players with CP in preparation for the 2007 World Championships (Boyd and Goosey-Tolfrey, 2008). This work enabled the coaching and support staff to determine the effectiveness of training and development of these individuals for a major competition, which was then modified accordingly for the Paralympics the following year. No published information exists regarding the physiological and biomechanical impact of the six disability categories on soccer match-play and training. However, on-going investigations by the present authors and colleagues are examining a programme of study that includes the workload and match-analysis demands of the CP game, the effects of muscle stretching on performance and the influence of game-related fatigue on running economy, balance and coordination in CP soccer players. Unpublished findings from our laboratories have suggested that fatigue has a significant impact on dynamic balance. What seems to be an integral part of disability soccer research is the need to examine differences between athletic disability classifications so as to endorse and/or inform changes to the current classification systems.

## SOCCER FOR ATHLETES WITH CEREBRAL PALSY (CP) AND ACQUIRED BRAIN INJURY

### Classification of players

The 7-a-side version of disability soccer combines speed, agility and impressive ball skills (IPC [International Paralympic Committee], 2010). Athletes with varying degrees of CP or acquired brain injury (stroke, brain haemorrhage, Parkinson's disease and related conditions) participate together based on an individual athlete classification system (IPC, 2007; Table 14.1).

For equality of participation in competition players are placed into classification categories determined by the severity of their disability. *Classification* is a process whereby a group of entities are systematically ordered into a number of smaller groups (or classes) on the basis of

Table 14.1 Cerebral palsy terminology.

| Topographical | Definition |
| --- | --- |
| Diplegia | More involvement in lower limbs than upper limbs, may be asymmetric. |
| Hemiplegia | Involvement in upper and lower limb and trunk on same side. |
| Monoplegia | Involvement in only one limb. |

the observable attributes that they have in common. Specifically, classification is an integration of classification used in two fields; The International Classification of Functioning, Disability and Health (ICF) is the most widely used classification in this field. The Paralympic movement uses language and concepts that are common to ICF, and also a sport classification which attempts to reduce one-sided or unfair competition. It is important to mention here that the sport classification assessments should not penalise athletes who enhance their physical performances through training, and this should not promote changes in their classification (Tweedy and Vanlandewijck, 2009).

The Cerebral Palsy International Sports and Recreation Association (CPISRA) classifies all ambulatory disabled athletes in soccer from 5 (most affected by CP or related condition) to 8 (least affected by CP or related condition). The classification assessment takes the form of: (1) an individual medical examination determining a clinical diagnosis of the degree and range of disability; (2) a field-based test observation of the physical and coordinative capabilities; and (3) a match-based observation of each individual's movement characteristics in competitive match situations (Table 14.2).

### Rules of CP soccer

In order to match teams fairly, at least one C5 or C6 athlete per team must play throughout the match and no more than two players from category C8 are allowed to play at the same time. There are seven players per team on the field, rather than 11, and the pitch dimensions are smaller than for the 11-a-side game (~50 m–70 m), with the pitch markings and goals proportional to a full size pitch. A notable difference between this game and the able-bodied equivalent is that the match consists of two halves of 30 min, making it 30 min shorter than the full form of the game. However, there is no off-side rule, and so the shorter duration is offset by the playing dimensions of a pitch that is not limited by the defensive lines of the playing teams (CPISRA, 2010). Unlike the full form of the game, current published literature has not quantified the workload demands of the modified game for players with CP, and so at present we can only speculate as to the demands of this form of the game.

## SOCCER FOR ATHLETES WITH VISUAL IMPAIRMENT (B1: BLIND)

### Classification of players

Blind players are classified from B1 to B3, depending on the degree to which they are impaired. This chapter will focus upon the B1 athletes. The B1 category athletes are totally or almost totally blind, ranging from no light perception to light perception but with an inability to make out the shape of a hand.

### Rules of Blind Soccer (modified Futsal)

In order to match teams fairly, all players wear blindfolds, with the exception of the goal keepers, who are sighted and qualify if they are non-professional players. There are many

**Table 14.2** Cerebral palsy soccer classification categories.

| | |
|---|---|
| **Class 5** | These athletes are diplegic but are fully ambulatory without assistance. They have a noticeable hip and shoulder rotation when walking, inwardly rotated hips, knees and feet in standing/walking. There is only minimal difficulty with upper limbs. |
| | During soccer, exertion will increase tone and decrease function. The athletes will have difficulty in turning, pivoting and stopping, usually running only short distances, due to involvement in both lower limbs. Stride length is reduced/decreased with exertion. |
| **Class 6** | These athletes also walk without any assistive devices but have involvement in all four limbs. They have particular problems in trying to control their movements. Walking is laboured and uncoordinated, often rolling head movement during running. |
| | During soccer, the player will have trouble stopping and changing direction quickly with and without the ball. Coordination and timing problems will be seen when tackling, trapping and kicking the ball. |
| | The player will have difficulty dribbling or controlling the ball when running. Explosive movements are difficult to perform. |
| **Class 7** | These athletes are generally hemiplegic but walk without assistive devices although a marked limp is often noticed. The dominant upper limb should have normal strength and movement. The affected upper limb is usually more apparent during activity, possibly flat footed on affected side when running, often tilts head to one side during exertion. |
| | The player will walk with a noticeable limp, but may appear to have a smoother stride when running but will not have a heel strike. The player has difficulty when pivoting and balancing on the impaired side and therefore often pivots on the unaffected side and consequently this limits kicking ability while executing such tasks, as the affected side is not often used for kicking. The player's affected arm muscles will have an increase in tone when running and appear bent when walking. There are many patterns in the lower limb demonstrating spasticity in the hemiplegic limb. Training does not change these patterns; it only changes the quality of the movement of functional ability. |
| **Class 8** | These athletes are minimally affected diplegic, hemiplegic, monoplegic or have minimal movement control problems. They will run without noticeable limp, but disability is more evident on exertion; must demonstrate evidence of a functional disability during testing. |
| | Players with minimal involvement may appear to have near-normal function when running but the player must demonstrate a limitation in function to classifiers, based on evidence of spasticity (increased tone), ataxic, athetoid or dystonic movements while performing on the field of play or in training. |
| | In some players with an acquired brain injury, the dominant side may be the impaired side. If the player is unable to balance or has insufficient support on the impaired side, they may choose to stand on the less affected side and kick with the impaired leg. |

notable differences between this game and the able-bodied 11-a-side version, but the game has many similarities to the Futsal version of soccer. There are 5 players per team on the field, rather than 11, and the pitch dimensions are smaller than for the 11-a-side game (~40 m–60 m), with the goal keeper restricted to a 2 m x 1 m penalty area keeping a Futsal goal, while outfield players may travel anywhere on the hard court. The team coach/manager is positioned behind the opposition goal and communicates with his team in order to more efficiently direct the players toward goal. The ball is a size 4 ball and contains ball bearings to create a 'rattle' sound when in rolling motion. Sound boards up to waist height run down the entire length of

C. Boyd and V. Goosey-Tolfrey

the court to keep the ball in play and permit the players to gain their bearings on the court through auditory information. There are no throw-ins and there is no off-side rule. The match consists of two halves of 25 min, once again considerably shorter than the full form of the game. Unlike the full form of the game, current published literature has not quantified the workload demands of the modified game for B1 players and so, like CP soccer, we can only speculate as to the demands of this form of the game, based upon an extensive qualitative evaluation of the sport and data collected in the supporting role of sport science, as a substitute for empirical research (IBSA, 2009).

## ISSUES IN THE APPLICATION OF EFFECTIVE TRAINING FOR PLAYERS WITH CP AND VI

Soccer entails high-intensity intermittent activity where players continually switch between performing different activities, with and without the ball. There is a wealth of literature and research on the physical and physiological demands of soccer (Ekblom, 1986; Bangsbo, 1994), though the majority of these data describe the work-rate of elite male players. Published information regarding the characteristics of the disabled player is not readily available. In consequence, the lack of such information, in addition to the lack of quantified match-play demands, means that the requirements of training are often adapted from literature that relates to male, often elite, populations.

These assumptions are undoubtedly inaccurate, as the physical capabilities of non-disabled players will in most cases exceed those of their disabled counterparts. In addition, the modified versions of soccer that are employed for athletes with disabilities are significantly different from the full form of the game. These observations would suggest that disabled players will be unable to cover the same distances and reproduce the same absolute intensities as able-bodied players during matches, and in all likelihood will not be required to undertake the same quantity or type of workload in the modified versions of the game. On-going research in disability soccer from a multi- and interdisciplinary perspective can only seek to enable a better understanding of the demands of the game played by different disability groups, as well as provide a framework for the development of optimal preparation strategies for competition.

Exercise physiology research in these populations, in particular CP, has been predominantly limited to paediatric studies (Butler, Scianni and Ada, 2010). Although specific soccer research and elite performance research is somewhat lacking, it is still pertinent to outline some of the issues that should be considered when administering soccer-based physical programmes for the players.

The most significant aspects of disability posed by CP are outlined in Table 14.2. From a training perspective, issues of muscle balance, range of motion (ROM) and early onset of fatigue need to be carefully considered when administering any physical training. For most CP athletes, physical load and fatigue exacerbate the impairments and can lead to observed changes in posture, gait, balance and coordination. Without due attention to the consideration of the physical impairment, it is possible to place the athlete at risk of overtraining, injury, worsened states of spasticity, loss of ROM and greater muscle imbalances.

263

It may be possible to enhance the capabilities of an otherwise impaired limb or body segment through effective training. Unilateral exercises for the affected side and the use of adapted equipment for impaired hands should be considered in order to develop balanced physical strength. Increased recovery time between work activities will also reduce the amount of technique deterioration that is due to fatigue. In our opinion, flexibility training is a fundamental aspect of conditioning to increase ROM and not only to enhance performance but to increase the capacity to train more extensively in other aspects of training, by developing the capacity for improved technical form.

In contrast to CP athletes, B1 athletes possess no musculoskeletal impairments. However, a number of issues arise with regard to their ability to train effectively. Training alone poses significant problems. Gym-based exercise using treadmills, resistance equipment and free weights are almost impossible to complete safely. Consequently, paired training with a sighted partner is essential.

It is common to observe differences between congenital and acquired blind athletes when examining gait mechanics. Congenitally blind athletes tend to develop a 'shuffling' gait, while acquired blind athletes tend to possess a gait more akin to sighted individuals, as they have learned through previous sighted experience. Consequently, consideration has to be given to any attempt to alter gait and the impact that it may have upon the musculoskeletal system. Often it may be advisable to retain the natural gait of the athlete if it is not causing any risk of injury or impairing performance. Alterations in gait can increase the risk of musculoskeletal and joint injuries if they are not well managed.

Overall, the impact that a loss or absence of sight can have upon the day-to-day activities of an individual is overarching and poses significant barriers to participation and adherence to effective training and, in conclusion, all the issues impacting upon CP and B1 players illustrate that the type and severity of impairment will be key determinants of training effectiveness.

The elite programme for the Paralympic disciplines of CP and Blind Soccer has led to the development of an extensive programme of training and physiological testing and support, while on-going research attempts simultaneously to inform the interventions. Tables 14.3 and 14.4 highlight the range of tests that have been undertaken and, more importantly, the considerations for adapted versions of these tests for the unique populations they serve.

## PHYSICAL PREPARATION OF ELITE DISABILITY PLAYERS: A CASE STUDY INVOLVING THE CP ENGLAND SQUAD

Research in paediatric CP populations has suggested that aerobic fitness gains can be made through training over a prolonged period (Butler et al., 2010). However, the magnitude of the adaptation is somewhat ambiguous. This case study presents data from the assessment sessions over the final 9-month preparation period for the 2007 World Championships for the England CP national team and illustrates the adaptations made through physical preparation and education of the squad players. Data were collected over a period of 9 months, from February to October 2007. The results are taken from the final squad selected for the championships (n=12; age: 22±4.5yrs; height: 178.7±10.6cm). A battery of well-established anthropometric and field-based tests were undertaken to monitor progression of the squad. Tests assessed aerobic power (predicted $\dot{V}O_{2max}$), speed (10 m and 20 m) and explosive power (vertical

C. Boyd and V. Goosey-Tolfrey

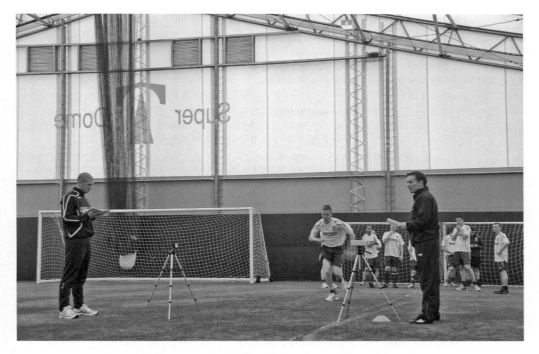

**Figure 14.1** Field testing for sprint performance with the CP England squad (photograph courtesy of Craig Boyd).

jumping). Assessments were undertaken on the water-based artificial surface at Lilleshall National Sports Centre, Shropshire, England. Environmental conditions on all occasions were favourable, dry, still and mild (temp. 15–20°C).

The results indicate a trend and, in some cases, a significant positive adaptation to the training programmes set out for the squad. Body mass and aerobic performance steadily improved. While the improvement in more explosive activities was less apparent, a common trend can be observed in all three related data sets where interventions of related training activities were introduced in the latter stages of the training cycle.

Overall, it has been noticeable that the development of aerobic power ($\dot{V}O_{2max}$) has been more effective than the anaerobic components of fitness. It is not thought that this is a physiological issue, but more of a training implementation and adherence issue for players working independently when off training camp.

### Special considerations – thermoregulation and jet lag in CP soccer players

Hutlzer, Meckel and Berzen (2011) suggested that heat transfer and regulation in persons with CP is impaired, and consequently is a factor that requires careful attention while designing training sessions and the use of cooling methods. Unpublished findings from the authors have shown rapid rises in core temperature of up to 40°C after just 30 min of game play under

**Table 14.3** Considerations for physiological assessments for players with CP.

| Physiological parameter | Considerations/tips |
|---|---|
| Body composition | Postural disorders develop in affected body segments that may prevent individuals holding the anatomical reference position. |
| | For DEXA (dual energy x-ray absorptiometry) scans where movement during the scan must be avoided, problems may occur, as some individuals may show continuous shaking and trembling. |
| | If bioelectrical impedance (BIA) is used, then it has been shown that the degree of spasticity in the limbs may influence the reproducibility, and it has been recommended to allow sufficient time (15–20 s) for stability of these measures (Bhambhani, 2011). |
| | Affected and non-affected segments differ considerably in muscle development, tone and adipose storage and therefore 'Sum of Skin Folds' is preferred to algorithmic determination of percentage body fat. It is either recommended to use the non-affected side as the reference aspect or to take the measurements on both sides in order to evaluate the changes over time. |
| | Girth measurements on both sides to monitor imbalances. |
| Sprint/agility testing | Adapt tests to assess change of direction on both sides of the body. |
| | Recovery time should be lengthened to counter earlier onset of fatigue. |
| | Warm-up requires significant time spent in static stretching followed by dynamic activity to enhance muscle activation. |
| | Identify the 'affected side' of the athlete to examine differences in the left and right dominance. |
| | Adapt tests to assess change of direction on both sides of the body. |
| Jump and balance tests | The use of a force plate to assess dynamic and static balances. |
| | Left- and right-side dominance should be identified. |
| | Bi- and unilateral jumps and balances should be conducted. |
| Laboratory-based testing | Individuals with mild CP (who have minimal motor control deficits) can be tested on a treadmill or cycle ergometer – careful monitoring of the player's balance is required during treadmill running. |
| | Discontinuous protocols (stopping the treadmill) must be employed to allow the safe transition between stages when blood lactate profiling, due to issues with hemiplegia. |
| Pre-test requirements and medical considerations | Stretching is critical to the success of players with CP, so this practice should be part of both the pre- and post-practice routine as well as before and after competition (Hutlzer, Meckel and Berzen, 2011). |
| | Some players with CP may take antispastic medications (e.g., Baclofen or Botex injections) that can influence muscle function and improve performance (Bhambhani, 2011). Moreover, if anticonvulsive medications are being taken, then these should be documented, as they may influence mental alertness and gross movement patterns. |

C. Boyd and V. Goosey-Tolfrey

**Table 14.4** Considerations for physiological assessments for players with VI (B1).

| Physiological parameter | Considerations/tips |
|---|---|
| Aerobic field tests | For 'Bleep Test' style assessments: prevention of disorientation. |
| | The use of sighted runners between each player to act as guides. |
| | The use of verbal instructions from guides at each end of the short track. |
| | The use of ropes held the length of the short track at waist height to provide tactile sensory information to guide the players. |

The most significant aspect of testing is the clarity and continual verbal instruction/supervision given by the testers to the athlete. Rehearsals will also allow the performer to become confident and familiar with the protocols, which may require additional space around the performer in order for safe execution of the activity.

**Table 14.5** England National Team physiological variations over 9-month preparation for CPISRA World Championships Brazil 2007.

| Parameter/date | February | May | July | October |
|---|---|---|---|---|
| Mass (kg) | 75.4 | 75.1 | 74.8 | 74.4 |
| ±SD | 9.21 | 9.13 | 9.41 | 9.70 |
| MSFT | 9.7 | 10.2* | 10.2 | 10.7* |
| ±SD | 1.0 | 1.1 | 0.6 | 1.1 |
| VJ (cm) | 35.9 | No data | 35.7 | 36.2 |
| ±SD | 5.6 | | 6.8 | 6.3 |
| 10m Sprint (s) | 1.95 | No data | 1.98 | 1.92** |
| ±SD | 0.18 | | 0.12 | 0.14 |
| 20m Sprint (s) | 3.38 | No data | 3.41 | 3.36 |
| ±SD | 0.22 | | 0.20 | 0.24 |

Notes:
* Significant difference from February assessment ($P < 0.04$); ** Significant difference from July assessment ($P < 0.015$); MSFT = multistage fitness test; VJ = vertical jump.

conditions of 35.3°C–39.1°C (in the shade and sunlight, respectively) and 57% relative humidity. Through heat and acclimatisation work conducted with the FA in collaboration with ParalympicsGB, it was recommended that the CP soccer players should follow recommendations advocated for able-bodied individuals to minimise their risks of heat stress during competition (Marino, 2002; Price, Boyd and Goosey-Tolfrey, 2009). Using an ice vest during the warm-up or at half time, as shown in Figure 14.2, is just one example of these methods.

The information gathered during the ParalympicsGB's simulation and holding camps (2007 and 2008) in Macau suggested that jet lag recovery for the squad took approximately 3–4 days, which is in line with the average data for all the Paralympic athletes in attendance at the camp. Athlete well-being scores were depressed during the first days of the camp but recovered once symptoms of jet lag had resided (Figure 14.3). These data support the fact that the body of knowledge on heat stress and acclimatisation may be directly transferrable from able-bodied athletes to the CP squad.

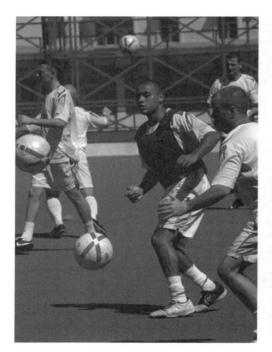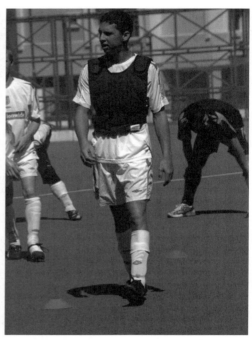

Figure 14.2 Great Britain players warming up whilst wearing ice vests under conditions of 35.3°C–39.1°C and 57% relative humidity (photographs courtesy of Dr Jim House).

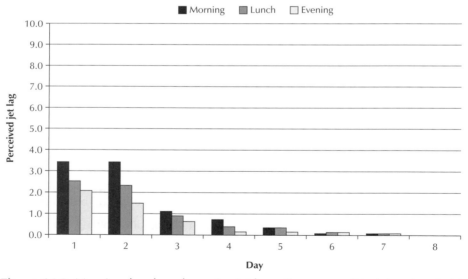

Figure 14.3 Morning, lunch and evening jet lag ratings across 7 training days in Macau for the Great Britain CP squad.

*Source*: Unpublished data from the ParalympicsGB simulation camp, 2007.

268

C. Boyd and V. Goosey-Tolfrey

## FUTURE DEVELOPMENTS

The scope for research in special-population soccer is vast and is on-going in several academic institutions. The authors are currently approaching the area from a number of perspectives. In order to better understand the demands placed upon the players, match analysis of elite competitive CP and B1 soccer will provide a greater understanding of the performance capabilities of the players and, in the case of CP, a greater insight into the performance characteristics of the classifications 5–8.

It is certain that in the years that have passed since the 2007 case study the conditioned status of the elite players has progressed and a detailed picture of the attributes of elite players is becoming ever clearer, with more extensive laboratory and field-based testing. From a physiological standpoint, the response of spastic muscle to training is of great interest and colleagues are currently investigating the muscle–tendon responses of CP-impaired individuals with regard to elastic properties and force generation. A greater understanding of match analysis and the physical characteristics of CP and B1 players is of paramount importance for training interventions. It will be possible to examine the inherent issues of fatigue in these population groups, in particular the effect of CP and the impact that congenital and acquired forms of blindness may have upon running economy and consequent performance.

## SUMMARY

The sport scientist faces an extremely complex challenge in advising on what training strategies may be the most effective and what type of field and laboratory tests should be conducted with disabled players, as this depends very much on the specific disability. It is clear, from this chapter, that in general we can employ the same underpinning training principles as for able-bodied players, yet with subtle but significant alterations. In order to achieve this aim, an understanding of the disability is essential and assessment of the needs of the individual must be completed thoroughly. Part of this process may be driven by the soccer classification categories, yet it is debatable whether the classes should be seen as the only discriminating factor when prescribing training. It is clear that, like their able-bodied counterparts, CP and blind players are also individuals and must be treated as such.

## ACKNOWLEDGEMENTS

Thanks to the British Paralympic Association Beijing Acclimatisation Group in Macau. Also, thanks to the Football Association for their continued support of football for athletes with Cerebral Palsy and visual impairments.

## REFERENCES

Andrade, M., Fleury, A.M., and de Silva, C. (2005). Isokinetic muscular strength of paralympic athletes with cerebral palsy (CP) from the Brazilian soccer team. *Revista Brasileira de Medicina do Esporte* 11(5), 263–266. English version.

Bangsbo, J. (1994). The physiology of soccer – with special reference to intense intermittent exercise. *Acta Physiologica Scandinavica* Suppl. 619, 1–155.

Bhambhani, Y. (2011). Physiology. In Y.C. Vanlandewijck and W.R. Thompson (eds), *The Paralympic Athlete* (pp. 51–73). Chichester, West Sussex: Wiley-Blackwell.

Boyd, C. and Goosey-Tolfrey, V.L. (2008). Variations in the physiological profile of the National CP squad over a 9 month preparation period leading to the CPISRA Football World Championships Brazil 2007. *British Paralympic Association Sport Science and Medicine Conference, March 2008, Loughborough*.

Butler, J.M., Scianni, A. and Ada, L. (2010). Effect of cardiorespiratory training on aerobic fitness and carryover to activity in children with cerebral palsy: a systematic review. *International Journal of Rehabilitation Research* 33(2), 97–103.

CPISRA (2010). www.cpisra.org/files/manual10p/CPISRA_Sports_Manual_10th_Edition_2009_Section_B_Sports_Rules_Football_7-a-side.pdf.

da Silva Gomes, A.I., Ribeiro B.G., and de Abreu Soares, E. (2006). Nutritional profile of the Brazilian Amputee Soccer Team during the precompetition period for the world championship. *Nutrition* 22(10), 989–995.

Ekblom, B. (1986). Applied physiology of soccer. *Sports Medicine* 3(1), 50–60.

FA (2010). Disability Football Strategy 2010–2012. http://www.thefa.com/TheFA/WhatWeDo/Equality/DisabilityFootball.

Ferrara, M.S. and Peterson, C.L. (2000). Injuries to athletes with disabilities – identifying injury patterns. *Sports Medicine* 30(2), 137–143.

Hutlzer, Y., Meckel, Y., and Berzen, J. (2011). Aerobic and anaerobic power. In Y.C. Vanlandewijck and W.R. Thompson (eds), *The Paralympic Athlete* (pp. 137–155). Chichester, West Sussex: Wiley-Blackwell.

IBSA (2009). www.ibsa.es/eng/deportes/football/IBSA_Futsal_Rulebook_2009–2013.pdf.

IPC (International Paralympic Committee) (2007). *IPC Classification Code and International Standards*. Bonn, Germany.

IPC (2010). www.paralympic.org/Sport/IOSD_Sports/Football_7-a-side/

Macbeth, J.L. (2009). Restrictions of activity in partially sighted football: experiences of grassroots players. *Leisure Studies* 28(4), 455–467.

Marino, F. (2002). Methods, advantages, and limitations of body cooling for exercise performance. *British Journal of Sports Medicine* 36(2), 89–94.

Price, M.J., Boyd, C., and Goosey-Tolfrey, V.L. (2009). The physiological effects of pre-event and midevent cooling during intermittent running in the heat in elite female soccer players. *Applied Physiology, Nutrition and Metabolism* 34 (5), 942–949.

Steenbergen, B., and van der Kamp, J. (2008). Attentional processes of high-skilled soccer players with congenital hemiparesis: differences related to the side of the hemispheric lesion. *Motor Control* 12(1), 55–66.

Tweedy, S.M., and Vanlandewijck, Y.C. (2009). International Paralympic Committee position stand – background and scientific rationale for classification in paralympic sport. *British Journal of Sports Medicine*. doi:10.1136/bjsm.2009.065060.

Wilson, D. (2002). Sport science support for the England amputee team. *Insight: The FA Coaches Association Journal* 5(2), 31–33.

**C. Boyd and V. Goosey-Tolfrey**

# CHAPTER 15

## MATCH OFFICIALS

M. Weston and W. Helsen

### INTRODUCTION

Soccer is a hugely popular sport that is played worldwide and the rules of the game need to be interpreted and applied in a highly consistent manner, irrespective of match location. Each match is controlled by a referee, who is assisted by two assistant referees. It is the duty of the match referee to enforce the laws of the game and to safeguard match integrity. Assistant referees help the referee to control the match in accordance with the laws of the game, and this is achieved via verbal and non-verbal communication.

The interpretation of match incidents and the awarding of correct decisions during soccer matches is a complex task. However, this task would be expected to be made easier were match officials in close proximity to incidents and had optimal viewing angles of incidents. The need to have a clear view of each incident dictates that officials should keep up with play at all times, regardless of match tempo. Consequently, the perceptual-cognitive demands of officiating are superimposed onto a high level of match physical strain.

In this chapter, the match and training performances of soccer match officials are considered. These include the physical and physiological demands of match play, the validity of fitness training and testing protocols, and the demands and training of the perceptual-cognitive abilities of match officials in soccer.

### MATCH PHYSICAL DEMAND

#### Match activity profiles

Soccer match officials are required to keep up with play at all times so as to ensure optimal positioning when viewing incidents. Consequently, the physical demands of officiating matches are as high as, if not higher than, the demands imposed upon players. These match demands have received increased focus in the scientific literature over recent years and can be quantified as physical, measured by distances covered, and physiological, as measured by heart rates, perceived exertion and blood lactate.

An early investigation into the total distance covered by match referees revealed distances of less than 10 km (Catterall et al., 1993). More recently, the total distance covered during top-level national matches has been reported to be in excess of 11 km; a distance similar to that covered by midfield players and greater than that of attackers and defenders. The total match distances of referees in the English Premier League (11.3 km) are greater than the mean player distance for the same match (10.8 km) (Weston et al., 2011a). The total distance covered during a match, however, is a poor indicator of physical match demand, as referees spend a substantial amount of time engaged in standing, walking and jogging, all of which can be classified as low-intensity. It is therefore the amount of high-speed activity that best reflects the physical demands of soccer, and researchers have focused on the distribution of high-speed (or intensity) running profiles in order to evaluate an official's ability to keep up with play and explore the possible occurrence of fatigue, especially during the later stages of matches. High-speed thresholds ranging from 13.0 to 19.8 km.h[1] make between-study comparisons difficult, and consequently, high-speed running as a percentage of total match distance ranges from 7 to 17% in referees. Of the limited available data, assistant referees cover ~7.5 km per match, with high-speed running constituting approximately 4% of total match distance (Krustrup et al., 2002; 2009).

An understanding of match-related fatigue in officials increases in importance when one considers the link between physical workload and decrements in cognitive functioning (Reilly and Smith, 1986). Several researchers have examined between-half differences in high-speed running distances in an attempt to determine fatigue, as determined by lower distances in the second half. However, equivocal findings have been reported. When analysing within-match activity profiles to explore the possible occurrence of fatigue, between-half comparisons will offer little, as maximal efforts during the first half cannot be assumed and this approach lacks intricacy. Consequently, researchers have categorised matches into 6 equal 15-min periods in order to evaluate within-match activity profiles. Reduced high-speed running distances, and non-orthodox activities (i.e., backwards and sideways running), during the later phases of matches have been reported both for national (Krustrup and Bangsbo, 2001) and international (Mallo et al., 2007) referees and assistant referees (Krustrup et al., 2009; Krustrup et al., 2002), respectively.

Reductions in the most physically demanding match activities, namely high-speed running and sprinting, toward the end of matches may provide evidence for chronic fatigue across the duration of matches. However, using a more intricate design whereby total distance, high-speed running and sprinting distances were evaluated for 18 x 5-min match periods, Weston et al. (2011a) reported only minor rates of decline in high-speed running and sprinting across the duration of matches, when compared to total distance covered (Figure 15.1). As suggested by Castagna and Abt (2003), referees 'moderate their competitive behaviour, reducing useless activity in order to perform at high-intensity, particularly at the end of the match when game intensity often reaches its peak' (p. 388).

Mallo et al. (2007; 2009) reported a decrease, when compared to the match average, in referees' high-speed running in the 5-min period that immediately followed the peak 5-min period of high-speed running. This finding could well provide evidence of acute fatigue during the match, although it is acknowledged that these observations could have been the result of natural variation in match play, due to team tactics and the effective playing time (i.e., ball in play). Whilst strong evidence has been presented for impaired muscle function, as determined by reduced sprint and repeated-sprint ability, in assistant referees at the end of competitive

272

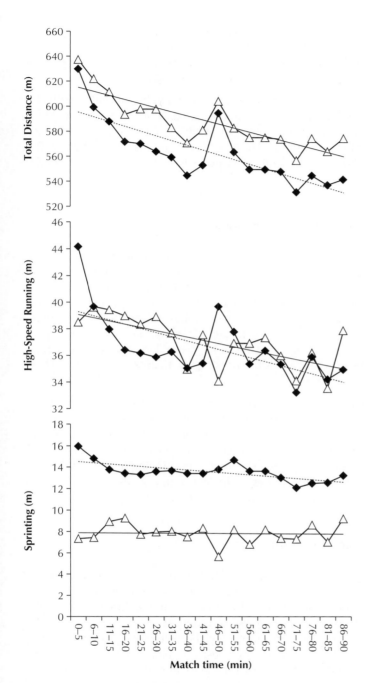

**Figure 15.1** Total distance, high-speed running and sprinting for referees (open symbols) and players (closed symbols) across the 18 x 5-min match periods.

*Source*: Adapted from Weston *et al.* (2011a).

matches (Krustrup et al., 2002), Tessitore and colleagues (2007) observed no post-match reduction in vertical jump performance in young (23±3 years) soccer referees during competitive matches played at the highest level of regional soccer in Italy. Therefore, the available reports provide equivocal evidence for match-related fatigue.

Any suppositions of acute and chronic match-related fatigue need to be supported with data on the underlying mechanisms and should be linked to the accuracy of an official's decisions. Yet, the collection of physiological data in competitive contexts is limited by restricted access to elite sports performers and the rules and regulations of competitions (Drust et al., 2007). Further research examining the potential for acute and chronic fatigue on performance during matches is warranted.

## Positioning with respect to foul play and offsides

Soccer referees are required to keep up with play in order to ensure that they make correct decisions. The ability to keep up with play can be evaluated via the analyses of distances from the ball and fouls (i.e., foul play, handball, simulation). Weston et al. (2010) reported a mean distance from the ball and fouls for English referees of 19.3 and 14.4 m, respectively. Krustrup et al. (2009) reported that the average distance from fouls was 12 m in the middle zone of the field of play and up to 16 m in the attacking zones in a selection of international and European matches. The distance from fouls in the attacking zones has been demonstrated to increase during the later stages of matches (Mallo et al., 2007; Krustrup et al., 2009), which could have implications for decision-making accuracy.

The primary role of the assistant referee is to award offside decisions. Their positioning should therefore be in-line with the second last defender at all times. Catteeuw et al. (2010) calculated that assistants in the Premier League were, on average, closer than 1 m to the line during offside situations, whereas in Denmark assistant referees were typically 2 (1–3) m from the offside line (Krustrup et al., 2002). Although the exact role of positioning on correct decision making has yet to be effectively explored in referees, slight deviations from the offside line have a significant influence on decisions regarding whether or not to raise the flag.

## Factors influencing match activity profiles

Several factors have been reported to influence the match demands of soccer officiating and these must be given due consideration when evaluating the physical performance of officials during matches. The total match distances covered by referees and assistant referees vary across both playing standard and country. There is also substantial between-match variability in performances, with this variability being high for the crucial activities of high-speed running and sprinting (Weston et al., 2011b). As such, care must be taken when evaluating and interpreting physical performances in matches from a single or limited number of games.

International referee governing bodies enforce age-related retirement (45 years), although this procedure has been successfully challenged in several countries, as it contravenes employment law. Elite officials are now refereeing into their mid-50s and an age effect has

274

been reported for match activity profiles. Weston et al. (2010) reported large negative correlations between referee age and physical performance in matches. Yet, these reduced distances did not impair the older referees' ability to keep up with play, as indicated by similar average distances from the ball and fouls when compared to younger referees.

Given the nature of soccer match-play and the integrated roles of officials and players, it makes sense that the central factor influencing the physical performance of referees in matches is the activity profile of the players. Weston et al. (2011a) demonstrated that the total high-speed running and sprinting distances recorded by elite referees are interrelated with those of the mean player response on the same match (Figure 15.1). Such experimental evidence indicates that referees are able to keep pace with the players and that their physical performance in matches should be evaluated alongside that of the players. If referees' match activity profiles are driven by the players, then this could account for the previously reported reductions in high-speed activities toward the end of matches, as the same observation has been reported for players (Mohr et al., 2003; Bradley et al., 2009).

## Match physiological demand

### Heart rates

The activity of officiating is non-contact, and this provides researchers with the unique opportunity to measure physiological strain during competitive matches – something which is not often possible for players. Krustrup and Bangsbo (2001) reported mean match heart rates of 85% maximal heart rate ($HR_{max}$) for elite soccer referees in the top two leagues in Denmark. A mean match heart rate of 85% $HR_{max}$ was confirmed by Helsen and Bultynck (2004) for soccer referees during the final round of the 2000 European Championship. Match standard has been reported to influence heart rates, however, as the same referees recorded higher heart rates for Premier League (83.6% $HR_{max}$) when compared to Football League matches in England (81.5% $HR_{max}$) (Weston et al., 2006).

Although competitive match heart rates overestimate the actual exercise intensity, these data demonstrate that soccer refereeing imposes a significant strain on the aerobic energy system during matches. This substantial aerobic demand is evidenced further by Krustrup and Bangsbo (2001) and Weston and Brewer (2002), who, using the laboratory-determined heart rate– $\dot{V}O_2$ relationship, estimated the mean match $\dot{V}O_2$ to be approximately 80% of $\dot{V}O_{2max}$ for top-level Danish and English referees, respectively. Lower mean match heart rates have been reported for assistant referees, with values of 77% $HR_{max}$ (65% $\dot{V}O_{2max}$) recorded during both national and international matches. Whilst this figure is reflective of the lower match physical demand imposed upon assistant referees, it is still evidence of substantial aerobic loading.

### Ratings of perceived exertion

Ratings of perceived exertion are a valid and accurate means of evaluating exercise intensity, yet there are limited data available describing the perceived match demands of soccer referees. Typically, referees rate the overall demand of their matches from 'hard' to 'very hard'. In keeping with the application of ratings of perceived exertion as a global measure of exercise

275

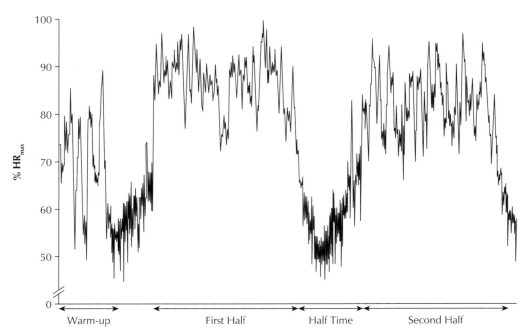

**Figure 15.2** Illustration of a referee's heart rate response during an English Premier League match.

intensity that encompasses physical and mental workloads, both technical and physical match demand influence ratings, as the number of yellow and red cards, mean distance from the ball and total high-speed running for referees and players explain 76% of the variance in the match ratings (Weston *et al.*, 2011d). Match standard has also been reported to influence perceived demand, as the same referees reported higher perceived exertion scores for Premier League as compared to Football League matches in England (Weston *et al.*, 2006).

### Blood lactate

Alongside a high aerobic demand, blood lactate measures have demonstrated that officials experience frequent bouts of anaerobic activity. Krustrup and Bangsbo (2001) reported mean blood lactate concentrations of 4.8 and 5.1 mmol after the first and second halves, respectively, in elite referees in Denmark. Moreover, values of 3.4 and 4.6 mmol were recorded after the first and second halves, respectively, for referees officiating in a selection of international and European matches (Krustrup *et al.*, 2009). The same trend has been observed in elite assistant referees (Krustrup *et al.*, 2002; 2009). These differences could be a result of natural variations in overall match intensity, differences in the fitness levels of the officials involved, or a combination of both.

*M. Weston and W. Helsen*

## Injury profiles

The high volume and intensity of match running undertaken by officials could well predispose them to a high incidence of match injuries, especially when considering their age. Wilson and colleagues (2011) reported an incidence of match injury in elite soccer referees of 16.4 injuries per 1000 h. The majority of these match injuries were muscular (55%) and to the lower leg (76%). A higher incidence of match injuries was reported for the 2006 FIFA World Cup referees (31.3 injuries per 1000 h), with the muscle strains of the lower leg accounting for the majority of the match injuries (Bizzini et al., 2009a). The same authors reported a lower incidence of match injuries for assistants (15.6 injuries per 1000 h) at the same tournament. The risk of non-contact match injuries for soccer officials appears to be similar to, if not higher than, that for players.

## FITNESS TRAINING

Soccer officials have a strong culture of fitness training. Research into their training practices has demonstrated that most training sessions are fitness based, with very little skill practice (MacMahon et al., 2007; Catteeuw et al., 2009). Given the match demands imposed upon officials, a good level of aerobic fitness, combined with the ability to perform single and repeated bouts of high-intensity exercise, is a physiological prerequisite. Therefore, it is recommended that high-intensity aerobic running and sprint training are an integral part of a weekly training routine.

Of the limited research available into the effects of training interventions on the fitness of match officials, Krustrup and Bangsbo (2001) and Weston et al. (2004) reported that high-intensity (90% $HR_{max}$) training sessions elicited significant fitness improvements, as determined by a soccer-specific fitness test. The referees also improved their match high-speed running distance after a 12-week training intervention of 3–4 high-intensity training sessions per week. Consistent with the training studies performed on soccer players, high-intensity training protocols appear to be an effective means of improving match-related fitness in officials.

High-intensity training is a time-efficient mode of training, as similar or greater improvements in measures of aerobic and anaerobic fitness are observed following intensive short-duration, low-volume interval training, as compared to medium-intensity, high-volume routines (Gibala et al., 2006). Since only a small number are full-time professionals, most officials have to balance their career with a full-time job and this can reduce the time available to train. Therefore, high-intensity interval training is crucial, given that it is both time-efficient and an effective means of eliciting training-induced exercise adaptations. The nature of this type of training is appealing from a specificity perspective, as it is consistent with the match demands of officiating, that is, frequent bouts of intense exercise followed by longer bouts of recovery.

Very often, sprinting is the vital activity performed by match officials immediately preceding important events (e.g., when teams break quickly and the attack results in penalty kicks, offsides or a red card for a challenge from the last defender). Consequently, a high demand has been evidenced in the literature, with referees performing on average 30 sprints (>25.2 km.h$^{-1}$)

per match (Weston et al., 2011b), which equates to a maximal sprint every 3 min. Therefore, short (~10 m) and long (~40 m) sprint distances should be an integral part of a training routine.

A change in match activity every 5–6 seconds (Krustrup and Bangsbo, 2001) necessitates good agility, and this should be trained accordingly. An ideal breakdown of training activities is provided in Figure 15.3. This training routine helped an elite referee to progress from part-time status in 2002 to refereeing the 2010 FIFA World Cup and UEFA Champions League finals (Weston et al., 2011c). A gradual increase in short-term, explosive training activities was observed across the training period, and during this time the referee made substantial improvements in his ability to perform the most physically demanding match activities, namely high-speed running and sprinting. A training routine of this type may help to offset the age-related reductions in sprinting performance reported for elite soccer referees (Castagna et al., 2005; Casajus and Castagna, 2007).

The high volume of training and match loads performed each season by match officials, along with their advancing years, necessitates that training activities are carefully monitored. Data collected on the incidence of training injuries has demonstrated that the proportion of match officials reporting at least one complaint in their career ranged from 60% to 90% (Bizzini et al., 2009b). Therefore, exercises focusing on injury prevention are recommended and these can be successfully integrated into regular warm-up routines.

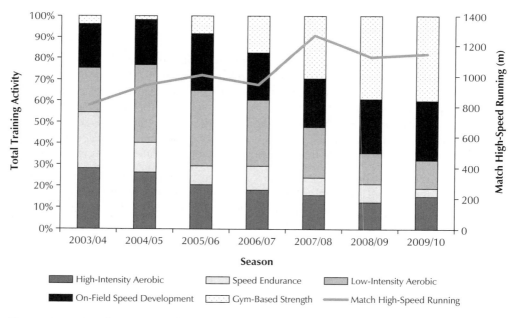

Figure 15.3 An elite soccer referee's typology of training sessions performed across a period of seven consecutive soccer seasons (2003/4–2009/10).

*Source*: Adapted from Weston et al. (2011c).

M. Weston and W. Helsen

## FITNESS TESTING

Fitness testing is part of the selection process for governing bodies, as they routinely assess officials across all levels of the professional game. Only those officials who meet the minimum criteria are available for match appointments. FIFA recently introduced two new fitness tests: a high-intensity, athletics track-based 150 m interval test; and a repeated 6 x 40 m sprint test. FIFA established minimum criteria for both of these tests and referees have to achieve the minimum criteria before they are awarded matches to officiate. However, only a single 40 m sprint test has demonstrated acceptable construct validity as a measure of match-related fitness in soccer referees (Weston et al., 2009). Therefore, modifications to the test protocols should be considered in order to verify the construct and content validity.

Fitness tests possess good content validity only if they adequately represent the domain of the physical task. Given the strong association between match running capacity and distance covered on the Yo-Yo intermittent recovery test, consideration should be given to the worldwide use of this test as the measure of match-related aerobic fitness in officials. However, this factor does not overcome the difficulty in establishing a valid and robust minimum criterion for the test. The threat of legal action from referees increases the need for a rigorous, scientific validation of any proposed minimum standards threshold.

## DECISION MAKING

A team of officials is typically made up of one referee and two assistant referees (plus a fourth official). Although their declarative knowledge and perceptual-cognitive skills may be similar, as their common goal is to ensure that the match is played in accordance with the laws they have to make decisions on different types of rule infringements. Referees are primarily involved in the assessment of foul play and assistant referees in the assessment of offside. Whilst the referee has the final responsibility, more than 60% of their decisions are based on communication with the assistant referees and/or fourth official (Helsen and Bultynck, 2004).

Following a video analysis of all 31 matches played at the 2000 European Championship, Helsen and Bultynck (2004) reported that referees make approximately 137 observable decisions per match. It was estimated that the number of non-observable decisions increased this overall count to ~200 match decisions; which equates to 3–4 decisions each minute of actual playing time, with the majority of referee decisions being free kicks (85%). The majority of assistant referee decisions related to the awarding of throw-ins (48%), goal kicks (23%), corner kicks (12%) and offsides (8%).

### Referees and foul play

It is the referee's role to interpret and apply the laws consistently in order to protect the players from the risk of injury due to unfair challenges (Fuller et al., 2004), which have a causative role in player injuries (Gilis et al., 2006). Fuller et al. (2004), Gilis et al. (2006) and Andersen et al. (2004) compared match referee decisions against the consensus decision of a panel of expert referees and reported agreement rates of 70%, 77% and 85%, respectively, for decisions relating to foul play. The latter study concluded that match referees' judgments are consistent with the interpretation of the laws of the game.

According to the rules and regulations of the game, referees should evaluate each individual match incident in isolation, separately from the score and playing time remaining (Plessner and Haar, 2006), so that a decision is not influenced by the context of the match. However, whilst panel reference decisions are very often made in isolation and not in the context of the match, there will always be some variation in match circumstances preceding the assessment of foul play that will cause match referees to observe, interpret and judge the same events in slightly different ways on different occasions (Fuller *et al.*, 2004). The awarding of a penalty kick to one team increases the probability of the other team's being awarded a penalty kick (Plessner and Betsch, 2001), whereas the awarding of decisions that are less likely to have a direct influence upon match outcome, such as free kicks, was not influenced in the same way. It appears that referees make assessments of foul play in the context of a match. This notion was reinforced by Unkelbach and Memmert (2008), who reported that referees who judged foul play in the context of the match awarded fewer yellow cards than referees who observed the same incidents in a random order. Also, in a controlled experiment, whereby referees were informed that a team had an aggressive reputation, referees were more likely to award this team red and yellow cards, as compared to referees who were not provided with prior knowledge (Jones, Paull and Erskine, 2002).

Along with the perception of foul play, external factors have been examined with regard to their influence on decision making. Nevill and co-authors (1996) reported that the frequency of red cards and penalty kicks – decisions that impact significantly upon match outcome – favoured the home team. Whilst the authors acknowledged that a large home support could provoke away team players into reckless foul play, they raised the possibility that the home crowds could influence the referee into believing that away team players committed more fouls. Similarly, Nevill, Balmer and Williams (2002) reported that referees are more lenient when awarding foul play sanctions to players from the home team when influenced by crowd noise.

## Assistant referees and offsides

The offside law is one of the most debated laws. Catteeuw *et al.* (2010) performed a detailed performance analysis of Premier League assistant referees. They observed 4,960 potential offside situations in 165 matches, with on average 30 situations per match. An error rate of 17.5% was found, with bias toward non-flag errors (i.e., keeping the flag down when an attacking player is offside), as compared to flag errors (i.e., raising the flag when an attacker is onside). Analysis of offsides in the 2002 FIFA World Cup demonstrated that one in four offside situations was judged incorrectly (Helsen *et al.*, 2006). The error percentage of the flag signals decreased to 10% in an analysis of the 2006 FIFA World Cup (Helsen *et al.*, 2006). In contrast to the data from Premier League assistant referees, data collected during the FIFA World Cups demonstrated a bias toward flag errors (Helsen *et al.*, 2006; Catteeuw *et al.*, 2010).

A range of explanations for incorrect offside judgments has been proposed. Such explanations focus on the positioning of the assistant referees in relation to the offside line and incorrect offside judgments due to poor positioning (Oudejans et al., 2000; Oudejans et al., 2005). For example, an assistant referee closer to the goal line than the second-last defender will make a flag error for an attacker on the opposite side of the second-last defender and a non-flag error for an attacker on the near side (see Figure 15.4a). In contrast, an assistant referee trailing the second-last defender will commit a flag error for an attacker on the near side of the second-last defender and a non-flag error for an attacker on the opposite side (see Figure 15.4b).

Some researchers propose the flash-lag effect as a more plausible explanation. In the context of offside decision making, the flash-lag effect occurs when the attacker receiving the ball (moving object) is perceived to be ahead of his/her actual position at the moment of the pass (flash). This illusion results in an overall bias toward flag errors, in comparison with non-flag errors (Baldo et al., 2002; Gilis et al., 2008). Consequently, assistant referees misjudge offside

**(a)**

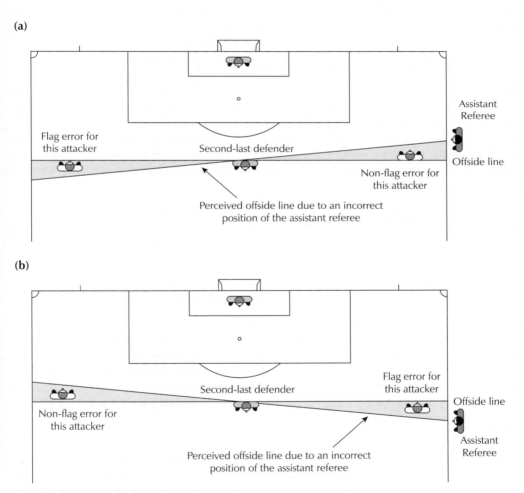

**(b)**

**Figure 15.4a and b** Illustration of flag and non-flag error scenarios.

*Source*: Adapted from Gilis et al. (2008).

situations because of a positioning error relative to the second-last defender and a perceptual error associated with the flash-lag effect. This latter suggestion explains the previously reported bias toward flag errors. In the Premier League, assistant referees tend not to signal in doubtful situations, as they have specific instructions to give the benefit of any doubt to the attacker.

## Expertise and perceptual-cognitive training

As officials work together to ensure that the match is played in accordance with the laws, it would be expected that their declarative knowledge and perceptual-cognitive skills will be similar. Yet, referees and assistant referees are required to make decisions on a different types of infringements, and Catteeuw et al. (2009) examined to what extent it is possible to capture specific expertise in both roles. Foul play and offside decision-making tasks were used to investigate role-specific differences, with referees outperforming assistant referees on a foul play task, and assistant referees outperforming referees on an offside decision-making task.

The development of role-specific skills results from years of practice (Ericsson et al., 1993) and this applies to both referees and assistant referees (MacMahon et al., 2007; Catteeuw et al., 2009). An analysis of practice history profiles established a positive correlation for years of officiating, hours of practice per week and number of matches officiated with skill. To achieve international standard, referees and assistant referees officiated ~600 matches over a career of 20 years and more. At this level, they practised approximately 8 hours per week, with a principal focus on physical training sessions. Match officials indicated the relevance of decision making; albeit they acknowledged that access to any form of training relating to this skill was limited.

There have been repeated calls for the development of effective perceptual-cognitive training methods to improve decision making (Schweizer et al., 2011). Some encouraging preliminary findings have been presented for the efficacy of video-based training methods in both referees (Schweizer et al., 2011) and assistant referees (Catteeuw et al., 2010). However, there is a paucity of research examining the transfer of video-based training methods to the field of play, and the need to employ some measure of transfer is frequently highlighted in the literature (Williams and Grant, 1999; Williams and Ward, 2003).

Considering the importance of effective transfer to on-field performances, researchers interested in improving the decision-making skills of officials should attempt to develop and apply ecologically valid training tools. As the training environment becomes more professional, sport scientists, coaches and governing bodies should give more attention to the development of role-specific perceptual-cognitive training tools.

## SUMMARY

In this chapter we have provided an overview of the physical and perceptual-cognitive demands of soccer officiating. It is clear that match officials have to cope with considerable physical demands. These demands are predominantly volume based, given the distances covered, and the aerobic energy system is heavily taxed during matches. Combined with a high rate of aerobic energy expenditure, match officials are required to perform frequent

M. Weston and W. Helsen

bouts of brief, intensive running, which adds further to the demands of match-play. The officials are required to keep pace with the match from the first to the final whistle; unlike players, they can be replaced only if they are unable to continue due to injury. It is vital that referees are able to meet the physical demands of the game, as match-related fatigue could negatively impact on positioning and, ultimately, decision making.

The physical performances of officials during matches would appear to be driven predominantly by the workload of players who are younger athletes with a far greater capacity for physical work. If the match activity profiles of referees are not evaluated alongside those of the players it is difficult to determine whether fluctuations in match activities are a consequence of fatigue or pacing strategies, or a response to changes in the overall match tempo, as determined by player activity.

An understanding of match demands, combined with knowledge of the effectiveness of valid fitness training protocols, suggests that high-intensity intervals and bouts of single and repeated sprints should dominate the weekly training routine. To help minimise match- and training-related injury, the implementation of specific injury prevention exercises should be considered by those responsible for the design and delivery of training programmes. The effectiveness of any training programme can be evaluated by regular fitness testing. However, at present, fitness tests for officials lack construct and content validity.

The high volume of decisions made during a match advocates the need for a highly developed perceptual-cognitive skill set as a prerequisite for match officials, especially when considering that their decisions can be crucial to the outcome of the match. Such training may enhance decision-making performance, although the ecological validity of any training programmes requires careful evaluation. Referees and assistant referees should, however, be provided with perceptual-cognitive skill training in an attempt to reduce decision-making errors and increase consistency of rule interpretation.

## REFERENCES

Andersen, T.E., Engebretsen, L., and Bahr, R. (2004). Rule violations as a cause of injuries in male Norwegian professional football: are the referees doing their job? *American Journal of Sports Medicine* 32, S62–S68.

Baldo, M.V., Ranvaud, R.D., and Morya, E. (2002). Flag errors in soccer games: the flash-lag effect brought to real life. *Perception* 31, 1205–10.

Bizzini, M., Junge, A., Bahr, R., Helsen, W., and Dvorak, J. (2009a). Injuries and musculoskeletal complaints in referees and assistant referees selected for the 2006 FIFA World Cup: retrospective and prospective survey. *British Journal of Sports Medicine* 43, 490–7.

Bizzini, M., Junge, A., Bahr, R., and Dvorak, J. (2009b). Injuries and musculoskeletal complaints in referees – a complete survey in the top divisions of the Swiss football league. *Clinical Journal of Sport Medicine* 19, 95–100.

Bradley, P.S., Sheldon, W., Wooster, B., Olsen, P., Boanas, P., and Krustrup, P. (2009). High-intensity running in English FA Premier League soccer matches. *Journal of Sports Sciences* 27, 159–68.

Casajus, J.A., and Castagna, C. (2007). Aerobic fitness and field test performance in elite Spanish soccer referees of different ages. *Journal of Science and Medicine in Sport* 10, 382–9.

Castagna, C., and Abt, G. (2003). Intermatch variation of match activity in elite Italian soccer referees. *Journal of Strength and Conditioning Research* 17, 388–92.

Castagna, C., Abt, G., D'Ottavio, S., and Weston, M. (2005). Age-related effects on fitness performance in elite-standard soccer referees. *Journal of Strength and Conditioning Research* 19, 785–90.

Catteeuw, P., Gilis, B., Wagemans, J., and Helsen, W. (2010). Offside decision making of assistant referees in the English Premier League: impact of physical and perceptual-cognitive factors on match performance. *Journal of Sports Sciences* 28, 471–81.

Catteeuw, P., Helsen, W.F., Gilis, B., and Wagemans, J. (2009). Decision-making skills, role specificity, and deliberate practice in association football refereeing. *Journal of Sports Sciences* 27, 1125–36.

Catterall, C., Reilly, T., Atkinson, G., and Coldwells, A. (1993). Analysis of the work rates and heart rates of association football referees. *British Journal of Sports Medicine* 27, 193–6.

Drust, B., Atkinson, G., and Reilly, T. (2007). Future perspectives in the evaluation of the physiological demands of soccer. *Sports Medicine* 37, 783–805.

Ericsson, K.A., Krampe, R.T., and Tesch-Romer, C. (1993). The role of deliberate practice in the acquisition of expert performance. *Psychological Review* 100, 363–406.

Fuller, C.W., Junge, A., and Dvorak, J. (2004). An assessment of football referees' decisions in incidents leading to player injuries. *American Journal of Sports Medicine* 32, S17-S22.

Gibala, M., Little, J.P., van Essen, M., Wilkin, G.P., Burgomaster, K.A., Safdar, A., Raha, S., and Tarnoplosky, M.A. (2006). Short-term interval versus traditional endurance training: similar initial adaptations in human skeletal muscle and exercise performance. *Journal of Physiology* 575, 901–11.

Gilis, B., Helsen, W., Catteeuw, P., and Wagemans, J. (2008). Offside decisions by expert assistant referees in association football: perception and recall of spatial positions in complex dynamic events. *Journal of Experimental Psychology: Applied* 14, 21–35.

Gilis, B., Weston, M., Helsen, W.F., Junge, A., and Dvorak, J. (2006). Interpretation and application of the laws of the game in football incidents leading to player injuries. *International Journal of Sport Psychology* 37, 121–38.

Helsen, W., and Bultynck, J.B. (2004). Physical and perceptual-cognitive demands of top-class refereeing in association football. *Journal of Sports Sciences* 22, 179–89.

Helsen, W., Gilis, B., and Weston, M. (2006). Errors in judging 'offside' in association football: test of the optical error versus the perceptual flash-lag hypothesis. *Journal of Sports Sciences* 24, 521–8.

Jones, M.V., Paull, G.C., and Erskine, J. (2002). The impact of a team's reputation on the decisions of association football referees. *Journal of Sports Sciences* 20, 991–1000.

Krustrup, P., and Bangsbo, J. (2001). Physiological demands of top-class soccer refereeing in relation to physical capacity: effect of intense intermittent exercise training. *Journal of Sports Sciences* 19, 881–91.

Krustrup, P., Mohr, M., and Bangsbo, J. (2002). Activity profile and physiological demands of top-class assistant refereeing in relation to training status. *Journal of Sports Sciences* 20, 861–71.

Krustrup, P., Helsen, W., Randers, M.B., Christensen, J.F., MacDonald, C., Rebelo, A.N., and Bangsbo, J. (2009). Activity profile and physical demands of football referees and assistant referees in international games. *Journal of Sports Sciences* 27, 1167–76.

*M. Weston and W. Helsen*

MacMahon, C., Helsen, W., Starkes, J.L., and Weston, M. (2007). Decision-making skills and deliberate practice in elite association football referees. *Journal of Sports Sciences* 25, 65–78.

Mallo, J., Navarro, E., Garcia-Aranda, J.M., and Helsen, W. (2009). Activity profile of top-class association football referees in relation to fitness-test performance and match standard. *Journal of Sports Sciences* 27, 9–17.

Mallo, J., Navarro, E., Garcia-Aranda, J.M., Gilis, B., and Helsen, W. (2007). Activity profile of top-class association football referees in relation to performance in selected physical tests. *Journal of Sports Sciences* 25, 805–813.

Mohr, M., Krustrup, P., and Bangsbo, J. (2003). Match performance of high-standard soccer players with special reference to development of fatigue. *Journal of Sports Sciences* 21, 519–528.

Nevill, A.M., Balmer, N.J., and Williams, A.M. (2002). The influence of crowd noise and experience upon refereeing decisions in football. *Psychology of Sport and Exercise* 3, 261–72.

Nevill, A.M., Newell, S.M., and Gale, S. (1996). Factors associated with home advantage in English and Scottish soccer matches. *Journal of Sports Sciences* 14, 181–6.

Oudejans, R.R., Bakker, F.C., Verheijen, R., Gerrits, J.C., Steinbruckner, M., and Beek, P.J. (2005). How position and motion of expert assistant referees in soccer relate to the quality of their offside judgments during actual match play. *International Journal of Sport Psychology* 36, 3–21.

Oudejans, R.R.D., Verheijen, R., Bakker, F.C., Gerrits, J.C., Steinbrucken, M., and Beek, P.J. (2000). Errors in judging 'offside' in football. *Nature* 404, 33.

Plessner, H., and Betsch, T. (2001). Sequential effects in important referee decisions; the case of penalties in soccer. *Journal of Sport and Exercise Psychology* 23, 200–5.

Plessner, H., and Haar, T. (2006). Sports performance judgments from a social cognitive perspective. *Psychology of Sport and Exercise* 7, 555–75.

Reilly, T., and Smith, D. (1986). Effect of work intensity on performance in a psychomotor task during exercise. *Ergonomics* 29, 601–6.

Schweizer, G., Plessner, H., Kahlert, D., and Brand, R. (2011). A video-based method for improving soccer referees' intuitive decision-making skills. *Journal of Applied Sport Psychology* 23, 429–42.

Tessitore, A., Cortis, C., Meeusen, R., and Capranica, L. (2007). Power performance of soccer referees before, during, and after official matches. *Journal of Strength and Conditioning Research* 21, 1183–7.

Unkelbach, C., and Memmert, D. (2008). Game-management, context-effects, and calibration: the case of yellow cards in soccer. *Journal of Sport and Exercise Psychology* 30, 95–109.

Weston, M., and Brewer, J. (2002). An investigation into the physiological demands of soccer refereeing. *Journal of Sports Sciences* 20, 59–60.

Weston, M., Drust, B., and Gregson, W. (2011a). Intensities of exercise during match-play in FA Premier League referees and players. *Journal of Sports Sciences* 29, 527–32.

Weston, M., Drust, B., Atkinson, G., and Gregson, W. (2011b). Variability of soccer referees' match performances. *International Journal of Sports Medicine* 32, 190–4.

Weston, M., Gregson, W., Castagna C., Breivik, S., Impellizzeri, F.M., and Lovell, R.J. (2011c). Changes in a top-level soccer referee's training, match activities and physiology over an

8-year period: a case study. *International Journal of Sports Performance and Physiology* 6, 281–6.

Weston, M., Castagna, C., and Batterham, A.M. (2011d) Factors influencing referees' ratings of perceived exertion during competitive soccer matches. Presentation at 16th Annual Congress of the Europe College of Sport Science (ECSS), Liverpool, UK, 6–9 July 2011, in Cable, T. N. and George, K. (eds) *Book of Abstracts*, European College of Sport Science, p. 248.

Weston, M., Castagna, C., Helsen, W., and Impellizzeri, F.M. (2009). Relationships among field-test measures and physical match performance in elite-standard soccer referees. *Journal of Sports Sciences* 27, 1177–84.

Weston, M., Helsen, W., MacMahon, C., and Kirkendall, D. (2004). The impact of specific high-intensity training sessions on football referees' fitness levels. *American Journal of Sport Medicine* 32, S54-S61.

Weston, W., Bird, S., Helsen, W., Nevill, A., and Castagna, C. (2006). The effect of match standard and referee experience on the objective and subjective match workload of English Premier League referees. *Journal of Science and Medicine in Sport* 9, 256–62.

Weston, M., Castagna, C., Impellizzeri, F.M., Rampinini, E., and Breivik, S. (2010). Ageing and physical match performance in English Premier League soccer referees. *Journal of Science and Medicine in Sport* 13, 96–100.

Williams, A.M., and Grant, A. (1999). Training perceptual skill in sport. *International Journal of Sport Psychology* 30, 194–220.

Williams, A.M., and Ward, P. (2003). Perceptual expertise: development in sport. In J.L. Starkes and K.A. Ericsson (eds), *Expert Performance in Sports: Advances in Research on Sports Expertise* (pp. 219–50). Champaign, IL: Human Kinetics.

Wilson, F., Gissane, C., and Byrne, A. (2011). A prospective study of injuries in elite soccer referees and assistant referees. *British Journal of Sports Medicine* 45, 383–4.

*M. Weston and W. Helsen*

# PART V

# TALENT IDENTIFICATION AND YOUTH DEVELOPMENT

# CHAPTER 16

## IDENTIFYING YOUNG PLAYERS

R. Vaeyens, M. Coelho e Silva, C. Visscher,
R.M. Philippaerts and A.M. Williams

### INTRODUCTION

The attainment of excellence is the ambition of many individuals across a variety of domains. Expert performance in sports can be defined as consistent superior athletic performance over an extended period of time (Starkes, 1993). As it is the most popular sport worldwide, millions of children aspire to become a professional world-class soccer player, benefitting from the accompanying fame and fortune. On street corners across the world many young players attempt to imitate the skills of Messi, Ronaldo or Rooney, hoping one day to realise their dream of becoming an elite player. Unfortunately, the reality is that for the vast majority of these youngsters, playing at the highest level will remain only a dream.

The domain of sport, and of soccer in particular, has been transformed in recent decades. For instance, club teams have become much more commercialised. Since achievements on the field of play safeguard financial success, the attainment of high performance levels is essential to professional clubs. In many countries elaborate, science-based support systems are employed in an effort to realise this goal (e.g., match analysis, psychological and social counselling, training and fitness programmes; Williams and Reilly, 2000a). Also, the 'Bosman Ruling' (European Court of Human Rights, 1995), which precludes professional soccer clubs from withholding a player's registration at the completion of a contract, led to an escalation in wages and transfer fees. This development reduced the likelihood for many, especially less affluent clubs, of recruiting high-quality players. To maintain their status, professional clubs are more aware of the importance of identifying and developing their own talented youth players for the senior team. Players are identified so that they receive specialised coaching and training to accelerate the talent development process (Williams and Franks, 1998; Williams and Reilly, 2000b). The reliable identification of future elite players guarantees effective financial investment, focusing limited resources on the development of a smaller number of players (Morris, 2000). However, existing talent identification programmes have a relatively flimsy scientific foundation (Moore, Collins, Burwitz et al., 1998; Williams and Franks, 1998; Williams and Reilly, 2000b).

In this chapter, we present some key research findings that can help to inform practitioners, scouts and coaches involved in the talent identification (and development) process. We provide a conceptual backdrop for this area of study and discuss some of the difficulties in identifying 'gifted' players. Moreover, the need for a multidisciplinary approach is highlighted and potential new avenues to facilitate transition from youth to adult soccer are explored.

Finally, we present some suggestions for future research that can help to increase knowledge on talent identification.

## TALENT: A COMPLEX ITEM

Talent is an extremely complex concept, which is hard to define and lacks a clear theoretical framework. A key factor in the lack of consensus is the perennial debate about the relative contribution of nature and nurture in the development of talent. The importance of both innate and environmental characteristics has been highlighted, suggesting that neither account can exclusively describe talent (Durand-Bush and Salmela, 2001; Csikszentmihalyi, 1998). Williams and Reilly (2000b) suggested that it could perhaps be best described as 'the potential to attain expertise'. In this regard, the Differentiated Model of Giftedness and Talent (DMGT) developed by Gagné (2003) offers a valuable contribution. The model recognises that the rate of learning is more important than a level of ability. The DMGT presents a constructive conceptual framework encompassing six components that bring together in a dynamic way all the recognised determinants of talent and describes how it emerges from natural gifts through a complex choreography between various causal influences (Figure 16.1).

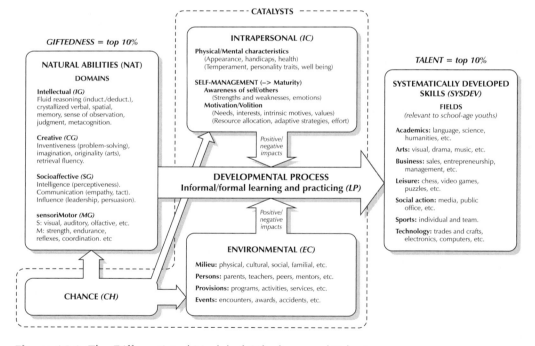

**Figure 16.1** The Differentiated Model of Giftedness and Talent.

*Source*: Gagné (2003).

*R. Vaeyens et al.*

## Stages in the talent identification process

Williams and Reilly (2000b) defined four key stages on the road to excellence. Talent *detection* refers to the discovery of potential performers who are currently not involved in the sport in question. In comparison with minority sports, talent detection in soccer may not be a significant issue, given the popularity and high number of children participating in the game (Williams and Reilly, 2000b). Talent *identification* (TID) alludes to the process of recognising current participants with the potential to become elite players. According to Régnier, Salmela and Russell (1993), it refers to the attempt to match a variety of performer characteristics, either innate or (and) amenable to learning or training, to the specific task requirements to ensure the highest probability of maximum performance outcome. Talent *selection* involves the on-going process of identifying at various stages players who demonstrate qualification levels of performance for inclusion in a particular team. It is focused on choosing the most appropriate individual or group of individuals who can best carry out the task within a specific situational context. Talent selection is perceived as 'very short-term talent detection', as it is related to determining the players who will perform best 2 weeks, 2 months (or even 2 years) from now (Régnier et al., 1993). In this regard, soccer is a special environment, as the best team is not necessarily comprised of the 11 best players or individuals. A coach may be more likely to choose players to balance the needs of the team as a whole and to ensure good results. Talent *development* implies that players are provided with a suitable learning environment so that they have the opportunity to realise their potential. Talent identification is often the start of, and a necessity for, access to talent development processes and resources (Reilly, Williams, Nevill and Franks, 2000; Tranckle and Cushion, 2006).

## The relative age effect: a confounding factor

In soccer, late-maturing boys are systematically excluded in favour of average and early-maturing boys as chronological age and sport specialisation increases (Cacciari, Mazzanti, Tassinari et al., 1990; Panfil, Naglak, Bober and Zaton, 1997; Peña Reyes, Cardenas-Barahona and Malina, 1994; Malina, Peña Reyes, Eisenmann et al., 2000). Consequently, youth players advanced in biological maturity receive more opportunities to employ their potential, and dominate youth soccer. In their review of research investigating the physiological (e.g., power) and technical (e.g., dribbling) characteristics of players varying in maturity status, Meylan, Cronin, Oliver and Hughes (2010) concluded that early maturers had a tendency to perform better in these tests and were likely to be more influential in matches and to be recognised as more talented. Moreover, players born early in the selection year can benefit more from past experience, leading to enhanced perceptual-cognitive or 'game intelligence' skills (Toering, Elferink-Gemser, Jordet et al., 2011; Jonker, Elferink-Gemser, Toering et al., 2010).

Sports governing bodies generally allocate participants to chronological age groups based on a specific cut-off date, presumably to ensure developmentally equitable competition and opportunity (Barnsley, Thompson and Legault, 1992; Musch and Grondin, 2001). This grouping has been generally set in the context of an activity year (Barnsley et al., 1992). Youth teams are selected from individuals born within the same 12-month period. As a result, there are age differences among youth of the same age born shortly after the cut-off date relative to those born almost one year after the cut-off date. For example, with a 1 January cut-off date, those born shortly after this date (e.g., 5 January) are chronologically older than those born almost one year after the cut-off date (e.g., 30 December); yet the two sub-sets are included in the same chronological age group. However, differences in the timing and tempo of maturation indicate that chronological age is a poor index of physical potential (Caine and Broeckhoff, 1987) and can lead to the misclassification of children in relation to their biological maturity (Baxter-Jones, 1995).

The consequences of this 'relative age' phenomenon for sports participation and talent identification are significant. The comparisons of birth dates among youth and professional-level athletes in several sports have revealed skewed birth date distributions, favouring individuals born early in the selection year (see Musch and Hay, 1999; Cobley, Baker, Wattie and McKenna, 2009). Consequently, those children benefit from selection policies and enhanced practice opportunities. In soccer there is a significant over-representation of players born in the early part of the selection year among youth (Barnsley et al., 1992; Brewer, Balsom, Davis and Ekblom, 1992; Baxter-Jones, 1995; Brewer, Balsom and Davis, 1995; Helsen, Starkes and Van Winckel, 1998; Vincent and Glamser, 2006; Jiménez and Pain, 2008; Mujika, Vaeyens, Matthys et al., 2009; Williams, 2010; Augste and Lames, 2011), as well as senior and professional players (Barnsley et al., 1992; Verhulst, 1992; Dudink, 1994; Helsen et al. 1998; Musch and Hay, 1999; Cobley et al., 2009; Mujika et al., 2009).

The bias towards players born early in the year is likely even more pronounced than is reported in the literature. In a recent study involving French U14 youth academy soccer players, Carling, le Gall, Reilly and Williams (2009) reported few differences across players born in each of the four quarters of the year on any of the physical (other than height) and physiological measures of performance. These findings suggest that players selected for elite academies in France who are born later in the year are likely to be relatively more mature biologically, as compared to their peers born earlier in the year. It appears that players who are born later in the selection year and who are average or below average in regard to their biological maturity are far less likely to be recruited into specialised training academies.

Published reports of the relative age effect are typically based on the distributions of birth dates and do not include variables that might be indicative of actual game involvement. In a quasi-longitudinal study, Vaeyens, Philippaerts and Malina (2005a) collected official match data of second and third national division league games for four competitive seasons (1998–99 through 2001–02). Variables indicative of match involvement, such as number of selections for matches and time played, were examined retrospectively in relation to the relative age effect for 2,138 semi-professional and amateur soccer players. In contrast to the equal distribution of the general population (circa. 25% per quarter), semi-professional and amateur senior soccer players born in the first quarter of the selected age band were significantly over-represented. The observation that more players from the first months of the selection year 'survived' the youth development stage and reached senior level is in line with recent findings from Delorme, Boiché and Raspaud (2010), who detected significantly higher drop-out rates in French youth players born late in the selection year. Comparisons of birth date distributions with match-related variables gave similar, though not entirely consistent, results. In absolute (total) terms, there was a skewed distribution for the game involvement parameters (selections and minutes played). However, on an individual basis there were no differences among adult soccer players born throughout the selection year (Figure 16.2). The lack of differences in mean playing opportunities at senior level demonstrates that soccer talent is equally distributed

292

throughout the year, regardless of the presence of a relative age effect. These data suggest that children disadvantaged by birth date or physical maturity might have become equally skilled senior athletes if they were afforded equivalent developmental opportunities. Moreover, Ford and Williams (2011) recently reported that award-winning athletes in soccer, ice hockey, baseball and American football were more likely to be born late than early in the selection year. Previously, researchers reported that relatively younger male athletes received higher salaries (Ashworth and Heyndels, 2007) and were over-represented in early draft picks (Baker and Logan, 2007). Consequently, the talent identification procedures currently applied by teams need to be questioned and objective measures are recommended to at least complement the subjective opinions of coaches.

## TALENT IDENTIFICATION PROCEDURES

The identification process in soccer is hindered by various factors, including the dynamic nature of talent (e.g., adolescents who possess the required characteristics will not necessarily retain these attributes throughout maturation), the absence of objective performance indicators such as time or distance, and the difficulty of evaluating an individual performance in a team setting (for a review, see Vaeyens et al., 2008). Traditionally, professional clubs rely on scouts who subjectively assess players during a game. Although the game may be the ideal environment in which to evaluate a player, there are several confounders that influence

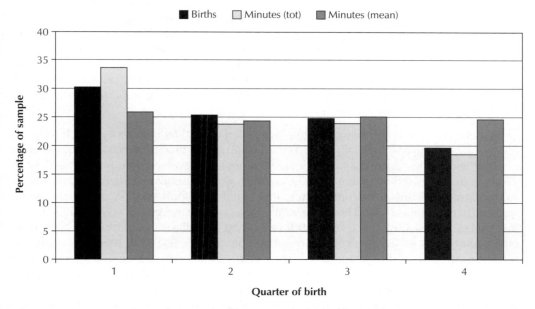

**Figure 16.2** Soccer players born in the first quarters of the selection year are over-represented both in number of births and total playing minutes but the mean number of playing minutes is equal for adult players.

*Source*: Vaeyens and Philippaerts (2007).

a player's performance (e.g., teammates, opponents, tactics/system of play, game-to-game variability). Rampinini and colleagues (2007; 2009) demonstrated that the activity profile of the opponent team or the competition phase (seasonal variations) affects running performance in matches. In addition, various researchers have highlighted that match running performance is position-specific (e.g., Bradley, Sheldon, Wooster et al., 2009; Di Salvo, Baron, Tschan et al., 2007). In a study with youth soccer players, Buchheit, Mendez-Villanueva, Simpson and Bourdon (2010a) revealed match running performance to be (small to moderately) related to most physical capacities. However, the magnitude of this relationship depended on the physical capacity and playing position. The 'position effect' was more apparent in match parameters than in physical capacity tests, implying that players cannot always display their maximal physical/physiological capacities due to other (technical/tactical) restrictions.

There is limited information available on how scouts approach talent identification and on what grounds they base their decisions. Scouts may base their evaluation on a select number of criteria that are expressed in an acronym such as TIPS: technique; intelligence; personality; and speed (Williams and Reilly, 2000b). However, the rationale for these selection criteria is unclear. The challenge is therefore to objectively capture soccer using appropriate performance criteria (Cronbach, 1971). A typical (academic) approach to identifying the determinants underlying successful performance is to compare a group of elite soccer players with sub-elite and/or non-elite counterparts. Meylan et al. (2010) reported that, when compared to recreational youth and future non-professional players, elite youth and future professional players scored better in physiological and technical testing, independently of maturity status. However, these testing procedures were not sensitive enough to distinguish youth elite from sub-elite or future national team from professional club players. It is apparent that soccer requires a multitude of skills and attributes. The multifaceted nature of expertise in soccer therefore necessitates that the process must be multidisciplinary. Williams and colleagues (Williams and Franks, 1998; Williams and Reilly, 2000b) highlighted some potential predictors of talent in soccer from various disciplinary perspectives including anthropometry, physiology, psychology and sociology (Figure 16.3).

The Ghent Youth Soccer Project has employed such a multidisciplinary approach to talent identification (Vaeyens, Malina, Janssens et al., 2006). It examines the relationships between physical and performance characteristics and competitive level in youth players aged 12 to 16 years, using a mixed-longitudinal design controlling for variation related to skeletal maturity. Anthropometry, skeletal maturity status, functional and sport-specific parameters were assessed in elite, sub-elite and non-elite youth players in four age groups: U13 (n=117), U14 (n=136), U15 (n=138) and U16 (n=99) years. The elite players outperformed their non-elite counterparts on aerobic endurance, anaerobic power, flexibility, speed, strength and technical skill. Overall, the performance scores of the sub-elite players were in-between, with no apparent consistent distinction from the elite players. A crucial discovery was that the parameters discriminating youth soccer players appeared to differ by age group, and while running speed and technical skill were the most discriminating features in the younger age groups (U13–U14), cardiorespiratory endurance became more influential in late adolescence (U15–U16). Similarly, adolescent changes in functional capacities were shown to vary, corresponding to the moment of peak height velocity (Philippaerts, Vaeyens, Janssens et al., 2006). This inconsistent pattern of discriminating factors reflects the dynamic aspect of talent

294

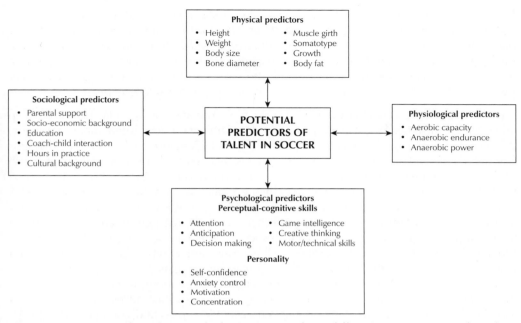

**Physical predictors**
- Height
- Weight
- Body size
- Bone diameter
- Muscle girth
- Somatotype
- Growth
- Body fat

**Sociological predictors**
- Parental support
- Socio-economic background
- Education
- Coach-child interaction
- Hours in practice
- Cultural background

**POTENTIAL PREDICTORS OF TALENT IN SOCCER**

**Physiological predictors**
- Aerobic capacity
- Anaerobic endurance
- Anaerobic power

**Psychological predictors
Perceptual-cognitive skills**
- Attention
- Anticipation
- Decision making
- Game intelligence
- Creative thinking
- Motor/technical skills

**Personality**
- Self-confidence
- Anxiety control
- Motivation
- Concentration

**Figure 16.3** Potential predictors of talent in soccer from different sports science discipline areas.

*Source*: Adapted from Williams and Franks (1998).

identification and has similarly been reported in studies with gymnasts, field hockey and rugby players, although these studies did not account for maturity level (Abbott and Easson, 2002; Nieuwenhuis, Spamer and van Rossum, 2002; Pienaar and Spamer, 1998; Régnier and Salmela, 1987). It was suggested that the differential timing and rate of the adolescent growth spurt may account for the observed variation in discriminating factors among youth players.

Coelho e Silva *et al.* (2010) examined positional differences in Portuguese U14 players. Although they observed significant differences in skeletal maturation, body size, functional capacities, skills and goal orientation by competitive level (with regional players outperforming their local peers), position and the interaction of position and competitive level were not a consistent source of variation among players. In each position, those selected as regional players were advanced in skeletal maturation, heavier and taller than local players. At this age, variation by position was negligible. Midfielders had a slightly higher ego orientation compared to defenders and forwards. Players in the competitive groups at each position did not differ in agility, aerobic endurance, soccer skills (except for ball control in forwards) and in task orientation. A discriminant function analysis indicated a linear function of six variables (height, ego orientation, repeated sprint ability, 10 x 5 m agility test, squat jump and years of training) that successfully predicted 86% of players by competitive level. The discriminant function analysis by position successfully distinguished regional and local players, but predictors did not substantially vary for each position. Similarly, Buchheit, Mendez-Villanueva, Simpson and

Bourdon (2010b) observed that between-position differences varied as a function of the physical capacities considered (e.g., weak differences for CMJ and cardiorespiratory fitness but no differences for acceleration). These authors proposed performance tests that can reveal the between-position differences observed in games. On the other hand, one could question the need for position-specific talent identification in youth soccer. It is possible that soccer players benefit from the experience in different playing positions in early phases.

There is a need for research that can provide valuable information on how elite players develop and what are the crucial steps in this process. In longitudinal studies carried out in Groningen, gifted youth soccer players from two Eredivisie (i.e., the highest level in the Netherlands) clubs have been followed over the last 10 years to gain insight into the characteristics that distinguish players who eventually reached professional level in adulthood from those who tried but failed to reach this level. Players were followed in their evolution and transition from youth to adult stage (Huijgen, Elferink-Gemser, and Visscher, 2009). In this study, players were tested twice a year on a variety of measures, including anthropometry, physical performance, technical and tactical aspects, and psychological characteristics (Elferink-Gemser, Visscher, Lemmink and Mulder, 2004; Elferink-Gemser, Jordet, Coelho e Silva and Visscher, 2011). The successful players had acquired better dribbling skills by the age of 14 years (Huijgen, Elferink-Gemser, Post and Visscher, 2010), developed better interval endurance capacity from the age of 15 years (Roescher, Elferink-Gemser, Huijgen and Visscher, 2010) and outscored less successful players on tactical skills at the age of 17 years (Kannekens, Elferink-Gemser and Visscher, 2009; 2011). Nevertheless, one has to be careful in interpreting scores based on only one test. It is possible to reach professional level while scoring worse than the predicted curves for professionals. This has been referred to as the 'compensation phenomenon'; weaknesses in one area can be compensated for by strengths in other areas (Williams and Ericsson, 2005). Therefore, it is of utmost importance to present the total picture of a gifted player's scores on multidimensional performance characteristics as well as on maturation, learning and training, to coaches and staff (Phillips, Davids, Renshaw and Portus, 2010).

Various researchers (e.g., Vaeyens et al., 2006; Figueiredo, Coelho e Silva and Malina, 2011) have demonstrated the need to use estimates of (biological) maturity status and subsequent appropriate analysis of data obtained from physical, physiological and technical testing. Ideally, tests should not be used as a marker of selection before full maturity is attained. When maturity is taken into account, these testing procedures can provide an indication of responsiveness to training load in youth players and an evaluation of potential to become a successful soccer player (Meylan et al., 2010).

## NEW AVENUES FOR TID: PERCEPTUAL-COGNITIVE SKILLS

When compared to anthropometric and physiological profiles, perceptual-cognitive and technical skills may be more likely to discriminate performers as they progress (Elferink-Gemser et al., 2004; Williams and Reilly, 2000b). The skilled athlete's superior performance is underpinned by a number of perceptual-cognitive skills that are seamlessly integrated during task performance across a range of domains (Williams and Ward, 2007). However, psychological (personality and perceptual-cognitive skills) and technical predictors are frequently ignored in TID programmes (Abbott and Collins, 2004; Morris, 2000).

## 296

The number of scholars studying perceptual-cognitive expertise in sport is increasing, presumably because of the growing awareness that skilled perception precedes and determines appropriate action in sport (Abernethy, Thomas and Thomas, 1993; Starkes and Allard, 1993; Janelle and Hillman, 2003). The complex and rapidly changing environment in team ball sports requires players to pick up information from the ball, teammates and opponents ahead of making an appropriate decision. In soccer, when compared with less skilled counterparts, skilled players: (a) are faster and more accurate in recognising and recalling patterns of play (Helsen and Pauwels, 1993; Williams, Hodges, North, and Barton, 2006; Williams and Davids, 1995); (b) are superior in picking up contextual cues based on an opponent's postural orientation (Williams and Burwitz, 1993); (c) have enhanced knowledge of situational probabilities (Williams, 2000; Ward and Williams, 2003); and (d) display more efficient and effective visual search strategies (Helsen and Starkes, 1999; Williams and Davids, 1998). However, the majority of researchers have relied almost exclusively on adult sample groups.

Although the testing of perceptual-cognitive skills has been suggested as a promising avenue for talent identification, these measures have hardly ever been applied for this objective. Only a few exceptions exist in the literature. Reilly et al. (2000) revealed that, within a group of 16 elite and 15 sub-elite youth soccer players (15–16 years of age), the ability to anticipate an opponent's action appeared to be one of the most discriminating variables in a multivariate test battery.

Vaeyens, Lenoir, Williams, Mazyn and Philippaerts (2007a) examined differences in decision-making skill and visual search behaviours across five categories of small-sided, offensive game simulations in soccer (2 vs. 1, 3 vs. 1, 3 vs. 2, 4 vs. 3, and 5 vs. 3). A total of 87 male adolescents (13.0–15.8 yrs) were recruited and assigned to one of four subgroups (elite, sub-elite, regional and control) according to their experience and playing level. The three groups of soccer players demonstrated superior decision-making skills, as compared to non-players (controls) across all the microstates of offensive play. Generally, the soccer players were more accurate and faster in making decisions than their non-playing counterparts (Figure 16.4). As a result of extensive exposure to the domain over many years of practice, skilled performers develop elaborate task-specific knowledge structures, coupled with efficient encoding and retrieval processes, which provide them with a significant advantage over less skilled players when attempting to make appropriate decisions under time constraint (see Ericsson and Delaney, 1999; Ericsson and Kintsch, 1995).

The elite and sub-elite players generally performed better than the regional level players, although the three groups of soccer players were reasonably well matched in relation to the amount of playing experience. It appears that national (sub-elite) and international (elite) level youth soccer players develop more refined and sophisticated knowledge structures than do regional players of comparable age and experience level (cf., Ward and Williams, 2003). The differences in decision-making skill across groups suggest that the elite and sub-elite players are able to benefit more than regional players from their exposure to the task domain (Williams and Davids, 1995). Alternatively, it is feasible that the quality of the practice/match-play experience and the level of instruction provided by significant others, such as coaches and mentors, may be equally responsible for the differences in decision-making skill across groups (Ward, Hodges, Williams and Starkes, 2004).

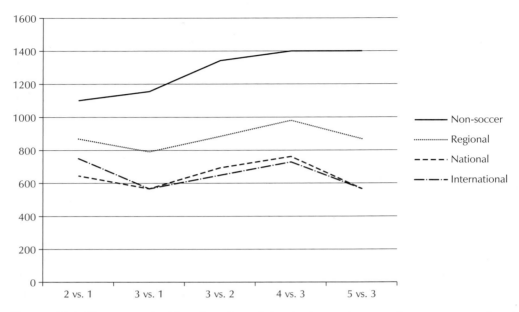

**Figure 16.4** The mean decision time (in ms) for the four subgroups (non-soccer, regional, national and international) according to the playing condition (2 vs. 1, 3 vs. 1, 3 vs. 2, 4 vs. 3 and 5 vs. 3).

The decision-making test employed was sufficiently sensitive to discriminate national and international level players from regional level players. In most previous studies, researchers have employed groups differentiated on the basis of both their playing skill (i.e., skilled vs. less skilled) and experience level (experienced vs. inexperienced). The lack of differences between the national- and international-level players may reflect the fact that such measures are not sensitive enough to discriminate between players who are relatively close together on the skill continuum. It is also feasible that not all elite players are exceptional decision makers. A player who is not an exceptional decision maker may be able to compensate by being quick and agile or by developing excellent technical skills. This latter issue was addressed methodologically in a follow-up study in which 40 youth soccer players were allocated to successful or less successful groups based on their performance in the laboratory-based test of tactical skill (Vaeyens, Lenoir, Williams and Philippaerts, 2007b). The results showed that film-based tests can be used to discriminate soccer players of comparable experience and playing level on the basis of their decision-making skills (see also Savelsbergh, Haans, Kooijman and van Kampen, 2010).

## TRANSITION TO FIRST TEAM CULTURE

The primary aim of talent identification and development programmes in soccer is to 'deliver home-grown' players who can be integrated into the first team at adulthood. However, young adult soccer players often experience difficulties when making the transition to open-age

R. Vaeyens *et al.*

competition (Kuhn, 2002; Vaeyens et al., 2005a). Large first team squads can significantly reduce opportunities for players to transition from young professional to first team player (Richardson, Littlewood and Gilbourne, 2005). According to these authors, the progress from a nurturing and supportive youth environment to a less socially supportive first team culture, alongside a reduced tolerance of failure and heightened expectations for performance, is the most critical period in a player's career. Feelings of uncertainty and reduced self-confidence may influence demoralised young players to give up. Also, self-regulation and self-reflection are crucial in this transition phase (Toering et al., 2011). Self-regulated learning is reflected in taking responsibility for learning, monitoring progress, managing emotions, focusing on self-improvement and seeking help and support from others when necessary (Toering et al., 2011). Jonker and colleagues (Jonker, Elferink-Gemser, Toering, Lyons and Visscher, 2010; Jonker, Elferink-Gemser and Visscher, 2010) concluded that successful players are more: (a) willing to invest effort in training and competition; (b) able to set clearer and more realistic goals that focus on progression; (c) aware of their strengths and weaknesses; (d) capable of adapting their learning strategies to the practice/game requirements.

Abandonment of the quota limiting the number of foreign players in domestic European Union leagues has led to changes in the structure of the game. The identification and selection of elite senior players has produced migration patterns that appear to be having a negative impact on indigenous player development (Littlewood, Richardson, Lees and Peiser, 2001; Maguire and Pearton, 2000). For instance, analysis of match statistics in the Premier League suggests that English players are no longer in the majority (Voetbal International, 2007). After four months into the 2007–8 competitive season, English players had played for only 99,186 minutes out of a total of 270,766 minutes, in comparison to 171,580 minutes for their foreign colleagues or 37% as compared to 63%, respectively. Only one in three players were English and there were only four teams that gave more playing opportunities to English than foreign players.

Authorities are now more aware of this problem and are considering introducing new laws to support the development of home-grown players. The Royal Belgian Football Association now requires national division teams to include at least two players younger than 21 years in their match selection ('under-21 rule'). Vaeyens, Coutts and Philippaerts (2005b) evaluated the effectiveness of the under-21 rule over four seasons. They analysed 2,138 semi-professional and amateur second and third division soccer players aged 16–39 years. The following measures were recorded: (a) number of times a player was selected to be in the first team squad; (b) number of times a player was selected to play in the starting line-up; and (c) the number of minutes played. Although the teams had complied with the new selection regulations (95% of the games were played in conformity with the rule), individual player data revealed no increase in the number of playing minutes or selections in the under-21 group. Many teams had complied with the new regulations by selecting young players as substitutes (especially goalkeepers, who almost never played), using a rotation system (36% of the U21 players were selected for 5 or fewer games, while 48% of them played in a maximum of 5 games) and/or transferring U21 players from higher-level league teams. Inadequate player development and short-term selection policy are plausible reasons for the limited playing opportunities afforded to young soccer players.

Alternative strategies are needed to resolve this problem. In recent years, the UEFA has revealed proposals for the inclusion of a minimum of home-grown players in the match selection or club squad. However, in keeping with the results of the under-21 rule (Vaeyens *et al.*, 2005b), it remains unclear whether such amendments will increase playing opportunities and facilitate the transition from youth to senior level. Systematic competition with lower-level senior teams, as is the case in, for example, France and Spain, may be beneficial for young players in bridging the gap to high-level soccer. The true challenge facing federations and club teams is to change attitude in favour of nurturing and providing opportunities for home-grown players to optimise their potential. It is evident that clubs must invest more effort and resources in talent development so that promising young players can optimise their performance in a stimulating environment.

## SUMMARY

It is clear that there is no simple mechanistic solution that can adequately predict talent in soccer. While there are without doubt excellent scouts who successfully identify talent, there is research evidence to suggest that the talent identification procedures used in clubs are not always successful. Science can therefore provide valuable complementary information. For instance, objective assessments are very useful in identifying strengths and weaknesses to be remedied. Although access to technology has improved markedly in recent years, difficulties remain in trying to adequately capture the demands of competition under controlled laboratory conditions (Williams and Ericsson, 2005). It is recommended that researchers develop performance measures that better simulate the demands of actual competition. This move towards more realistic test protocols should improve the predictive utility of the measures employed. However, due to the endless number of formulae for talent in any domain, models that attempt to correlate success in a domain with individual component scores may be largely unsuccessful (Abbott and Collins, 2004; Simonton, 2001). The challenge is to create a device that can objectively evaluate 'total' performance in the competitive setting. The advent of increasingly more sophisticated measurement systems may enable such developments at some stage in the future.

Contemporary research in youth soccer suggests that perceptual-cognitive measures success-fully discriminate between various skill levels (Reilly *et al.*, 2000; Savelsbergh *et al.*, 2010; Vaeyens *et al.*, 2007a; 2007b). Clearly, these skills need to be included in any parsimonious and reliable model of talent identification, as these measures may have practical utility for testing and training in soccer. In future, research is needed to identify the practical utility of such measures in the talent identification process.

It is clear that the transition period between youth and adult soccer requires more attention. Players who excel at youth level are not necessarily those who strive at the highest levels of the adult game, and vice versa. The use of interviews with elite players and those who eventually failed to reach the elite level may help in understanding the discriminating factors. Moreover, longitudinal research designs are particularly useful, as they offer insight into how players with different success rates vary in their development profiles. To date, longitudinal changes in relationships between growth and technical, tactical, physical and physiological characteristics of young players are limited. It is clear that it is inappropriate to extrapolate data on adult players when prescribing performance criteria (and training) for children. In future, researchers need to examine the demands experienced during match play as a function of

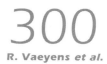

300

age, maturity status (and playing position). Match analysis data on adolescent players is scarce and may facilitate understanding of the demands on youth players, which in turn could provide valuable information for talent identification and development. On the other hand, efforts are needed to explore how young adult players can be better prepared for integration into the first team culture, as current applied methods often fail to help these youngsters.

# REFERENCES

Abbott, A. and Collins, D. (2004). Eliminating the dichotomy between theory and practice in talent identification and development: considering the role of psychology. *Journal of Sports Sciences* 22(5), 395–408.

Abbott, A. and Easson, B. (2002). The mental profile. In B.D. Hale and D. Collins (eds), *Rugby Tough* (pp. 17–33). Champaign, IL: Human Kinetics.

Abernethy, B., Thomas, K.T. and Thomas, J.T. (1993). Strategies for improving understanding of motor expertise (or mistakes we have made and things we have learned!!). In J.L. Starkes and F. Allard (eds), *Cognitive Issues in Motor Expertise* (pp. 317–356). Amsterdam, Netherlands: Elsevier.

Ashworth, J. and Heyndels, B. (2007). Selection bias and peer effects in team sports: the effect of age grouping on earnings of German soccer players. *Journal of Sport Economics* 8, 355–377.

Augste, C. and Lames, M. (2011). The relative age effect and success in German elite U-17 soccer teams. *Journal of Sports Sciences* 29(9), 983–987.

Baker, J. and Logan, A.J. (2007). Developmental contexts and sporting success: birth date and birthplace effects in national hockey league draftees 2000–2005. *British Journal of Sports Medicine* 41, 515–517.

Barnsley, R.H., Thompson, A.H. and Legault, P. (1992). Family planning: football style. The relative age effect in football. *International Review of Sport Sociology* 27, 77–87.

Baxter-Jones, A.D.G. (1995). Growth and development of young athletes: should competition levels be age related? *Sports Medicine* 20(2), 59–64.

Bradley, P.S., Sheldon, W., Wooster, B., Olsen, P., Boanas, P. and Krustrup, P. (2009). High-intensity running in English FA Premier League soccer matches. *Journal of Sports Sciences* 27, 159–168.

Brewer, J., Balsom, P. and Davis, J. (1995). Seasonal birth distribution amongst European soccer players. *Sports, Exercise and Injury* 1, 154–157.

Brewer, J., Balsom, P., Davis, J. and Ekblom, B. (1992). The influence of birth date and physical development on the selection of a male junior international soccer squad. *Journal of Sports Sciences* 10, 561–562.

Buchheit, M., Mendez-Villanueva, A., Simpson, B.M. and Bourdon, P.C. (2010a). Match running performance and fitness in youth soccer. *International Journal of Sports Medicine* 31, 818–825.

Buchheit, M., Mendez-Villanueva, A., Simpson, B.M. and Bourdon, P.C. (2010b). Repeated-sprint sequences during youth soccer matches. *International Journal of Sports Medicine* 31, 709–716.

Cacciari, E., Mazzanti, L., Tassinari, D., Bergamaschi, R., Magnani, D., Zappula, F., Nanni, G., Cobianchi, C., Ghini, T., Pini, R. and Tani, G. (1990). Effects of sport (football) on growth: auxological, anthropometric and hormonal aspects. *European Journal of Applied Physiology* 61(1–2), 149–158.

Caine, D.J. and Broeckhoff, J. (1987). Maturity assessment: a viable preventive measure against physical and psychological insult to the young athlete? *Physician and Sportsmedicine* 15(3), 67–80.

Carling, C., le Gall, F., Reilly, T. and Williams, A.M. (2009). Do anthropometric and fitness characteristics vary according to birth date distribution in elite youth academy soccer players? *Scandinavian Journal of Medicine and Science in Sports* 19(1), 3–9.

Cobley, S., Baker, J., Wattie, N. and McKenna, J. (2009). Annual age-grouping and athlete development: a meta-analytical review of relative age effects in sport. *Sports Medicine* 39(3), 235–256.

Coelho e Silva, M.J., Figueiredo, A.J., Simões, F., Seabra, A., Natal, A., Vaeyens, R., Philippaerts, R., Cumming, S.P. and Malina, R.M. (2010). Discrimination of U-14 soccer players by level and position. *International Journal of Sports Medicine* 31, 790–796.

Cronbach, L.J. (1971). Test validation. In R.L. Thorndike (ed.), *Educational Measurement*, 2nd edn (pp. 443–507). Washington, DC: American Council on Education.

Csikszentmihalyi, M. (1998). Fruitless polarities. *Behavioral and Brain Sciences* 21(3), 411.

Delorme, N., Boiché, J. and Raspaud, M. (2010). Relative age and drop-out in French male soccer. *Journal of Sports Sciences* 28(7), 717–722.

Di Salvo, V., Baron, R., Tschan, H., Calderon Montero, F.J., Bachl, N., Pigozzi, F. (2007). Performance characteristics according to playing position in elite soccer. *International Journal of Sports Medicine* 28, 222–227.

Dudink, A. (1994). Birth date and sporting success. *Nature* 368(6472), 592.

Durand-Bush, N. and Salmela, J. (2001). The development of talent in sport. In R.N. Singer, H.A. Hausenblas and C.M. Janelle (eds), *Handbook of Sport Psychology*, 2nd edn (pp. 269–289). New York: Wiley.

Elferink-Gemser, M.T., Jordet, G., Coelho e Silva, M.J. and Visscher, C. (2011). The marvels of elite sports: how to get there? *British Journal of Sports Medicine* 45(9), 683–684.

Elferink-Gemser, M.T., Visscher, C., Lemmink, K.A.P.M. and Mulder, T.W. (2004). Relation between multidimensional performance characteristics and level of performance in talented youth field hockey players. *Journal of Sports Sciences* 22(11–12), 1053–1063.

Ericsson, K.A. and Delaney, P.F. (1999). Long-term working memory as an alternative to capacity models of working memory in everyday skilled performance. In A. Miyake and P. Shah (eds), *Models of Working Memory: Mechanisms of Active Maintenance and Executive Control* (pp. 257–297). Cambridge, UK: Cambridge University Press.

Ericsson, K.A. and Kintsch, W. (1995). Long-term working memory. *Psychological Review* 102, 211–245.

European Court of Human Rights (1995). Case C-415/93. *European Court Reports*, p. I-04921.

Figueiredo, A.J., Coelho e Silva, M.J. and Malina, R.M. (2011). Predictors of functional capacity and skill in youth soccer players. *Scandinavian Journal of Medicine and Science in Sports* 21, 446–454.

Ford, P. and Williams, A.M. (2011). No relative age effects in the birth dates of award-winning athletes in male professional team sports. *Research Quarterly for Exercise and Sport* 82(3), 570–573.

Gagné, F. (2003). Transforming gifts into talents: the DMGT as a developmental theory. In N. Colangelo and G.A. Davis (eds), *Handbook of Gifted Education*, 3rd edn (pp. 60–74). Boston: Allyn & Bacon.

Helsen, W.F. and Pauwels, J.M. (1993). The relationship between expertise and visual information processing in sport. In J.L. Starkes and F. Allards (eds), *Cognitive Issues in Motor Expertise* (pp. 109–134). Amsterdam: North-Holland.

Helsen, W.F. and Starkes, J.L. (1999). A multidimensional approach to skilled perception and performance in sport. *Applied Cognitive Psychology* 13(1), 1–27.

Helsen, W.F., Starkes, J.L. and Van Winckel, J. (1998). The influence of relative age on success and drop out in male soccer players. *American Journal of Human Biology* 10(6), 791–798.

Huijgen, B., Elferink-Gemser, M.T. and Visscher, C. (2009). Soccer skill development in professionals. *International Journal of Sports Medicine* 30, 585–591.

Huijgen, B.C., Elferink-Gemser, M.T., Post, W., Visscher, C. (2010). Development of dribbling in talented youth soccer players aged 12–19 years: a longitudinal study. *Journal of Sports Sciences* 28(7), 689–698.

Janelle, C.M. and Hillman, C.H. (2003). Expert performance in sport: current perspectives and critical issues. In J.L. Starkes and K.A. Ercisson (eds), *Expert Performance in Sports. Advances in Research on Sport Expertise* (pp. 19–47). Champaign, IL: Human Kinetics.

Jiménez, I.P. and Pain, M.T. (2008). Relative age effect in Spanish association football: its extent and implications for wasted potential. *Journal of Sports Sciences* 26(10), 995–1003.

Jonker, L., Elferink-Gemser, M.T. and Visscher, C. (2010). Differences in self-regulatory skills among talented athletes: the significance of sport performance level and type of sport. *Journal of Sports Sciences* 8, 901–908.

Jonker, L., Elferink-Gemser, M.T., Toering, T.T., Lyons, J. and Visscher, C. (2010). Academic performance and self-regulatory skills in elite youth soccer players. *Journal of Sports Sciences* 28, 1605–1614.

Kannekens, R., Elferink-Gemser, M.T. and Visscher, C. (2009). Tactical skills of world-class youth soccer teams. *Journal of Sports Sciences* 27(8), 807–812.

Kannekens, R., Elferink-Gemser, M.T. and Visscher, C. (2011). Positioning and deciding: key factors for talent development in soccer. *Scandinavian Journal of Medicine and Science in Sports* 21(6), 846–852.

Kuhn, W. (2002). Changes in professional soccer in Germany since 1990. In W. Spinks, T. Reilly and A. Murphy (eds), *Science and Football IV: Proceedings of the Fourth World Congress of Science and Football* (pp. 421–430). London: Routledge.

Littlewood, M., Richardson, D., Lees, A. and Peiser, B. (2001). Migration patterns in top level English football. *Insight – The FA Coaches Association Journal* 3(4), 40–41.

Maguire, J. and Pearton, R. (2000). The impact of elite labour migration on the identification, selection and development of European soccer players. *Journal of Sports Sciences* 18, 759–769.

Malina, R.M., Peña Reyes, M.E., Eisenmann, J.C., Horta, L., Rodrigues, J. and Miller, R. (2000). Height, mass and skeletal maturity of elite Portuguese soccer players aged 11–16 years. *Journal of Sports Sciences* 18(9), 685–693.

Meylan, C., Cronin, J., Oliver, J. and Hughes, M. (2010). Talent identification in soccer: the role of maturity status on physical, physiological and technical characteristics. *International Journal of Sports Science & Coaching* 5(4), 571–592.

Moore, P.M., Collins, D.J., Burwitz, L., Tebbenham, D., Abbott, A. and Arnold, J. (1998). Identification and development of talent in selected UK sports. *Journal of Sports Sciences* 16(1), 23.

Morris, T. (2000). Psychological characteristics and talent identification in soccer. *Journal of Sports Sciences* 18(9), 715–726.

Mujika, I., Vaeyens, R., Matthys, S.P., Santisteban, J., Goiriena, J. and Philippaerts, R. (2009). The relative age effect in a professional football club setting. *Journal of Sports Sciences* 11(27), 1153–1158.

Musch, J. and Grondin, S. (2001). Unequal competition as an impediment to personal development: A review of the relative age effect in sport. *Developmental Review* 21(2), 147–167.

Musch, J. and Hay, R. (1999). The relative age effect in soccer: cross-cultural evidence for a systematic discrimination against children born late in the competition year. *Sociology of Sport Journal* 16(1), 54–64.

Nieuwenhuis, C.F., Spamer, E.J. and van Rossum, J.H.A. (2002). Prediction function for identifying talent in 14- to 15-year-old female field hockey players. *High Ability Studies* 13(1), 21–33.

Panfil, R., Naglak, Z., Bober, T. and Zaton, E.W.M. (1997). Searching and developing talents in soccer: A year of experience. In J. Bangsbo, B. Saltin, H. Bonde, Y. Hellsten, B. Ibsen, M. Kjaer and G. Sjøgaard (eds), *Proceedings of the 2nd Annual Congress of the European College of Sport Science* (pp. 649–650). Copenhagen, Denmark: HO + Storm.

Peña Reyes, M.E., Cardenas-Barahona, E. and Malina, R.M. (1994). Growth, physique, and skeletal maturation of soccer players 7–17 years of age. *Auxology, Humanbiologia Budapestinensis* 25, 453–458.

Philippaerts, R.M., Vaeyens, R., Janssens, M., Van Renterghem, B., Matthys, D., Craen, R., Bourgois, J., Vrijens, J., Beunen, G. and Malina, R.M. (2006). The relationship between peak height velocity and physical performance in youth soccer players. *Journal of Sports Sciences* 24(3), 221–230.

Phillips, E., Davids, K., Renshaw, I. and Portus, M. (2010). Expert performance in sport and the dynamics of talent development. *Sports Medicine* 40, 271–283.

Pienaar, A.E. and Spamer, E.J. (1998). A longitudinal study of talented young rugby players as regards their rugby skills, physical and motor abilities and anthropometric data. *Journal of Human Movement Studies* 34(1),13–32.

Rampinini, E., Coutts, A.J., Castagna, C., Sassi, R. and Impellizzeri, F.M. (2007). Variation in top level soccer match performance. *International Journal of Sports Medicine* 28, 1018–1024.

Rampinini, E., Impellizzeri, F.M., Castagna, C., Coutts, A.J. and Wisloff, U. (2009). Technical performance during soccer matches of the Italian Serie A league: effect of fatigue and competitive level. *Journal of Science and Medicine in Sport* 12, 227–233.

Régnier, G. and Salmela, J. (1987). Predictors of success in Canadian male gymnasts. In B. Petiot, J.H. Salmela and T.B. Hoshizaki (eds), *World Identification Systems for Gymnastic Talent* (pp 143–150). Montreal: Sport Psyche Editions.

Régnier, G., Salmela, J.H. and Russell, S.J. (1993). Talent detection and development in sport. In R.N. Singer, M. Murphey and L.K. Tennant (eds), *Handbook of Research in Sport Psychology* (pp. 290–313). New York: Macmillan.

Reilly, T., Williams, A.M., Nevill, A. and Franks, A. (2000). A multidisciplinary approach to talent identification in soccer. *Journal of Sports Sciences* 18(9), 695–702.

Richardson, D., Littlewood, M. and Gilbourne, D. (2005). Homegrown or nationals? Some considerations on the local training debate. *Insight Live*, https://ice.thefa.com/.

Roescher, C.R., Elferink-Gemser, M.T., Huijgen, B.C. and Visscher, C. (2010). Soccer endurance development in professionals. *International Journal of Sports Medicine* 31(3), 174–179.

Savelsbergh, G.J.P., Haans, S.H.A., Kooijman, M.K. and van Kampen, P.M. (2010). A method to identify talent: visual search and locomotion behavior in young football players. *Human Movement Science* 29, 764–776.

Simonton, D.K. (2001). Talent development as a multidimensional, multiplicative, and dynamic process. *Current Directions in Psychological Science* 10, 39–43.

Starkes, J.L. (1993). Motor experts: opening thoughts. In J.L. Starkes and F. Allard (eds), *Cognitive Issues in Motor Expertise* (pp. 3–16). Amsterdam, Netherlands: Elsevier.

Starkes, J.L. and Allard, F. (eds) (1993). *Cognitive Issues in Motor Expertise*. Amsterdam, Netherlands: Elsevier.

Toering, T., Elferink-Gemser, M., Jordet, G., Jorna, C., Pepping, G.J. and Visscher, C. (2011). Self-regulation of practice behavior among elite youth soccer players: an exploratory observation study. *Journal of Applied Sport Psychology* 23, 110–128.

Tranckle, P. and Cushion, C.J. (2006). Rethinking giftedness and talent in sport. *Quest* 58(2), 265–282.

Vaeyens, R. and Philippaerts, R. (2007). Oma's aan de top! In M. Lenoir and R. Philippaerts (eds), *Bewegingswetenschap in beweging: een bloemlezing uit 100 jaar sportwetenschappelijk onderzoek aan de Universiteit Gent* (pp. 74–76). Gent: Vakgroep Bewegings- en Sportwetenschappen.

Vaeyens, R., Coutts, A. and Philippaerts, R.M. (2005b). Evaluation of the 'under-21 rule': do young adult soccer players benefit? *Journal of Sports Sciences* 23(10), 1003–1012.

Vaeyens, R., Philippaerts, R.M. and Malina, R.M. (2005a). The relative age effect in soccer: a match-related perspective. *Journal of Sports Sciences* 23(7), 747–756.

Vaeyens, R., Lenoir, M., Williams, A.M., Mazyn, L. and Philippaerts, R.M. (2007a). The effects of task constraints on visual search behaviour and decision-making skill in youth soccer players. *Journal of Sport and Exercise Psychology* 29(2), 147–169.

Vaeyens, R., Lenoir, M., Williams, A.M. and Philippaerts, R.M. (2007b). The mechanisms underpinning successful decision-making in skilled youth soccer players: analysis of visual search behaviors. *Journal of Motor Behavior* 39(5), 395–408.

Vaeyens, R., Lenoir, M., Williams, A.M. and Philippaerts, R.M. (2008). Talent identification and development programmes in sport: current models and future directions. *Sports Medicine* 38(9), 703–714.

Vaeyens, R., Malina, R.M., Janssens, M., Van Renterghem, B., Bourgois, J., Vrijens, J. and Philippaerts, R.M. (2006). A multidisciplinary selection model for youth soccer: the Ghent Youth Soccer Project. *British Journal of Sports Medicine* 40(11), 928–934.

Verhulst, J. (1992). Seasonal birth distribution of West European soccer players: a possible explanation. *Medical Hypotheses* 38(4), 346–348.

Vincent, J. and Glamser, F.D. (2006). Gender differences in the relative age effect among US Olympic development program youth soccer players. *Journal of Sports Sciences* 24(4), 405–413.

Voetbal International (2007). Engelsen zijn greep op Premier League kwijt. http://www.vi.nl/web/show/id=310011/langid=43/contentid=145855.

Ward, P. and Williams, A.M. (2003). Perceptual and cognitive skill development in soccer: the multidimensional nature of expert performance. *Journal of Sport and Exercise Psychology* 25(1), 93–111.

Ward, P., Hodges, N.J., Williams, A.M. and Starkes, J.L. (2004). Deliberate practice and expert performance: defining the path to excellence. In A.M. Williams and N.J. Hodges (eds),

*Skill Acquisition in Sport: Research, Theory and Practice* (pp. 231–258). London, UK: Routledge.

Williams, A.M. (2000). Perceptual skill in soccer: implications for talent identification and development. *Journal of Sports Sciences* 18, 737–750.

Williams, A.M. and Burwitz, L. (1993). Advance cue utilization in soccer. In T. Reilly, J. Clarys and A. Stibbe, *Science and Football II* (pp. 239–244). London, UK: E and FN Spon.

Williams, A.M. and Davids, K. (1995). Declarative knowledge in sport: a byproduct of experience or a characteristic of expertise? *Journal of Sport and Exercise Psychology* 17, 259–275.

Williams, A.M. and Davids, K. (1998). Visual search strategy, selective attention, and expertise in soccer. *Research Quarterly for Exercise and Sport* 69(2), 111–128.

Williams, A.M. and Ericsson, K.A. (2005). Perceptual-cognitive expertise in sport: some considerations when applying the expert performance approach. *Human Movement Science* 24(3), 283–307.

Williams, A.M. and Franks, A. (1998). Talent identification in soccer. *Sports, Exercise and Injury* 4(4), 159–165.

Williams, A.M. and Reilly, T. (2000a). Searching for the stars. *Journal of Sports Sciences* 18(9), 655–656.

Williams, A.M. and Reilly, T. (2000b). Talent identification and development in soccer. *Journal of Sports Sciences* 18(9), 657–667.

Williams, A.M. and Ward, P. (2007). Anticipation and decision making: exploring new horizons. In G. Tenenbaum and R.C. Eklund (eds), *Handbook of Sport Psychology*, 3rd edn (pp. 203–223). Hoboken, NJ: Wiley.

Williams, A.M., Hodges, N.J., North, J. and Barton, G. (2006). Perceiving patterns of play in dynamic sport tasks: Investigating the essential information underlying skilled performance. *Perception* 35(3), 317–332.

Williams, J.H. (2010). Relative age effect in youth soccer: analysis of the FIFA U17 World Cup competition. *Scandinavian Journal of Medicine & Science in Sports* 20, 502–508.

# CHAPTER 17

## GROWTH AND MATURITY STATUS OF YOUTH PLAYERS

R.M. Malina, M. Coelho e Silva and A.J. Figueiredo

## INTRODUCTION

Given the popularity of soccer throughout the world, there is considerable interest in the growth and maturation of young players, both in general and in the context of talent development. In this chapter we summarize and evaluate the growth and maturity status of male soccer players between 9 and 18 years of age, and then consider several growth- and maturity-related issues in more detail. Implications of the data are discussed relative to selection and retention, age verification, size mismatches, relative age effect and injury risk.

Youth soccer has many participants and levels of competition. Many youth participate in soccer for one or several years and move to other activities as interests change, skill and training demands increase and competitive sport becomes more selective and exclusive. Samples of soccer players thus vary in composition from childhood through adolescence. Competitive levels of samples are accepted as described by authors of the papers cited in this chapter. Players are defined by level of competition (club, regional, elite) and on the basis of regional, national and international selections and competitions.

## GROWTH STATUS

Growth status refers most often to height and weight attained at a given chronological age (CA). Other indicators include physique and body composition. Mean ages, heights and weights of soccer players in Europe and the Americas are illustrated relative to selected percentiles of United States reference data (25th [P 25], median [P 50], and 75th [P 75]) in Figures 17.1 and 17.2, respectively. Mean heights generally fall between P 25 and P 75. Only one mean exceeds P 75, while 12 mean heights are just below P 25. The fourth degree polynomial fitted to mean heights of soccer players matches the reference median through the age range.

Most mean weights also fall within the bounds of P 25 and P 75. Nine mean weights are just above P 75, but one is well above P 75. In contrast, only four mean weights are just below P 25, although several are on P25. The fourth degree polynomial fitted to mean weights approximates the reference median from late childhood to about 13 years and is then above the reference through adolescence. The majority of mean weights of late adolescent players (15+ years) are at or above the reference median.

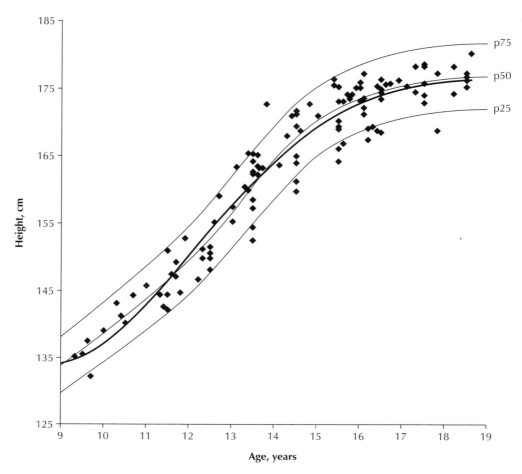

**Figure 17.1** Mean heights of young soccer players from Europe and the Americas plotted relative to United States reference data: 25th, 50th (median) and 75th percentiles (Centers for Diseases Control and Prevention, 2000).

*Sources:* Earlier data, primarily 1985 to 2002 (Malina, 2003); more recent data (Malina *et al.*, 2000, 2004b; Seabra *et al.*, 2001; Fragoso *et al.*, 2004; Vicente-Rodriguez *et al.*, 2003; Gissis *et al.*, 2006; Diniz da Silva *et al.*, 2008; Gravina *et al.*, 2008; Figueiredo *et al.*, 2009a; Le Gall *et al.*, 2010).
*Note:* The bold solid line is the fit of a fourth degree polynomial to the data points.

Mean heights of young Japanese soccer players fall close to the reference median for the general Japanese population, while mean weights are generally below the median (Malina, 1994, 2003). An exception is national youth team (17.5±0.7 years) players, who are taller and especially heavier. More recent data for players aged 9–14 years indicate mean heights consistently larger than the reference; mean weights are similar to the reference among younger players but above the reference in players aged 12–14 years (Hirose, 2009). There is a need for data for youth players in different areas of the world.

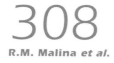

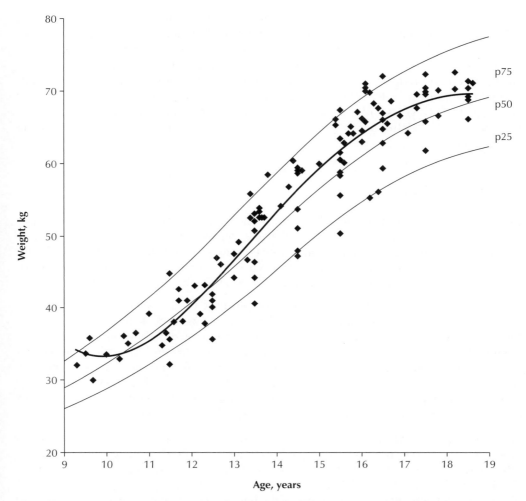

**Figure 17.2** Mean weights of young soccer players from Europe and the Americas plotted relative to United States reference data: 25th, 50th (median) and 75th percentiles (Centers for Diseases Control and Prevention, 2000).

*Sources:* As for Figure 17.1.
*Note:* The bold solid line is the fit of a fourth degree polynomial to the data points.

The overall trend for the body size of young soccer players suggests generally appropriate weight for height during childhood and early adolescence, but more weight for height in later adolescence. This finding is consistent with data for somatotype. Adolescent players are mesomorphic (Barbieri and Rodriguez Papini, 1996; Figueiredo *et al.*, 2005; Seabra *et al.*, 2004). Changes with age are relatively small, except for an increase in mesomorphy associated with the adolescent spurt in muscle mass. Mean somatotypes of late adolescent players generally fall within the ranges for national and international-calibre players (Carter *et al.*, 1998).

The proportionally high weight for height of adolescent players reflects a larger fat-free mass (FFM), specifically muscle mass. FFM follows a growth pattern similar to height and thus varies with body size. Mean % Fat (densitometry, total body water) of elite young adult soccer players in four studies ranges from $6.2 \pm 1.9\%$ to $9.7 \pm 3.0\%$ (Malina, 2007). Data for youth players are largely based on predictions from skinfold thicknesses, which tend to have relatively large standard errors. Mean % Fat of youth players fluctuates above and below reference values for youth aged 11–16 years and is higher than values for elite young adult players (Malina and Geithner, 2011). Relative fatness declines during adolescence, consistent with observations for males in general.

## MATURITY STATUS

Maturation refers to progress towards the biologically mature state, an operational concept, since maturity varies with body systems. All tissues, organs and systems of the body mature. Maturation, the process of maturing, can be viewed in two contexts: timing and tempo. Timing refers to when specific maturational events occur, while tempo refers to the rate at which maturation progresses. Timing and tempo vary considerably among individuals.

Studies of the biological maturation of soccer players have used skeletal age (SA); pubic hair (PH), genital (G) development and testicular volume; and age at peak height velocity (PHV). Methods of assessment and limitations of each are summarized elsewhere (Malina et al., 2004a; Malina, 2011). SA is applicable in childhood and adolescence. SA corresponds to the level of skeletal maturity attained by a player relative to the reference sample for each method. A player with a CA of 11.5 years may have an SA of 13.3 years; he has attained the skeletal maturity equivalent to a boy of 13.3 years in the reference sample. Secondary sex characteristics and age at PHV, by contrast, are useful only during adolescence.

Protocols for predicting age at PHV and mature (adult) height without the use of SA have been described. The former predicts maturity offset, time before PHV, from age, height, weight, sitting height and estimated leg length (Mirwald et al., 2002). Subtracting maturity offset from CA estimates age at PHV. The latter predicts mature height from age, height and weight of a player and midparent height, and average of the heights of the biological parents (Khamis and Roche, 1994). Current height is then expressed as a percentage of predicted mature height, which is an indicator of maturity status. Use of the protocols with athletes is increasing, but they need validation. Ages at PHV from maturity offset tend to have reduced standard deviations (Nurmi-Lawton et al., 2004; Malina et al., 2006; Sherar et al., 2007), as compared to estimates in longitudinal studies, usually about one year (Malina and Beunen, 1996b; Malina et al., 2004a). The protocols are based on samples of European ancestry, so that applications to other ethnic groups require care. Ethnic variation in proportions of sitting height and leg length is a potential concern with the maturity offset protocol.

Mean SAs ($\pm$standard deviations) from more recent studies of soccer players are plotted relative to mean CAs in Figure 17.3. The data include observations with the three commonly used methods of assessment and data for Japanese players. Mean SAs tend to approximate CAs among players aged 10–13 years. With increasing age, mean SAs tend to be in advance of CAs, so that boys advanced in skeletal maturity are more prevalent. Variation in SA is

# 310

reduced in later adolescence, as many players reach skeletal maturity and an SA is not assigned to individuals who are skeletally mature.

Studies of youth athletes in several sports commonly classify players into maturity categories based on the difference between SA and CA (Malina et al., 2004a; Malina, 2011). Distributions of soccer players by maturity categories within CA groups 11–16 years are summarized in Figures 17.4 and 17.5. Although there is variation among methods, similar numbers of late and early maturing players are represented in samples 11–13 years, while the majority is classified as on time (the difference between TW2 and TW3 is discussed below). Distributions shift towards players advanced in skeletal maturation with increasing CA during adolescence

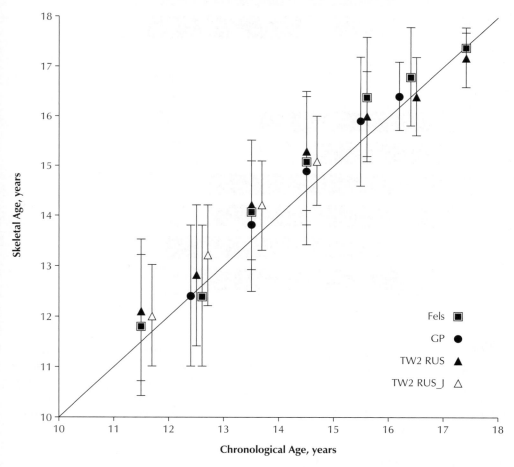

Figure 17.3 Skeletal ages (mean±standard deviations) plotted by mean chronological ages of youth soccer players assessed with the Fels (Portuguese, Spanish, Mexican), Greulich-Pyle (GP, French, Portguese), and Tanner-Whitehouse (TW2 RUS, Belgian, Italian, Portuguese, Spanish, Mexican) methods. Data are summarized in Malina (2011) and Malina et al. (2010). TW2 RUS_J data are for Japanese youth players (Hirose, 2009).

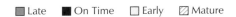

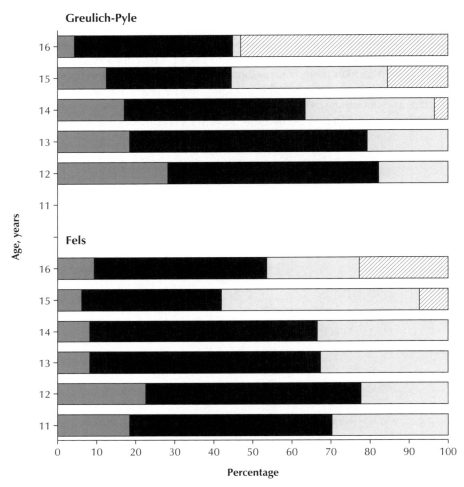

**Figure 17.4** Percentages of players classified as late, on time and early maturing and as mature in CA groups 11–16 years based on SA assessments with the Greulich-Pyle (French, Portuguese players) and Fels (Portuguese, Spanish players) methods. The cutoffs are as follows: on time (average), SA within ±1.0 year of CA; late, SA behind CA by more than 1.0 year; early, SA in advance of CA by more than 1.0 year. Players who have attained skeletal maturity are simply indicated as mature and no SA is assigned.

*Source*: Sources of data are summarized in Malina (2011) and Malina *et al*. (2010), which also include a discussion of the classification protocol.

**R.M. Malina** *et al.*

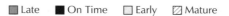

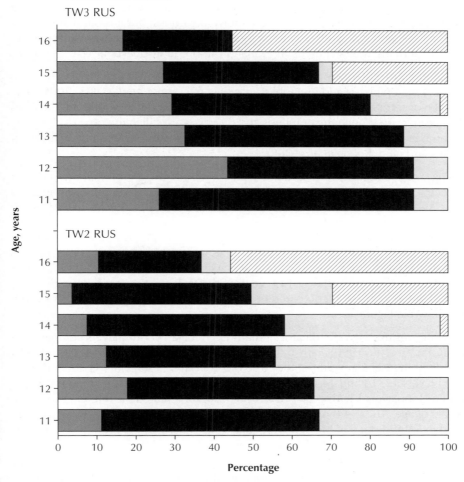

**Figure 17.5** Percentages of players classified as late, on time and early maturing and as mature in chronological age groups 11–16 years based on SA assessments with the Tanner-Whitehouse method (TW2 RUS and TW3 RUS; Belgian, Italian, Portuguese, Spanish, Mexican players). Cutoffs are as in Figure 17.4.

*Source*: Sources of data are summarized in Malina (2011).

– late maturing players decline while early maturing and skeletally mature players increase. Data are limited for 17-year-old players, but many are skeletally mature (Malina, 2011).

Differences in protocols influence variation in SAs among methods. The Greulich-Pyle method (Greulich and Pyle, 1959) calls for assessment of individual bones, but it is often applied by comparing the radiograph as a whole to the pictorial standards. It is necessary to interpolate between two and perhaps three standards and variation among individual bones is overlooked.

The Tanner-Whitehouse criteria for the final stage of maturity of the distal radius and ulna are simply, 'fusion of the epiphysis and metaphysis has begun' (Tanner et al., 1983, 2001). The time lag between onset and completion of union is not considered. Many youths are classified as skeletally mature even though the epiphysis and diaphysis are still in the process of fusing. The Fels method, in contrast, has specific criteria from beginning through complete fusion of the distal radius and ulna (Roche et al., 1988).

Age at attaining skeletal maturity for the radius-ulna-short bone (RUS) protocol was reduced in the most recent version of the method, TW3 (Tanner et al., 2001). Maturity was attained in boys at an SA of 18.2 years with TW2 RUS, but was reduced to 16.5 years in TW3 RUS. Stages of maturity of each bone and assigned maturity scores were not modified, but the scale for converting maturity scores to SAs was changed, especially for SAs 10 years and older. For example, a RUS maturity score of 316 was assigned a SA of 10.5 years with TW2 but was assigned a SA of 10.0 with TW3; a score of 602 was assigned an SA of 15.1 years with TW2 but a score of 603 was assigned a SA of 14.0 years with TW3. For the same maturity score, SAs were scaled down with TW3, compared to TW2 after about 10.0 years. This affects the distributions shown in Figure 17.5.

Testicular volume was used as an indicator of maturity in Italian youth players compared to non-athletes (Cacciari et al., 1990). Early pubertal players and non-athletes 10–11 and 12–13 years did not differ in testicular volume; they also did not differ in stage of PH, SA and body size. Pubertal players 12–13 and 14–16 years were advanced in testicular maturation. Mean testicular volume for players 14–16 years, 18.2±4.5 ml, approximated the reference for Swiss boys >17 years of age, 18.6±4.0 ml (Zachman et al., 1974). The players 14–16 years were also advanced in SA and stage of PH and were taller and heavier than non-athlete controls. A short-term longitudinal study of Danish players indicated advanced testicular maturation in elite as compared to non-elite youth at each of four observations between about 11 and 14 years (Hansen et al., 1999). The observations for both Italian and Danish youth players were consistent with SA, that is advanced sexual maturity compared to control subjects as adolescence progresses.

Distributions of stage of PH within CA groups of soccer players 11–18 years are summarized in Table 17.1. CA, height and weight of players by stage of PH within CA groups are also indicated. All five stages of PH are represented in players aged 13 years, while 4 stages are represented among players 12 and 14 years of age. Variability in PH is less in the youngest and oldest players.

Variation in body size by stage of PH within a CA group and among players of the same stage of PH in different CA groups should be noted, allowing for small sample sizes in some groups. Among players 11–15 years of age, those more advanced in stage of PH within a CA group tend to be, on average, taller and heavier. Older players tend to be taller and heavier than

**R.M. Malina et al.**

**Table 17.1** Distributions of youth soccer players by stage of pubic hair within chronological age groups and descriptive statistics for age, height and weight by stage within age groups.[1]

| | | Stages of Pubic Hair (PH) | | | | | | | | | | | | Mature | | |
| | | Prepubertal | | | | | | | | | | | | | | |
| | | PH 1 | | | PH 2 | | | PH 3 | | | PH 4 | | | PH 5 | | |
| Age, group | N | n | M | SD | n | M | SD | n | M | SD | n | M | SD | n | M | SD |
|---|---|---|---|---|---|---|---|---|---|---|---|---|---|---|---|---|
| **Age, yrs** | | | | | | | | | | | | | | | | |
| 11 | 71 | 43 | 11.5 | 0.3 | 27 | 11.5 | 0.3 | 1 | 11.6 | – | | | | | | |
| 12 | 45 | 16 | 12.5 | 0.3 | 14 | 12.5 | 0.2 | 13 | 12.6 | 0.3 | 2 | 12.9 | 0.0 | | | |
| 13 | 79 | 6 | 13.3 | 0.1 | 18 | 13.6 | 0.2 | 25 | 13.6 | 0.2 | 25 | 13.7 | 0.2 | 5 | 13.8 | 0.3 |
| 14 | 99 | | | | 6 | 14.3 | 0.2 | 20 | 14.5 | 0.4 | 53 | 14.4 | 0.3 | 20 | 14.6 | 0.3 |
| 15 | 50 | | | | | | | 2 | 15.2 | 0.0 | 25 | 15.4 | 0.4 | 23 | 15.5 | 0.3 |
| 16 | 32 | | | | | | | | | | 11 | 16.5 | 0.3 | 21 | 16.4 | 0.3 |
| 17–18 | 23 | | | | | | | | | | 6 | 17.6 | 0.4 | 17 | 17.9 | 0.4 |
| **Height, cm** | | | | | | | | | | | | | | | | |
| 11 | | | 141.1 | 5.0 | | 148.5 | 6.2 | | 145.8 | – | | | | | | |
| 12 | | | 144.5 | 6.7 | | 148.2 | 6.2 | | 156.4 | 4.9 | | 162.2 | 6.9 | | | |
| 13 | | | 155.8 | 3.1 | | 153.2 | 6.5 | | 163.9 | 7.0 | | 166.2 | 7.3 | | 172.2 | 2.8 |
| 14 | | | | | | 161.3 | 7.4 | | 163.1 | 8.1 | | 170.1 | 5.9 | | 175.7 | 6.4 |
| 15 | | | | | | | | | 167.5 | 2.8 | | 173.0 | 4.1 | | 176.0 | 3.6 |
| 16 | | | | | | | | | | | | 174.5 | 5.0 | | 174.1 | 5.2 |
| 17–18 | | | | | | | | | | | | 177.0 | 4.9 | | 176.5 | 4.7 |
| **Weight, kg** | | | | | | | | | | | | | | | | |
| 11 | | | 34.6 | 4.1 | | 42.0 | 5.4 | | 34.6 | – | | | | | | |
| 12 | | | 37.3 | 4.5 | | 41.9 | 7.7 | | 46.8 | 6.1 | | 50.7 | 5.3 | | | |
| 13 | | | 43.5 | 4.4 | | 42.8 | 6.7 | | 53.8 | 7.6 | | 56.3 | 7.4 | | 62.8 | 6.8 |
| 14 | | | | | | 53.1 | 9.5 | | 53.1 | 7.7 | | 60.1 | 6.1 | | 65.3 | 6.0 |
| 15 | | | | | | | | | 48.7 | 1.8 | | 65.3 | 7.0 | | 69.2 | 6.3 |
| 16 | | | | | | | | | | | | 67.3 | 5.5 | | 68.9 | 6.5 |
| 17–18 | | | | | | | | | | | | 70.6 | 4.0 | | 70.6 | 6.9 |

*Note:* [1] Calculated from data for Portuguese youth players reported by Horta (2003), Figueiredo *et al.* (2009a), Coelho e Silva *et al.* (2010) and Malina *et al.* (2000, 2004b).

younger players within a stage of PH. Among older adolescent players in PH 4 and PH 5 differences in body size are negligible. When CA is statistically controlled, none of the differences in height and weight among players within a stage of PH is significant (not shown). This finding reflects the fact that older players within a stage have had more time to grow, as compared to younger players.

Information on the age at PHV of soccer players is limited to three longitudinal studies. Estimates for 32 Welsh (Bell, 1993) and 8 Danish (Froberg et al., 1991) players are identical, 14.2±0.9 years, while that for 33 Belgian players (Philippaerts et al., 2006) is 13.8±0.8 years. The estimates are similar to those for European adolescents (Malina et al., 2004a). Although the results seemingly contrast trends in cross-sectional data for skeletal and sexual maturation, they are not entirely inconsistent. Advanced skeletal and sexual maturation is more apparent among players 14.0 years and older, ages when most have already passed PHV.

The 33 Belgian players were from a larger sample followed for 5 years. CAs varied from 10.4 to 13.7 years at the start of the study and PHV could not be estimated for 43 players. PHV was apparently attained by 25 early maturing players before the study started (SA=13.5±1.2 yrs; CA=12.6±0.5 yrs) and was not attained by 18 players during the study (SA=11.1±1.1 yrs; CA=11.5±0.8 yrs at the start). It should also be noted that models used to estimate PHV do not successfully fit longitudinal height records for all individuals.

Estimated ages at PHV based on the maturity-offset protocol in soccer players in Portugal were similar to the preceding, 13.9±0.4 years in players 11–12 years and 14.0 ±0.6 years in players 13–14 years (Malina et al., 2012). Reduced standard deviations with the offset protocol should be noted.

Estimated age at PHV for junior high school soccer players in Japan, 13.6±1.1 years (Nariyama et al., 2001), was later than estimates for boys and other school sport athletes (Malina et al., 2004a). The players participated in regional school competitions and were not at the level of elite youth players of the Japanese League Academy team, who were advanced in skeletal maturation at 13–15 years (Figure 17.3).

Relationships among two traditional (SA, stage of PH) and two more recent (PHV from maturity offset, percentage of predicted mature height) indicators of maturation were considered in Portuguese players 11–14 years (Malina et al., 2012). Factor analysis resulted in two components at 11–12 years, one suggesting maturity status (percentage of predicted mature height, stage of PH, explained variance 59%) and another suggesting maturity timing (SA/CA ratio, age at PHV, explained variance 26%). One component loading on all four indicators resulted for players 13–14 years (variance explained 68%). Results for soccer players were consistent with longitudinal data for boys in the US (Nicolson and Hanley, 1953) and Poland (Bielicki et al., 1984).

The players were also classified as late, on time and early maturing by SA, age at PHV and percentage of predicted mature height. Kappa coefficients were low for cross-tabulations (0.02 to 0.23) and Spearman rank order correlations were low to moderate (0.16 to 0.50). Although the maturity indicators were related, concordance of maturity classifications between SA and two more recent methods was relatively poor (Malina et al., 2012). Use of PH for classification is limited by lack of information on the age at which a stage is entered, duration of the stage, and lack of appropriate reference data. The results indicate a need for further cross-validation of maturity indicators and care in their application.

## MATURITY-ASSOCIATED VARIATION

### Size and performance

Heights and weights of players of contrasting skeletal maturity status (Fels SA) are illustrated in Figures 17.6 and 17.7, respectively. Gradients in size by maturity status were consistent from 11–14 years, early > on time > late. Among players 15–17 years, heights among the four groups overlapped considerably, consistent with the general population, while weights were

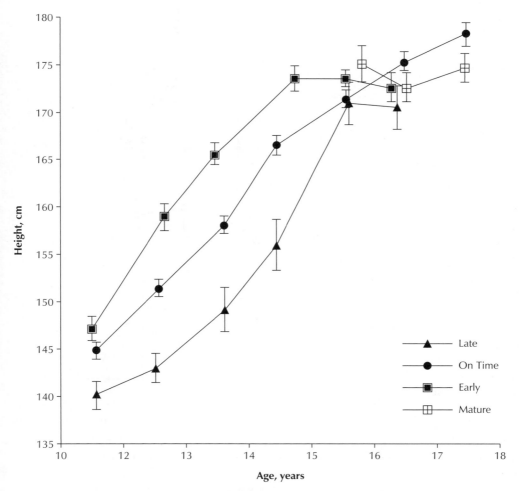

**Figure 17.6** Mean heights of Portuguese and Spanish soccer players classified as late, on time and early maturing and as mature in chronological age groups from 11 to 17 years based on SA (Fels method).

*Sources:* Heights and SAs are from Horta (2003), Figueiredo *et al.* (2009a), Malina *et al.*, 2000, 2007a). SAs are summarized in Malina (2011).

more variable but overlapped. The latter contrasted the general population, where the gradient early > on time > late persisted through 18 years (Malina *et al.*, 2004a). Variability in late adolescent players probably reflected small samples of mature and late maturing players.

Maturity-related performances of adolescent males tend to follow the gradient of early > on time > late for static and functional strength, power and running speed (Malina *et al.*, 2004a). A similar gradient is evident for maximal $O_2$ uptake (l/min), but expressing $O_2$ uptake per unit body mass (ml/kg/min) largely eliminates the differences among maturity groups (Malina *et al.*, 1997). Corresponding trends in soccer players are variable. Portuguese players 11–12

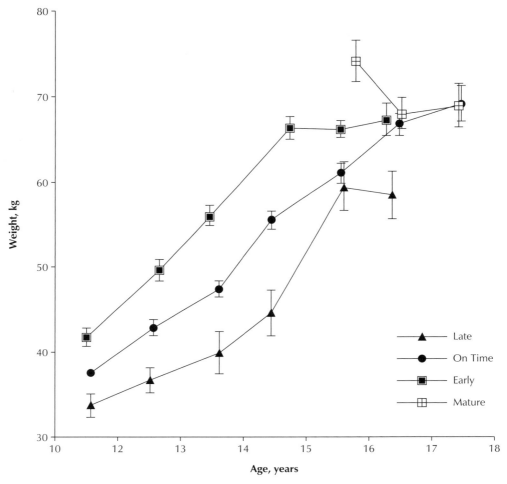

**Figure 17.7** Mean weights of Portuguese and Spanish soccer players classified as late, on time and early maturing and as mature in chronological age groups from 11 to 17 years based on SA assessments with the Fels method.

*Sources:* As for Figure 17.6.

R.M. Malina *et al.*

years of contrasting maturity status did not differ in speed (sprint), agility (shuttle run), power (counter movement jump) and four soccer skills (ball control, dribbling, passing, shooting); only aerobic capacity (endurance shuttle run) differed, late > on time = early. Results were identical in players 13–14 years of age with one exception; for the jump, early > on time > late (Figueiredo et al., 2009a). Among elite U14 French players, in contrast, the early > on time > late gradient was apparent for anaerobic power, strength, vertical jump and 40 m dash, while aerobic capacity (endurance shuttle run) did not differ among groups (Carling et al., no date). Corresponding comparisons among older adolescent players are limited. Comparisons of late (n=4), on time (n=27), early (n=29) and mature (n=6) Portuguese players 15–16 years showed no consistent differences in the standing long jump, dash and endurance shuttle run (Malina and Horta, unpublished).

Another way to address maturity-associated variation is through regression analysis. Multiple linear regressions were used to estimate the relative contributions of CA, SA and stage of PH, body size, adiposity and years of training to field tests of functional capacity and soccer skills among adolescent Portuguese players 11–15 years old (Malina et al., 2004b, 2005, 2007b; Figueiredo et al., 2011). More than one-half of the variance in functional capacities and most of the variance in soccer skills was not accounted for by the predictor variables. Maturity status explained a small though significant proportion of the variance. Maturity status appeared to be more relevant among players 13–15 years and interacted with training history, body size and body composition. This is no surprise, as functional capacities have adolescent spurts that vary in timing relative to PHV (Beunen et al., 1988; Malina et al., 2004a). Sport-specific skills, in contrast, are largely independent of maturation and body size. Other factors probably influence sport-specific skills. Individual differences in timing and tempo of maturation of neural control and perceptual-cognitive skills during adolescence, individual differences in responsiveness to instruction and training, and coach–athlete interactions are potential sources of variation. By inference, studies should be extended beyond growth and maturation to include perceptual-cognitive and behavioural characteristics of players and characteristics of coaches and training environments.

## Competitive level

Comparisons of players by level of competition or selection status are reasonably common. Regionally selected and non-selected U14 Portuguese players, for example, did not differ in CA, experience, adiposity, agility shuttle run, aerobic endurance, passing and shooting accuracy and dribbling. Selected players were advanced in SA, taller and heavier, and performed better in the squat jump, sprint and ball control (Coelho e Silva et al., 2010). No regionally select players were late maturing and about equal percentages were on time or early, while non-select players were predominantly on time in SA.

Belgian players 12–16 years were classified by competitive level: elite (1st and 2nd division clubs), sub-elite (3rd and 4th division clubs), and non-elite (regional teams), and compared in four age groups, U13 through U16 years (Vaeyens et al., 2006). Two soccer skills (juggling, lobbing) and two sprints (30 m dash, shuttle sprint) best discriminated U13 and U14 players by level. The shuttle tempo run (anaerobic) and endurance shuttle run (aerobic) also discriminated U13 and U14 players, respectively. Among U15 and U16 players, the endurance

319

shuttle run best discriminated by level; dribbling skill, two sprints and adiposity were additional discriminating variables in U15 players. Of interest, body size was not a discriminating variable in all groups. Although significant variables differed by age group, results highlighted the importance of technical skills and functional capacity, specifically cardiorespiratory endurance, in discriminating players by competitive level.

A retrospective analysis of the growth, skeletal maturation and functional characteristics of elite French youth players (Le Gall et al., 2010) compared them by playing status after leaving the programme: amateur (no professional contract); professional (contracted to a professional club); and international (full international professional). At programme entry (U14), players in the three groups did not differ in SA, height, weight, % Fat and functional capacities (strength, power, speed, aerobic, anaerobic). U15 amateurs were advanced in SA; all other variables did not differ among groups. As U16s, professionals and amateurs were advanced in SA and internationals were taller and had higher anaerobic power than amateurs; all other variables did not differ among the groups. Overall, differences were rather negligible, which perhaps reflected the highly select nature of the sample.

Players 15–16 years selected for the Portugal national team were, on average, slightly taller and heavier than non-selected players, 174.5±4.8 vs 172.2±6.5 cm and 67.5±6.3 vs 63.2±5.6 kg, respectively (Malina et al., 2000). Select and non-select players did not differ in SA and distribution by maturity status.

### Position

It is not clear when specific field positions are established among youth. Nevertheless, researchers have regularly compared players by position. Among Portuguese U14 players, defenders, midfielders and forwards (goalkeepers were not considered) did not differ in CA, SA, body size, adiposity, functional capacities and soccer skill, but regionally select and non-select players differed in several characteristics within position (Coelho e Silva et al., 2010). Regionally selected defenders and midfielders were advanced in SA, taller and heavier, and performed better in the squat jump and sprint, as compared to the non-select. Regionally select forwards were taller and heavier, and performed better in the squat jump, sprint and ball control.

Elite French youth players did not differ by position in CA and % Fat on entry to the Clairfontaine National Institute of Football (Carling et al., 2012). Goalkeepers were advanced in SA compared to midfielders, while goalkeepers and defenders were taller and heavier than midfielders and forwards. Field position players had higher aerobic capacity than goalkeepers, while midfielders had lower anaerobic power than players in the other positions. Forwards performed better in the jump and sprint, but comparisons by other positions were variable. The difference in SA among players by position was more apparent in distributions by maturity status. Most goalkeepers (78%) were on time and the remainder were early; no goalkeepers were late maturing. Defenders and forwards were similar. About one-half were on time (defenders, 55%; forwards, 52%), about one-third were early (defenders, 32%; forwards, 30%), and smaller percentages were late (defenders, 13%; forwards, 18%) maturing. Two-thirds of midfielders were on time in SA (67%), but proportionally more were late (23%) than early (10%) maturing.

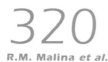

320

R.M. Malina et al.

Among 19 players 15–16 years on the Portuguese national team, forwards < midfielders < defenders in height, whereas defenders > forwards > midfielders in weight (Malina et al., 2000). Two goalkeepers were similar in height to defenders, but heavier. Forwards and defenders were advanced in SA compared to midfielders.

## IMPLICATIONS

Physical characteristics reflected in growth and maturity status are important, but are not the only determinants of successful soccer performance. They are part of a complex matrix of biobehavioural variables related to the demands of the sport. Several are discussed below.

### Selection and exclusion

Soccer apparently favours players on time and early in biological maturation, as CA and specialization increase during the transition into and during adolescence. This fact may reflect selection (self, coach, some combination), differential success of players advanced in maturation, changing nature of the game (more physical contact permitted with increasing CA), or some combination of these and other factors. It is also possible that late maturing boys selectively drop out.

Characteristics of soccer players who drop out or move up have not been systematically addressed. Baseline growth, maturation, functional capacities and soccer skills of Portuguese players at 11–12 (n=87) and 13–14 (n=72) years were compared on the basis of their follow-up status two years later: drop out – discontinued participation; club player – continued at the same level; or elite – moved to a higher level. Elite players were selected for the regional team or by elite clubs – SL Benfica, FC Porto and Sporting Lisbon (Figueiredo et al., 2009b). At baseline, a gradient of elite (n=12) > club (n=54) > drop out (n=21) was suggested among players 11–12 years for size and functional capacities, though differences were not consistent. Elite players performed better in two of four skills, dribbling and ball control. The gradient of elite (n=21) > club (n=36) > drop out (n=21) was more clearly defined among players 13–14 year at baseline. Elite players were older, advanced in SA and stage of PH, larger in body size and performed better in functional capacities and three skill tests than club players and drop outs. The results suggested a role for growth and maturity status, functional capacities and soccer skills as factors in attrition, persistence and moving up.

### Size and maturity mismatches

Recognition of potential size and maturity mismatches in youth sport has been in the literature for more than 100 years (Malina and Beunen, 1996a). Size and maturity variation are also indicated as risk factors for injury, especially in contact sports, but evidence relating the variation to risk of injury is not consistent (Emery, 2003; Malina, 2001). A study of ice hockey players 12.0–13.99 years was perhaps the first to draw attention to variation in impact forces associated with body size (Roy et al., 1989). The results highlighted the importance of size variation at the extremes within a competitive age group for injuries associated with body contact.

Functional and skill characteristics of soccer players at the extremes of size and maturity have apparently not been considered. Accordingly, the growth, maturation, functional capacities and soccer skills of the shortest and tallest, and of the least and most skeletally mature players 11–12 and 13–14 years (n=8 per group) were compared (Figueiredo et al., 2010). Among younger and older players, four and three boys, respectively, were represented in both the shortest and least mature groups, while two and no players, respectively, were included in both the tallest and most mature groups. In each group, the tallest players were older in CA, advanced in SA and PH, and heavier than the shortest players. At 11–12 years, the most mature players were younger in CA but advanced in PH, taller and heavier with more adiposity. At 13–14 years, the most mature were taller, heavier and advanced in PH than the least mature. Players at the extremes of height and skeletal maturity in the two age groups differed in speed and power (tallest>shortest; most mature>least mature), but did not differ consistently in aerobic endurance and soccer skills.

The preceding findings suggest that size and strength discrepancies among soccer players are not a major advantage or disadvantage to performances under standard test conditions. Application to game situations may be a different matter. Coaches and sport administrators may perceive players of greater size and power as being better in some facets of the game such as jumping to head a ball and in tackling, or for a specific position (e.g., defenders and goalkeepers). This factor may contribute to limited opportunities for smaller players. Although numbers were small, there was no size or maturity trend in dropout, club level or elite status two years after baseline in players 11–12 years (see Figueiredo et al., 2009b). However, five of eight shortest players 13–14 years dropped out, while four of eight tallest players moved to elite status. Five of the eight most mature players 13–14 years moved to elite status while five of the eight least mature remained at the club level. None of the tallest and most mature players 13–14 years dropped out of soccer, while five of the shortest and two of the least mature dropped out. The observations suggest that coaches and trainers should provide opportunities for or perhaps protect smaller, skilled players during the adolescent years.

## Age verification

SA was used for CA verification in the 1988 Asian Junior Youth Football Tournament (Tritrakarn and Tansuphasiri, 1991) and the 2001 Asian Youth U16 championship (CNN Sports Illustrated, 2001). Radiographs of players 15 (n=18) and 16 (n=32) years from 10 teams in the 1988 tournament were assessed with the Greulich-Pyle method. Thirty-nine players (78%) had SAs beyond the CA limit of 16 years (16.99 years) and 31 were skeletally mature (Tritrakarn and Tansuphasiri, 1991). The 39 players had SAs ≥ 17.0 years, thus exceeding the cut-off. If SA was used to verify CA, they would be eliminated from the competition even though CAs indicated age eligibility. Among the 217 soccer players 15–16 years of age for whom Greulich-Pyle SAs were available (Figure 17.4), 122 (56%) had SAs ≥ 17.0 years and 52 were skeletally mature. Though age eligible, the 122 players would be excluded from the competition.

TW3 RUS SA was used for age verification in the 2007 U15 Elite Cup for cricket (Asian Cricket Council, 2007). Eight out of 10 countries were disqualified for fielding overage players based on SA. According to the Council, 'Our Age-Verification protocols have been tested and proven to work. We stand by the results found and take heart that the integrity of our tournaments is assured.' How many age eligible youth (and teams) were disqualified because they were early maturing or skeletally mature with the TW3 RUS method? Ethnic variation among Asian populations relative to the reference is an additional concern (Malina, 2011).

MRI examination of the fusion of the distal radius diaphysis and epiphysis was used for age verification in FIFA international U17 competitions (Dvorak et al., 2007b; Fédération Internationale de Football Association, 2009). The MRI protocol describes six stages of fusion from non-union to complete union (Dvorak et al., 2007a; George et al., 2010), but it is not clear why stages were considered. Focus was primarily on identification (presumably elimination) of players deemed to be 'overage' on the basis of complete epiphyseal union of the distal radius: 'MRI of the wrist can identify players who are definitely above 17 years' (Fédération Internationale de Football Association, 2009).

Frequencies of players presenting complete fusion (union) of the distal radius in a normative sample of soccer players and in several U17 FIFA tournaments are summarized in Table 17.2. A number of eligible players 14–17 years presented complete fusion; 39 CA eligible players in the U17 competitions (21%) had complete union and would be considered overage. Of note, 75 of 85 players 18 years and 14 of 20 players 19 years in the normative sample presented incomplete fusion of the distal radius and would be eligible for competitions.

Use of the MRI protocol at the 2009 FIFA U17 World Cup was set in the context of fair play: 'In order to protect the integrity of the tournament and in the spirit of fair play, FIFA has decided to conduct MRI' (Fédération Internationale de Football Association, 2009). What is fair about denying an age eligible player the opportunity to participate in a tournament because he is skeletally mature?

Developers of the MRI protocol concluded that 'relying on the honesty of trainers and players . . . does not work' and use of MRI has curbed the number of 'completely fused' players (Dvorak et al., 2007c). This is a sad comment on the culture of international soccer and perhaps sport in general. More importantly, it misses the point. CA eligible players 14–17 years had complete fusion of the distal radius (Table 17.2) and would be eliminated by the FIFA protocol. The same applies to the use of SA for age verification. The range of SAs within a CA group can exceed four years and perhaps more. Cut-off dates implicitly require precision.

The use of SA to verify CA in competitions has a high risk of false negatives – athletes identified as older than a CA cut-off, due to advanced SA when they in fact have a valid CA. False positives are also possible – athletes identified as younger than a CA cut-off, due to delayed SA, while birth certificates indicate a CA older than the cut-off. Risks of false negatives and false positives apply as well to MRI assessment of fusion of the distal radius (Malina, 2011; Malina et al., 2010). SA provides only a crude approximation of CA with a large margin of error. SAs of the hand–wrist and MRI assessments of the distal radius are not valid indicators of CA. Methods for effective age verification need to be developed.

**Table 17.2** Frequencies of complete fusion of the distal radial epiphysis (skeletal maturity) based on MRI assessment in adolescent soccer players by age group.

| Age group | Normative[1] | | U17[2] | |
|---|---|---|---|---|
| | N | f | N | n |
| 14 | 21 | – | 8 | 3 |
| 15 | 125 | – | 27 | 4 |
| 16 | 130 | 1 | 85 | 15 |
| 17 | 115 | 11 | 66 | 17 |
| 18 | 85 | 10 | – | – |
| 19 | 20 | 6 | – | – |

Notes:
[1] Players were 'selected by the respective national football association or by regional football clubs' in Algeria, Argentina, Malaysia and Switzerland; adapted from Dvorak et al. (2007a).
[2] U17 – players from 2003 FIFA U17 World Cup in Finland, 2004 AFC U17 championship in Japan, 2005 FIFA U17 World Cup in Peru, and 2006 AFC U17 championship in Singapore; adapted from Dvorak et al. (2007b). Frequencies were interpolated from a bar graph showing percentages of players by age group and stage; absolute frequencies were not reported.

## Relative age effect (RAE)

The over-representation of players born in the first quarter of a selection year (RAE) is a focus of discussion in soccer (Helsen et al., 1998, 2005; Morris and Nevill, 2006). Explanations for the RAE often focus on size variation within a single chronological year; those born early in the year are, on average, taller and heavier than those born later in the year. Size per se may be a significant factor affecting success at young age levels where strength, speed and power are often at a premium, and bring successful players to the attention of coaches and trainers. The successful, in turn, may have enhanced opportunity for special attention, better coaching, and so on.

Size per se is only one factor and is confounded by variation in maturity status among players within a single year. A boy may be tall or short compared to peers because he is advanced or delayed, respectively, in biological maturation. He also may be tall or short because his parents are tall or short; size has a major genotypic component (Malina et al., 2004a). Behavioural characteristics associated with size and maturity variation also need consideration (Cumming et al., 2004).

Discussions of the RAE focus on records of birth dates within a selection year for relatively large samples. Field studies of young athletes, however, include relatively small samples; nevertheless, they may provide some insights. Among 62 players born in 1992 and observed in December 2003 (11 years), biological maturity status, body size, adiposity, functional capacities and soccer skills did not differ by birth quarter; similar results were noted among 50 players born in 1990 (13 years as of the cut-off date) but observed in April 2004 (Figueiredo et al., in preparation). Consistent with the preceding, aerobic endurance, anaerobic power,

324

vertical jump, speed and strength did not differ by birth quarter among elite U14 French players (Carling et al., 2009). Only two differences were noted; players born in the fourth quarter of the selection year were shorter and later in SA. Finally, in 39 players 14.0 to 14.99 years grouped by quartile of CA, there was no clear trend from youngest to oldest in experience, height and weight, functional capacities and a composite soccer skill score (Malina et al., 2007b). This finding may have reflected pubertal variation; none was prepubertal (PH 1), while most were nearing maturity (PH 4) or mature (PH 5). Of interest, the trend in mean heights paralleled the number of mature players in each quartile. Studies of the implications of the RAE for adolescent soccer players need to be expanded to include indicators of biological maturation, growth status, functional capacities, skills, and behavioural characteristics.

## Injury

Discussions of injuries generally enumerate factors related to characteristics of participants and conditions of the sport environment that might place an athlete at risk of injury (Malina, 2001). Risk factors related to the player include: physique; structural alignment; lack of flexibility and/or muscular strength; strength imbalance; adolescent growth spurt; maturity status; injury history; and behavioural factors. Risk factors in the sport environment include: inadequate rehabilitation from prior injury – loss of conditioning, flexibility and strength; training errors – improper technique, lack of adequate instruction, inappropriate drills, lack of conditioning; playing conditions – structural hazards (goal posts, fences, sprinklers), surfaces (uneven, wet), proximity to spectators; climate – heat/cold, humidity, lightning; multiple-year age groups – size, maturity, experience mismatches; coach behaviours – inappropriate drills and techniques, poor instruction, forced participation after injury or incomplete rehabilitation; parent behaviours – unrealistic expectations, pushing a youngster too fast, having a boy 'play-up' in an older age group; and sport organizations (coaches, officials, administrators) – focus on winning, tolerance for aggression and body contact. Interactions between player and sport environment risk factors are also important.

The adolescent growth spurt and maturity-associated variation are relevant to the present discussion. What is unique about the growth spurt that may place an adolescent at risk? An association between increased prevalence of injuries and the adolescent growth spurt has been long recognized (Dameron and Reibel, 1969; Peterson and Peterson, 1972; Burkhart and Peterson, 1979; Bailey et al., 1989). Peak velocity of bone mineral accrual occurs, on average, after PHV by more than one year (Iuliano-Burns et al., 2001). The lag in bone mineral accrual relative to linear growth may suggest a period of skeletal 'fragility' which might contribute to increased risk of injury (sport and non-sport) during the adolescent spurt. Other changes during the spurt need consideration. Range of motion of some joints increases during puberty, in contrast to the general suggestion that flexibility decreases. Flexibility is joint specific and highly individual. Loss of flexibility may be sport specific, for example, loss of quadriceps flexibility in soccer players (Kibler and Chandler, 1993). An imbalance between strength and flexibility may lead to abnormal mechanics, which may increase injury risk. This may reflect differential timing of growth spurts. On average, peak gain in flexibility (sit and reach) occurs before PHV, while peak gains in muscular strength and power occur after PHV and closer in time to peak velocity of body weight in non-athletes (Beunen et al., 1988; Malina et al.,

2004b). Limited data for soccer players are more variable. Estimated peak gains in trunk (sit-ups) and explosive (standing long and vertical jumps) strength occurred coincidently with PHV, while peak gain in flexibility (sit and reach) occurred after PHV in Belgian players (Philippaerts et al., 2006).

Injury in youth soccer is reasonably well documented (Emery et al., 2005; Kucera et al., 2005), but prospective data relating injuries to the growth spurt and maturation are very limited. Most injuries are minor, and associations with size, maturity and function have not been established. Baseline SA (Greulich-Pyle), BMI and functional capacities were not associated with risk of injury in elite U14 through U18 players (Le Gall et al., 2007). Incidence of injury was not associated with pubertal status in a mixed-longitudinal sample of elite players 8–15 years of age (Sports Council, 1992; Baxter-Jones et al., 1993) and with SA in elite players 9–16 years of age (Fels method, Johnson et al., 2009). On the other hand, 8 of 11 players 12.2–15.7 years presenting with epiphyseal injuries during a season had SAs (Sempé method) that would categorize them as late maturing (Vidalin, 1988).

A higher frequency of injuries in a summer camp was observed in boys classified as 'tall and weak' ('skeletally mature but muscularly weak'), as compared to the 'tall and strong' ('mature') or 'short and weak' ('immature'). Data were limited to height and grip strength (Backhous et al., 1988); biological maturity was not assessed. Height was assumed to be directly related to stage of puberty. The assumption is not valid and does not allow for individual differences in timing and tempo of growth and maturation, limitations of pubertal stages, and of course genotypic variation in height and maturation (Malina et al., 2004a).

## SUMMARY

The growth and maturity characteristics of youth soccer players may influence processes of exclusion and inclusion. Some boys will be excluded from participation and others may be included on the basis of growth and maturity status per se. Of relevance, what influence do the processes of inclusion and exclusion have on maximizing the possibility that boys with the greatest potential for success will still be participating in soccer and be available for selection to higher-level teams in their late adolescent or perhaps young adult years? The question is related to the identification of a select few participants who might bring local, regional and especially national recognition through the success of the respective teams at each level. The talented, later maturing boy who is smaller and muscularly weaker compared to age peers may be excluded. How can the small, later maturing boy who is exceptionally skilled be nurtured and in some cases protected so that he will persist in the sport? This youngster needs reassurance that he will eventually go through his growth spurt and sexual maturation, and catch up in height to the other boys.

The desire to win often drives the participatory process in sport. This is especially true in soccer, where national and international tournaments are available for youth at many ages. Many coaches, even at local levels, experience pressures to win. The pressures may influence coaches and programme administrators to directly or indirectly select early maturing players, who can help youth teams to win now, and exclude smaller and later maturing players, who might have the potential to become elite performers when they reach physical maturity.

326

# REFERENCES

Asian Cricket Council (2007) U-15 ACC elite age-verification results issued. Available from URL: http://www.asiancricket.org/h_1207_u15eageverification.cfm [Accessed 15 January 2008].

Backhous, D.D., Friedl, K.E., Smith, N.J., Parr, T.J., and Carpine W.D. (1988) Soccer injuries and their relation to physical maturity. *American Journal of Diseases of Children* 142, 839–842.

Bailey, D.A., Wedge, J.H., McCulloch, R.G., Martin, A.D., and Berhhardson, S.C. (1989) Epidemiology of fractures of the distal end of the radius in children as associated with growth. *Journal of Bone and Joint Surgery* 71A, 1225–1231.

Barbieri, C., and Rodriguez Papini, H. (1996) *Informe Final Proyecto Antropometrico Torneos Juveniles Bonaerenses Final Provincial 1996*. Buenos Aires, Argentina: Direccion de Impresiones del Estado y Boletin Oficial, Provinica de Buenos Aires.

Baxter-Jones, A.D.G., Maffulli, N., and Helms, P. (1993) Low injury rates in elite athletes. *Archives of Disease in Childhood* 68, 130–132.

Bell, W. (1993) Body size and shape: a longitudinal investigation of active and sedentary boys during adolescence. *Journal of Sports Sciences* 11, 127–138.

Beunen, G.P., Malina, R.M., Van't Hof, M.A., Simons, J., Ostyn, M., Renson, R., and Van Gerven, D. (1988) *Adolescent Growth and Motor Performance: A Longitudinal Study of Belgian Boys*. Champaign, IL: Human Kinetics.

Bielicki, T., Koniarek, J., and Malina, R.M. (1984) Interrelationships among certain measures of growth and maturation rate in boys during adolescence. *Annals of Human Biology* 11, 201–210.

Burkhart, S.S., and Peterson, H.A. (1979) Fractures of the prosimal tibial epiphysis. *Journal of Bone and Joint Surgery* 61A, 996–1002.

Cacciari, E., Mazzanti, L., Tassinari, D., Bergamaschi, R., Magnani, D., Zappula, F., Nanni, G., Cobianchi, C., Ghini, T., Pini, R., and Tani, G. (1990) Effects of sport (football) on growth: auxological, anthropometric and hormonal aspects. *European Journal of Applied Physiology* 61, 149–158.

Carling, C., Le Gall, F., and Malina, R.M. (2012) Body size, skeletal maturity and functional characteristics of elite U 14 academy soccer players between 1992 and 2003. *Journal of Sports Sciences*, in press.

Carling, C., Le Gall, F., Reilly, T., and Williams, A.M. (2009) Do anthropometric and fitness characteristics vary according to birth date distribution in elite youth academy soccer players? *Scandinavian Journal of Medicine and Science in Sports* 19, 3–9.

Carter, J.E.L., Rienzi, E.G., Gomes, P.S.C., and Martin, A.D. (1998) Somatotipo e tamaño corporal. In E. Rienzi and J.C. Mazza (eds), *Futbolista Sudamericano de Elite: Morfologia, Analisis del Juego y Performance*. Rosario, Argentina: Biosystem Servicio Educativo, pp. 64–77.

Centers for Disease Control and Prevention (2000) National Center for Health Statistics CDC growth charts: United States. http://www.cdc.gov/growthcharts.htm.

CNN Sports Illustrated (2001) 'Cheating does not pay': Asia bans teams, players for over-age infractions. http://sportsillustrated.cnn.com/soccer/news/2001/05/10/Asia [Accessed 14 June 2001].

Coelho e Silva, M.J., Figueiredo, A.J., Simões, F., Seabra, A., Natal, A., Vaeyens, R.,

Philippaerts, R., Cumming, S.P., and Malina, R.M. (2010). Discrimination of U-14 soccer players by level and position. *International Journal of Sports Medicine* 31, 790–796.

Cumming, S.P., Standage, M., and Malina, R.M. (2004) Youth soccer: a biocultural perspective. In M.J. Coelho e Silva and R.M. Malina (eds), *Children and Youth in Organized Sport*. Coimbra: University of Coimbra Press, pp. 209–221.

Dameron, T.B., and Reibel, D.B. (1969) Fractures involving the proximal humeral epiphyseal plate. *Journal of Bone and Joint Surgery* 51A, 289–297.

Diniz da Silva, C., Bloomfield, J., and Bouzas Marins, J.C. (2008) A review of stature, body mass and maximal oxygen uptake profiles of U17, U20 and first division players in Brazilian soccer. *Journal of Sports Science and Medicine* 7, 309–319.

Dvorak, J., George, J., Junge, A., and Hodler, A. (2007a) Age determination by MRI of the wrist in adolescent male football players. *British Journal of Sports Medicine* 41, 45–52.

Dvorak, J., George, J., Junge, A., and Hodler, A. (2007b) Application of MRI of the wrist for age determination in international U-17 soccer competitions. *British Journal of Sports Medicine* 41, 497–500.

Dvorak, J., George, J., Junge, A., and Hodler, A. (2007c) Re: Comment on age determination in adolescent male football players: it does not work! *British Journal of Sports Medicine* electronic letter 7 June 2007. Available at URL: www.bjsm.bjm.com [Accessed 29 May 2008].

Emery, C.A. (2003) Risk factors for injury in child and adolescent sport: A systematic review of the literature. *Clinical Journal of Sports Medicine* 13, 256–268.

Emery, C.A., Meeuwisse, W.H., and Hartmann, S.E. (2005) Evaluation of risk factors for injury in adolescent soccer. *American Journal of Sports Medicine* 33, 1882–1891.

Fédération Internationale de Football Association (2009) FIFA to introduce MRI screening at Nigeria 2009 to combat the fielding of over-age players. http://www.fifa.com/u17world cup/news/newsid=1096817.html [Accessed 22 September 2009].

Figueiredo, A.J., Coelho e Silva, M.J., and Malina, R.M. (2010) Size and maturity mismatch in youth soccer players 11- to 14-years-old. *Pediatric Exercise Science* 22, 596–612.

Figueiredo, A.J., Coelho e Silva, M.J., and Malina, R.M. (2011) Predictors of functional capacity and skill in youth soccer players. *Scandinavian Journal of Medicine and Science in Sports* 21, 446–454.

Figueiredo, A.J., Coelho e Silva, M.J., and Malina, R.M. (in preparation) Relative age effect: size, maturity, function, skill and goal orientation of youth soccer players by birth quarter.

Figueiredo, A.J., Coelho e Silva, M., Dias, J., and Malina, R.M. (2005) Age and maturity-related variability in body size and physique among youth male Portuguese soccer players. In T. Reilly, J. Cabri and D. Araujo (eds), *Science and Football V*. London: Routledge, pp. 448–452.

Figueiredo, A.J., Gonçalves, C.E., Coelho e Silva, M.J., and Malina, R.M. (2009a). Characteristics of youth soccer players who drop out, persist or move up. *Journal of Sports Sciences* 27, 883–891.

Figueiredo, A.J., Gonçalves, C.E., Coelho e Silva, M.J., and Malina, R.M. (2009b). Youth soccer players, 11–14 years: maturity, size, function, skill and goal orientation. *Annals of Human Biology* 36, 60–73.

Fragoso, I., Vieira, F., Canto e Castro, L., Oliveira Junior, A., Capela, C., Oliveira, N., and Barroso, A. (2004) Maturation and strength of adolescent soccer players. In M.J. Coelho e Silva and R.M. Malina (eds), *Children and Youth in Organized Sport*. Coimbra: University of Coimbra Press, pp. 199–208.

Froberg, K., Anderson, B., and Lammert, O. (1991) Maximal oxygen uptake and respiratory functions during puberty in boy groups of different physical activity. In R. Frenkl and I. Szmodis (eds), *Children and Exercise: Pediatric Work Physiology XV*. Budapest: National Institute for Health Promotion, pp. 265–280.

George, J., Nagendran, J., and Azmi, K. (2012) Comparison of growth plate fusion aging MRI versus plain radiographs as used in age determination for exclusion of overaged football players. *British Journal of Sports Medicine* 46, 273–278.

Gissis, I., Papadopoulos, C., Kalapotharakos, V.I., Sotiropoulos, A., Komsis, G., and Manolopoulos, E. (2006) Strength and speed characteristics of elite, subelite, and recreational young soccer players. *Research in Sports Medicine* 14, 205–214.

Gravina, L., Gil, S.M., Ruiz, F., Zubero, J., Gil, J., and Irazusta, J. (2008) Anthropometric and physiological differences between first team and reserve soccer players ages 10–14 years at the beginning and end of the season. *Journal of Strength and Conditioning Research* 22, 1308–1314.

Greulich, W.W, and Pyle, S.I. (1959) *Radiographic Atlas of Skeletal Development of the Hand and Wrist*, 2nd edn. Stanford, CA: Stanford University Press.

Hansen, L., Bangsbo, J., Twisk, J., and Klausen, K. (1999) Development of muscle strength in relation to training level and testosterone in young male soccer players. *Journal of Applied Physiology* 87, 1141–1147.

Helsen, W.F, Starkes, J.L., and van Winckel, J. (1998) The influence of relative age on success and dropout in male soccer players. *American Journal of Human Biology* 10, 791–798.

Helsen, W.F., van Winckel, J., and Williams, A.M. (2005) The relative age effect in youth soccer across Europe. *Journal of Sports Sciences* 23, 629–636.

Hirose, N. (2009) Relationships among birth-month distribution, skeletal age and anthropometric characteristics in adolescent elite soccer players. *Journal of Sports Sciences* 27, 1159–1166.

Horta, L. (2003) Factores de predicão do rendimento desportivo em atletas juvenis de futebol. Doctoral thesis, Faculdade de Medicina da Universidade do Porto.

Iuliano-Burns, S., Mirwald, R.L., and Bailey, D.A. (2001) The timing and magnitude of peak height velocity and peak tissue velocities for early, average and late maturing boys and girls. *American Journal of Human Biology* 13, 1–8.

Johnson, A., Doherty, P.J., and Freemont, A. (2009) Investigation of growth, development, and factors associated with injury in elite schoolboy footballers: prospective study. *British Medical Journal* 338, b490 (doi: 1136/bmj.b490).

Khamis, H.J., and Roche, A.F. (1994) Predicting adult stature without using skeletal age: The Khamis-Roche method. *Pediatrics* 94, 504–507 (erratum in *Pediatrics* 95, 457, 1995 for the corrected version of the tables).

Kibler, W.B., and Chandler, T.J. (1993) Musculoskeletal adaptations and injuries associated with intense participation in youth sports. In B.R. Cahill and A.J. Pearl (eds), *Intensive Participation in Children's Sports*. Champaign, IL: Human Kinetics, pp. 203–216.

Kucera, K.L., Marshall, S.W., Kirkendall, D.T., Marchak, P.M., and Garrett, W.E. (2005) Injury history as a risk factor for incident injury in youth soccer. *British Journal of Sports Medicine* 39, 462–466.

329

Le Gall, F., Carling, C., and Reilly, T. (2007) Biological maturity and injury in elite youth football. *Scandinavian Journal of Medicine and Science in Sports* 17, 564–572.

Le Gall, F., Carling, C., Williams, M., and Reilly, T. (2010) Anthropometric and fitness characteristics of international, professional and amateur male graduate soccer players from an elite youth academy. *Journal of Science and Medicine in Sport* 13, 90–95.

Malina, R.M. (1994) Physical growth and biological maturation of young athletes. *Exercise and Sports Science Reviews* 22, 389–433.

Malina, R.M. (2001) Injuries in organized sports for children and adolescents. In J.L. Frost (ed.), *Children and Injuries*. Tucson, AZ: Lawyers and Judges Publishing Company, pp. 199–248.

Malina, R.M. (2003) Growth and maturity status of young soccer (football) players. In T. Reilly and A.M. Williams (eds), *Science and Soccer*, 2nd edn. London: Routledge, pp. 287–306.

Malina, R.M. (2007) Body composition in athletes: assessment and estimated fatness. *Clinics in Sports Medicine* 26, 37–68.

Malina, R.M. (2011) Skeletal age and age verification in youth sport. *Sports Medicine* 41(11), 925–947.

Malina, R.M., and Beunen, G. (1996a) Matching of opponents in youth sports. In O. Bar-Or (ed.), *The Child and Adolescent Athlete*. Oxford, UK: Blackwell Science, pp. 202–213.

Malina, R.M., and Beunen, G. (1996b) Monitoring growth and maturation. In O. Bar-Or (ed.), *The Child and Adolescent Athlete*. Oxford, UK: Blackwell Science, pp. 647–672.

Malina, R.M., and Geithner, C.A. (2011) Body composition of young athletes. *America Journal of Lifestyle Medicine* 5, 262–278.

Malina, R.M., Bouchard, C. and Bar-Or, O. (2004a) *Growth, Maturation, and Physical Activity*, 2nd edn. Champaign, IL: Human Kinetics.

Malina, R.M., Beunen, G., Lefevre, J., and Woynarowska, B. (1997) Maturity-associated variation in peak oxygen uptake in active adolescent boys and girls. *Annals of Human Biology* 24, 19–31.

Malina, R.M., Chamorro, M., Serratosa, L., and Morate, F. (2007a) TW3 and Fels skeletal ages in elite youth soccer players. *Annals of Human Biology* 34, 265–272.

Malina, R.M., Ribeiro, B., Aroso, J., and Cumming, S.P. (2007b) Characteristics of youth soccer players aged 13–15 years classified by skill level. *British Journal of Sports Medicine* 41, 290–295.

Malina, R.M., Coelho e Silva, M.J., Figueiredo, A.J., Carling, C., and Beunen, G.P. (2012) Interrelationships among invasive and non-invasive indicators of biological maturation in adolescent male soccer players. *Journal of Sports Sciences*, in press.

Malina, R.M., Eisenmann, J.C., Cumming, S.P., Ribeiro, B., and Aroso, J. (2004b) Maturity-associated variation in the growth and functional capacities of youth football (soccer) players 13–15 years. *European Journal of Applied Physiology* 91, 555–562.

Malina, R.M., Cumming, S.P., Kontos, A.P., Eisenmann, J.E., Ribeiro, S., and Aroso, J. (2005) Maturity-associated variation in sport-specific skills of youth soccer players aged 13–15 years. *Journal of Sports Sciences* 23, 515–522.

Malina, R.M., Peña Reyes, M.E., Eisenmann, J.C., Horta, L., Rodrigues, J., and Miller, R. (2000) Height, mass, and skeletal maturity of elite Portuguese soccer players 11–16 years of age. *Journal of Sports Sciences* 18, 685–693.

Malina, R.M., Claessens, A.L., Van Aken, K., Thomis, M., Lefevre, J., Philippaerts, R., and

Beunen, G.P. (2006). Maturity offset in gymnasts: application of a prediction equation. *Medicine and Science in Sports and Exercise* 38, 1342–1347.

Malina, R.M., Peña Reyes, M.E., Figueiredo, A.J., Coelho e Silva, M.J., Horta, L., Miller, R., Chamorro, M., Serratosa, L., and Morate, F. (2010) Skeletal age in youth soccer players: Implications for age verification. *Clinical Journal of Sports Medicine* 20, 469–474.

Mirwald, R.L., Baxter-Jones, A.D.G., Bailey, D.A., and Beunen, G.P. (2002) An assessment of maturity from anthropometric measurements. *Medicine and Science in Sports and Exercise* 34, 689–694.

Morris, J.G., and Nevill, M.E. (2006) *A Sporting Chance. Enhancing Opportunities for High-level Sporting Performance: Influence of 'Relative Age'*. Loughborough, UK: Institute of Youth Sport, Loughborough University.

Nariyama, K., Hauspie, R.C., and Mino, T. (2001) Longitudinal growth study of male Japanese junior high school athletes. *American Journal of Human Biology* 13, 356–364.

Nicolson, A.B., and Hanley, C. (1953) Indices of physiological maturity: derivation and interrelationships. *Child Development* 24, 3–38.

Nurmi-Lawton, J.A., Baxter-Jones, A.D., Mirwald, R.L., Bishop, J.A., Taylor, R., Cooper, C., and New, S.A. (2004) Evidence of sustained skeletal benefits from impact-loading exercise in young females: a 3-year longitudinal study. *Journal of Bone Mineral Research* 19, 314–322.

Peterson, C.A., and Peterson, H.A. (1972) Analysis of the incidence of injuries to the epiphyseal growth plate. *Journal of Trauma* 12, 275–281.

Philippaerts, R.M., Vaeyens, R., Janssens, M., Van Renterghem, B., Matthus, D., Craen, R., Bourgois, J., Vrijens, J., Beunen, G., and Malina, R.M. (2006). The relationship between peak height velocity and physical performance in youth soccer players. *Journal of Sports Sciences* 24, 221–230.

Roche, A.F., Chumlea, W.C., and Thissen, D. (1988) *Assessing the Skeletal Maturity of the Hand-Wrist: Fels Method*. Springfield, IL: CC Thomas.

Roy, M-A., Bernard, D., Roy, B., and Marcotte, G. (1989) Body checking in Pee Wee hockey. *Physician and Sportsmedicine* 17, 119–126.

Seabra, A., Maia, J., and Garganta, R. (2001) Crescimento, maturação, aptidão fisica, força explosiva e habilidades motoros especificas. Estudo em jovens futebolistas e não futebolistas do sexo masculino dos 12 aos 16 anos de idade. *Revista Portuguesa de Ciencias do Desporto* 1, 22–25.

Seabra, A., Maia, J., and Garganta, R. (2004) Multivariate study of the somatotype of Portuguese young soccer players. *Biometrie Humaine et Anthropologie* 22, 171–178.

Sherar, L.B., Baxter-Jones, A.D.G., Faulkner, R.A., and Russell, K.W. (2007) Do physical maturity and birth date predict talent in male youth ice hockey players? *Journal of Sports Sciences* 25, 879–886.

Sports Council (1992) *TOYA and Sports Injuries*. London: The Sports Council.

Tanner, J.M., Healy, M.J.R., Goldstein, H., and Cameron, N. (2001) *Assessment of Skeletal Maturity and Prediction of Adult Height (TW3 Method)*, 3rd edn. London: Saunders.

Tanner, J.M., Whitehouse, R.H., Cameron, N., Marshall, M.A., Healy, M.J.R., and Goldstein, H. (1983) *Assessment of Skeletal Maturity and Prediction of Adult Height (TW2 Method)*, 2nd edn. New York: Academic Press.

Tritrakarn, A., and Tansuphasiri, V. (1991) Roentgenographic assessment of skeletal ages of

331

Asian junior youth football players. *Journal of the Medical Association of Thailand* 74, 459–464.

Vaeyens, R., Malina, R.M., Janssens, M., Van Renterghem, B., Bourgois, J., and Vrijens, J. (2006) A multidisciplinary selection model for youth soccer: the Ghent Youth Soccer Project. *British Journal of Sports Medicine* 40, 928–934.

Vicente-Rodriguez, G., Jimenez-Ramirez, J., Ara, I., Serrano-Sanchez, J.A., Dorado, C., and Calbert, J.A.L. (2003) Enhanced bone mass and physical fitness in prepubescent footballers. *Bone* 33, 853–859.

Vidalin, H. (1988) Football. Traumatismes et age osseux. Estude prospective de 11 cas. *Medecine du Sport* 62, 195–197.

Zachman, M., Prader, A., Kind, H.P., Hafliger, H., and Budliger, H. (1974) Testicular volume during adolescence: cross-sectional and longitudinal studies. *Helvetica Paediatrica Acta* 29, 61–72.

# PART VI

# INTEGRATION AND APPLICATION

# CHAPTER 18

## CONTEMPORARY ISSUES IN THE PHYSICAL PREPARATION OF ELITE PLAYERS

A.J. Strudwick

### INTRODUCTION

The key objective in this chapter is to provide a comprehensive account of the issues that impact upon the physical preparation of elite soccer players. The chapter details the demands of training and match-play, provides a systematic approach for working with elite players and discusses issues relating to the management of elite player performance. These observations are based on relevant experiences accumulated over the years in a high performance setting, together with contemporary applied research findings.

Throughout the past three decades there has been a shift towards systematic methods of preparing elite players for match-play. Contemporary coaches have been exposed to scientific approaches to preparing teams for competition. There are certainly a number of examples of 'good practice' in elite soccer. However, a worrying concern is that much of coaching practice is based largely on tradition, emulation and intuition, rather than on scientific evidence (Williams and Hodges, 2005). The potential over-reliance on historical precedence and traditional methods of physical preparation is perhaps surprising, in light of the ever-increasing professionalism within the game.

In general, clubs that have adopted a strategic approach have been rewarded with success by gaining an advantage over competitors. It has taken some time for the accumulation of scientifically based knowledge to be translated into a form usable by practitioners. Clearly, there has been a paradigm shift in contemporary high-performance sport. This shift has resulted in better-informed practitioners working with teams, stronger links with scientific institutes and more coaches being willing to accept the changing role of sports science in elite sport. Greater efforts are now being made to compile scientific information and make it accessible to the soccer world.

### CONTEMPORARY ELITE MATCH-PLAY

The physiological demands on modern players are more complex than in many individual sports and these demands on players vary, depending on the level of performance, positional role and style of play incorporated by a team (Bradley et al., 2009; Di Salvo et al., 2009; Gregson et al., 2010). Within the past few decades there has been increasing emphasis on work-rate during competitive play, with a requirement for mobility around the field (Strudwick,

335

2006; Di Salvo *et al.*, 2009). The modern game also includes more passes, runs with the ball, dribbles and crosses, which collectively suggest a significant increase in the 'tempo' of games. The increased physical demands of elite soccer, in accordance with an increase in the number of games per season, are placing increasing physiological and psychological demands on elite participants. The data presented in Tables 18.1 and 18.2 provide examples of seasonal match and training exposure of an elite soccer player.

On average, in men's soccer elite teams participate in approximately 220 training sessions and 60 competitive games over a season. This equates to 20 training sessions and 5.5 matches per month, yielding an average training:match ratio of 3.6 training sessions per match. However, these figures represent seasonal average values and there will be periods throughout the annual calendar where elite players are exposed to matches every 3.3 days over a 5-game period (refer to Table 18.2 for lowest period of days per game). When one factors in the confounding variation in kick-off times, travel commitments and international fixtures it is evident that the demands on elite soccer are intensive.

**Table 18.1** An example of seasonal match and training exposure for an elite male player.

| Month | Training | | | Match | | |
|---|---|---|---|---|---|---|
| | Number | Hours | Absent due to injury (N) | Number | Hours | Absent due to injury (N) |
| July | 21 | 31.5 | 0 | 0 | 0 | 0 |
| August | 18 | 27 | 0 | 7 | 13.2 | 0 |
| September | 20 | 30 | 0 | 6 | 3.6 | 0 |
| October | 20 | 30 | 0 | 5 | 4.2 | 0 |
| November | 15 | 22.5 | 0 | 8 | 6.1 | 0 |
| December | 18 | 27 | 2 | 7 | 6.7 | 1 |
| January | 14 | 21 | 0 | 9 | 12.5 | 0 |
| February | 21 | 31.5 | 2 | 4 | 6.2 | 1 |
| March | 18 | 27 | 0 | 6 | 9.3 | 0 |
| April | 16 | 24 | 0 | 8 | 10.1 | 0 |
| May | 14 | 21 | 0 | 7 | 8.0 | 0 |
| Average | 17.7 | 26.6 | 0.4 | 6.1 | 7.3 | 0.2 |
| Total | 195 | 292.5 | 4 | 67 | 79.9 | 2 |

**Table 18.2** An example of seasonal trainability and availability for an elite male player.

| | |
|---|---|
| Matches – total | 67 |
| Training sessions – total | 195 |
| Squad availability match (%) | 97 |
| Squad availability training (%) | 98 |
| Seasonal average days per game | 5.6 |
| Lowest period of days per game (over 5 competitive games ) | 3.3 |
| Match absence due to injury | 2 |
| Training absence due to injury | 4 |

*Notes: Where:*
Squad availability match = 100 – ((# of matches absent/Total no of matches) x 100).
Squad availability training = 100 – ((# of training sessions absent/Total no of training sessions) x 100).

A.J. Strudwick

In order to cope with these increased demands, players must have the necessary physical resources to perform the high work-rates and critical actions during match-play. Higher levels of strength and power are now required at an elite level to reproduce forceful bursts of energy and withstand the forces of physical impact. The observation that elite players perform 150–250 short, intense actions during a game indicates that the rate of anaerobic energy turnover is high during periods of match-play (Mohr et al., 2003). These activity patterns include maximal sprinting (30–40), turning (>700), tackling and jumping (30–40), as well as intense muscular bursts such as accelerations and decelerations (Bangsbo, 1994; Mohr et al., 2003; Bloomfield et al., 2007). All these efforts exacerbate the physiological strain imposed on players and contribute to high physical workloads during match-play.

Anaerobic actions are performed against a backdrop of aerobic energy supply. At the elite level, outfield players cover 10–13 km during the course of a match (Di Salvo et al., 2007; Rampinini et al., 2007; Di Salvo et al., 2009). Researchers have indicated that elite players perform 2–3 km of high-intensity running (>15km/h) and cover 1–1.5 km at very high intensity (>20 km/h) (Mohr et al., 2003; Rampinini et al., 2007; Bradley et al., 2009). Match analysis suggests that the distance covered in high-intensity running by elite players in the last 15 min of a game is 14–45% lower than in the first 15 min (Mohr et al., 2003). According to Mohr et al. (2003), this finding supports the notion that fatigue occurs towards the end of the game for players who play the full 90 min. These effects are observed independent of position. Accordingly, in the 5 min following the most demanding 5-min period of the game, the distance covered at high intensity is reduced by 6–12%, as compared with the game average. These findings suggest that at an elite level of play, players experience fatigue towards the end of the game, and temporarily following intense bursts.

## 'HIGH PERFORMANCE STATUS'

The intensive training and frequent competition in elite soccer induce a high degree of stress upon the player. An analysis of the stress and injuries that may result is helpful in identifying risk factors associated with soccer-related activities. In addition, players have to meet the requirements of the game with a demonstration of appropriate coping strategies. It is therefore prudent to focus on the 'High Performance Status' of individual participants so that appropriate strategies can be implemented to maximise performance.

The principal philosophy behind 'High Performance Status' is that coping strategy and overall success is reflected in a player's ability to sustain the load associated with training and match-play at the highest level. Clearly, the athlete and the environment per se are critical to achieving sustained success. Coaches and athletes need to understand the 'Performance v Cost/Benefit' profile of elite participation and how to manage/mitigate these risks on a team and individual basis through proactive monitoring and the implementation of preventative strategies.

In introducing this approach to monitoring high performance, it is important to identify the objectives most critical to success. Moreover, it is important to identify the critical few metrics to track high performance and alignment. 'High Performance Status' factors, along with metrics used to track these parameters are listed in Table 18.3. These parameters can also be used as individual and team selection criteria and form a basis for squad selection and rotation.

Additionally, there is a need to look at the 'Performance Reliability' of players, which is based on the following equation:

Performance Reliability = (Match Availability x Percentage time on pitch) / 1000

This equation has been introduced because it represents a player's ability to cope with the demands of training and games. That is, it reflects how constitutional factors in the athlete interact with how teams employ the player during matches. The fundamental point is that players can yield a high return in terms of match availability, but are not selected and hence not subjected to the high loads associated with match-play. To put these figures into perspective, figures of around 7 are expected from high performance athletes.

## SPORTS SCIENCE SUPPORT

The application of scientific support models has a self-evident part to play in improving elite performance. Important features of the model, such as devising training programmes, monitoring performance, establishing preparation for competition are informed by such knowledge. The primary role of sports science in elite soccer is to utilise scientific principles to maximise individual performance and player availability. Practitioners have to manipulate the training process effectively in order to achieve these objectives. Moreover, the dimensions of the training programme – intensity, frequency, duration and mode of exercise – have to be established and detailed planning carried out to positively influence both the coaching process and the resultant player performance risk management.

Table 18.3 'High Performance Status' of elite athletes.

| High performance factors | How the factor is measured |
| --- | --- |
| Remain injury free | Days missed through injury |
| Capable of sustaining high performance work rates | Work-rate profiles during elite match-play based on objective match analysis data. |
| Capable of playing 50 games per season. | Games played – percentage used during in-season competition. |
| Window of opportunity (22–30 years old). | Player age – number of playing seasons in premier league. |
| Capable of playing a game every 4 days over a 5-game period. | Number of days per game over 5-game period (90 min played). |
| Ability to demonstrate sound recovery on objective markers. | Objective markers as employed by sports science department. |
| Demonstrate seasonal match availability of 90%. | See equation below* |
| Demonstrate seasonal training availability of 85%. | See equation below** |

Notes:
Where:
* Squad availability match = 100 – ((# of matches absent/Total no of matches) x 100).
** Squad availability training = 100 – ((# of training sessions absent/Total no of training sessions) x 100).

A.J. Strudwick

Although a variety of sports science disciplines will impact upon sports performance and player availability, this chapter will focus specifically on the physiological aspects of performance planning and consider appropriate principles that should be incorporated into the coaching process.

## A SYSTEMATIC APPROACH FOR WORKING WITH ELITE PLAYERS

An elite player attempting to reach the highest level requires a systematic approach to all areas of performance management. Such an approach can be achieved by identifying critical component parts of the coaching process and the relationships between the sub-processes. There are several critical components that impact on player performance management, as detailed in Figure 18.1. Although many of the components overlap, successful implementation depends on a sound support structure being developed between players and staff. Each of the components will now be described.

### Data management

Information is the fuel that drives the performance management process. Planning, decision making, monitoring and performance analysis all depend on the availability of the necessary information. At an elite level of play, an enormous amount of data is generated about a player's performance, on a constant basis. For example, a single variable multiplied by 20 players multiplied by 52 weeks equals 1040 data points over the season. It is worth noting that at the height of AC Milan's biomedical research centre, the laboratory tracked 60,000 data points on each player to ensure optimal health and fitness. Potential data variables used to analyse

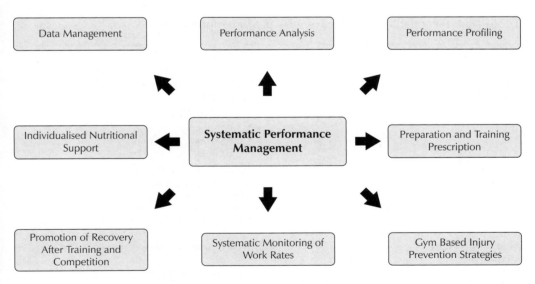

**Figure 18.1** A systematic performance management model for working with elite players.

and understand elite performance are provided in Table 18.4. Areas for critical data evaluation include Team Performance, Player Management, Sports Science/Medical and Talent Identification. All of these areas should be closely interrogated when planning fitness training for elite players.

Clearly, a key feature of the management process is the storage and retrieval of this range of information. High performance teams (those that substantially outperform their competitors) will adopt modern methods of electronic storage to enhance their decision making capabilities. There is a fine line between data and the practitioner's capacity to understand and make use of this information. It is therefore recommended that data management systems are developed in the preparation of elite players. These data management systems have the capacity to provide:

- a central means of storing information;
- programme planning for all staff;
- analysis of data;
- greater interaction between staff;
- executive-level communication;
- advanced mathematical modelling.

A critical concept in this process is distinguishing between which data are important and which are not. Data gathering for the sake of it can be very expensive, and is futile, unless it is used to drive action during the coaching process. While technology on its own cannot guarantee success at an elite level, a focus on developing robust analytical processes has great potential. Only recently has data begun to transform the management of professional soccer. Modern practitioners now have first-hand experience of how the intelligent use of 'analytics' can improve player acquisition and management, talent management and performance.

Table 18.4  Potential data variables for elite player performance.

| Team performance | Player management |
| --- | --- |
| Quantitative match analysis | Conditioning measures |
| Qualitative match analysis | Training details |
| Results of performance | Player monitoring: |
| | • readiness |
| | • recovery |
| | • wellness |
| Set targets for performance | Internal/external training load |
| Squad rotation | Competition loading |
| Objective performance scores | Lifecycle analysis |
| Sports science/medical | Talent identification |
| Medical screening | Recruitment analysis |
| Medical history | Test data |
| Performance assessments | Performance assessment |
| Performance profiling | Exposure hours |

A.J. Strudwick

Analytics are the extensive use of data, statistical and quantitative analysis, explanatory and predictive models and fact-based management to drive decisions and actions (Davenport and Harris, 2007). Potential questions that analytics can answer in soccer include:

- Which parameters are associated with successful performance?
- What is the probability of a player developing an injury?
- Where is the player's strength/weakness?
- How far is a player from the ideal state?
- How does a player's performance change over time?

## Performance analysis

In order to gain a correct impression of the physiological loads imposed on soccer players during competitive matches, observations have to be made during real match-play. Performance analysis entails determining work-rate profiles of players within a team and classifying activities in terms of intensity, duration and frequency (Reilly, 1994). In this way, an overall picture of the physiological demands of soccer can be gathered. The application of performance analysis to soccer has enabled the objective recording and interpretation of match events, describing the characteristic patterns of activity in soccer. An improvement in performance is the central purpose of the coaching process and a detailed knowledge at the behavioural level is essential for almost all stages of the performance management model – from promotion of recovery after training and competition to preparation and training programme.

The advent of computerised notation systems has facilitated sophisticated analysis of movement and patterns of play leading to key events during match-play. Used for real-time or post-event analysis, these systems provide qualitative and quantitative information. Moreover, these systems have great potential for assisting coaches and players alike in making decisions about future performance. The key here is to move the role of performance analysis from descriptive to prescriptive.

## Performance profiling

In order to ensure that elite players are well prepared, practitioners should use performance profiling as a means of providing information on current performance status. A performance profile of a player provides a benchmark of the overall state of his/her level of conditioning. A player's level of conditioning may vary due to stage of the season, the effectiveness of the training programme, game frequency or the maturity status of the player. Quite simply, performance profiling should provide information for analysis and subsequent action by both coach and player. In order to achieve this end, assessment needs to be built in to the training plan at regular and appropriate intervals. In this way, performance profiling will assist the design and regulation of a high-performance programme.

Performance profiles can be used to identify strengths and weaknesses of both individuals and teams, indicating any need for remedial action arising from injury, overreaching/overtraining or an inadequate training programme. They can also be used to set benchmarks for both individuals and groups and develop normative values on which assessments can be made. Profiles, therefore, provide valuable information to coaches regarding the physical condition of players and provide an aid in the evaluation, modification and prescription of training programmes. In addition, a performance management strategy can be provided on the basis of these evaluations to maximise player potential and guide individual players through their lifecycle. Moreover, targets should be implemented to manage this pathway effectively.

In the development of a performance profile, careful consideration must be taken when defining the factors to measure. It is important that tests are used for a purpose and that this is clearly identified. Suitable tests should be selected and their validity, reliability and feasibility taken into account. Care must be taken in the administration procedures used, and feedback should be given to all players and coaches. In any analysis players should not be ranked on the results obtained; it is more appropriate to compare personal results with personal standards, such as the percentage change from a previous test or the attained percentage of an individual's goal.

Figure 18.2 presents a typical performance profile. Clearly, performance profiles are not merely a means of collating relatively sophisticated data. Analysing and interpreting the results needs to be a process in which the sports scientist/physiologist is involved with the coach. The coach may then be responsible for appropriate modifications to the training plan. If this process is applied correctly, the resultant profile can be used to optimise the training plan and maximise the preparation of elite players.

## PREPARATION AND TRAINING PROGRAMME

In the preparation of elite players, it is important that the training programme is well planned. The training programme needs to be specific and objective, taking into consideration the player's potential and rate of development. Any training programme adopted should encompass relevant experiences accumulated over the years, together with applied research findings. A programme needs to be versatile, enabling it to be utilised as a model for training that can be easily applied to the specific characteristics and goals of individual players.

There are many components that need to be incorporated into a training programme. These include a full range of activities, such as activation modalities, injury prevention strategies, individual and team preparation (technical and tactical), match rehearsal and recovery strategies, in addition to the more obvious 'training session'. The design of the programme should be based on individual training philosophy and specificity to match performance per se. The need to isolate match performance components and to control workload intensity is achieved by a series of activities conducted within the training session. Training effects do not occur by coincidence. Not all training sessions automatically result in the appropriate physiological and performance adaptations. The specific activities that are performed place specific demands upon the body, resulting in structural and physiological changes.

All training sessions should incorporate elements of muscular activation and warming up to facilitate the appropriate recruitment of muscle fibres associated with the correct sequencing and timing of soccer-specific activities. Speed preparation should follow, with adequate

A.J. Strudwick

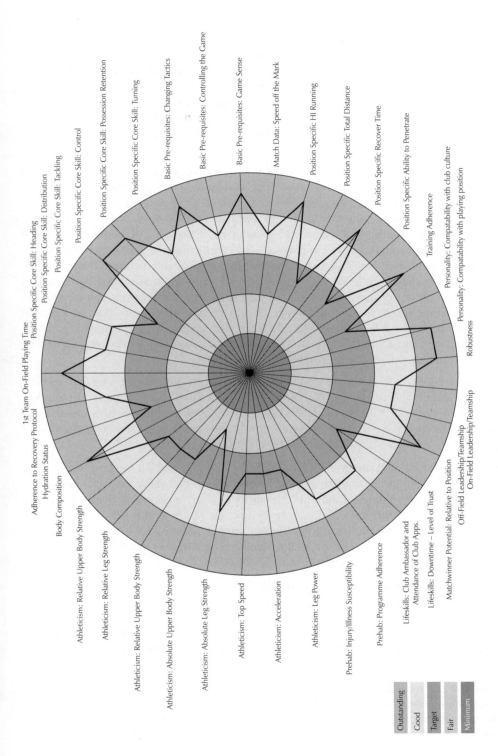

**Figure 18.2** Performance profile of an elite soccer player.

Position Specific Core Skill: Heading
1st Team On-Field Playing Time
Position Specific Core Skill: Distribution
Adherence to Recovery Protocol
Position Specific Core Skill: Tackling
Hydration Status
Position Specific Core Skill: Control
Position Specific Core Skill: Possession Retention
Body Composition
Position Specific Core Skill: Turning
Basic Pre-requisites: Changing Tactics
Athleticism: Relative Upper Body Strength
Basic Pre-requisites: Controlling the Game
Athleticism: Relative Leg Strength
Basic Pre-requisites: Game Sense
Athleticism: Absolute Upper Body Strength
Match Data: Speed off the Mark
Athleticism: Absolute Leg Strength
Position Specific HI Running
Athleticism: Top Speed
Position Specific Total Distance
Athleticism: Acceleration
Position Specific Recover Time
Athleticism: Leg Power
Position Specific Ability to Penetrate
Prehab: Injury/Illness Susceptibility
Training Adherence
Prehab: Programme Adherence
Personality: Compatability with club culture
Lifeskills: Club Ambassador and Attendance of Club Apps.
Personality: Compatability with playing position
Lifeskills: Downtime – Level of Trust
Robustness
Matchwinner Potential: Relative to Position
On-Field Leadership/Teamship
Off-Field Leadership/Teamship

Outstanding
Good
Target
Fair
Minimum

recovery time between repetitions and sets to allow continual energy resynthesis. Subsequent stimulation of the aerobic and anaerobic systems should then be performed via specific drills with the ball, involving changes of speed, direction and specific movement patterns typical of those performed during match-play. Appropriate recovery activities should be incorporated at the end of each training session, principally based upon adequate rest/sleep and relevant nutrition and hydration strategies. The application of a variety of other modalities may also confer some advantage (refer to section on promotion of recovery after training and competition).

In organising, designing and prescribing the training session, consideration must be given to major conditioning principles, particularly those associated with intensity, duration and specificity. The application of these principles in a planned progressive manner is the key to ensuring that the appropriate energy systems are stimulated during physiological preparation. In recent years there has been a shift towards using soccer-specific activities (small-sided games/drills) in the preparation of elite players (Little and Williams, 2006; Hill-Haas et al., 2011). Soccer-specific drills facilitate simultaneous physiological and technical development. A method for controlling the intensity during these drills is to manipulate variables such as field dimension and number of players involved, as well as to introduce specific rules (Bangsbo, 2008). This training mode has the advantage of enhanced player motivation and greater transfer to match-specific fitness. Therefore, when possible, small-sided games and/or position-specific drills containing tactical/technical components associated with the demands of elite match-play should be utilised by practitioners.

The variable nature of movement in conditioned games and drills means that control over intensity is potentially less precise. Nonetheless, with detailed planning and knowledge, practices with a moderate number of players or imposed high-intensity activities appear to be optimal for physiological development, as they consistently produce suitable work intensities (Rampinini et al., 2007; Kelly and Drust, 2009; Hill-Haas et al., 2011).

In the design of the training programme, practitioners should identify a methodology for the discrete activities used in the training session. These activities are based upon a number of components such as physiological stimulus, specificity to match performance, training mode, repetition duration, number of repetitions and work:rest ratios. These activities are based around the physiological stimulus of the different energy systems. Table 18.5 provides an appropriate methodology for a soccer-specific training programme that can be used with elite players. Please note that these guidelines refer specifically to field-based conditioning.

The consistency and knowledge of workloads during each of the training categories means that two of the most important training principles can be applied during field-based conditioning, namely, progression and periodisation. Progression refers to gradually increasing the training load over time as fitness gains are incurred. Periodisation can be defined as a logical, phasic method of manipulating training variables in order to increase the potential for achieving specific performance goals.

When planning fitness training for elite players, the annual cycle should be divided into three stages: transition; preparation; and in-season. The latter may be further divided into competition and peaking/maintenance. These phases have specific goals and require different levels of training variation. The use of a planned training programme can allow for tighter

344

**Table 18.5** Methodology for the main categories of field-based conditioning that can be used with elite players.

| Training category | Useful for | Physiological stimulus | Training mode | Repetition duration | Repetitions | Work:rest |
|---|---|---|---|---|---|---|
| Recovery training | Recovering from high intensity exercise | Recovery | Light aerobic running | 20–30 min | N/A | N/A |
| Aerobic moderate | Increasing the ability to exercise for prolonged periods of time | Aerobic moderate 8 v 8 – 10 v 10 games | Interval running | 4–30 min | 4–8 | 1:1– 1:0.5 |
| High-intensity endurance | Increasing the ability to sustain and perform repeated high-intensity exercise | Aerobic high 2 v 2 – 4 v 4 | Intermittent running | 1–4 min | 4–8 | 1–1.5 |
| Speed endurance | Increasing the ability to produce power rapidly and perform maximal runs repeatedly | Speed endurance | Straight shuttle and multi-directional specific runs –maximal or near-maximal runs | 10–30 s | 4–8 | 1:3 – 1:6 |
| Repeated sprint training | Increasing the ability to produce power rapidly and perform maximal runs repeatedly | Speed endurance | Straight shuttle and multi-directional specific runs –maximal runs | 5–8 s | 5–15 | 1:3 – 1.5 |
| Speed training | Increasing the ability to produce high speed muscular contraction and maximum sprinting speed | Speed | Straight shuttle and multi-directional specific runs –maximal runs | 2–10 s | 2–10 | 1:10 |

*Source:* Modified from F. M. Iaia (unpublished data).

control of training variables, superior performance adaptations and generally better perform-ance at the appropriate time.

## Preparation phase

This phase consists of moderate/high-volume, low-intensity training and is used as foundation training. The preparation phase is designed to increase exercise endurance, positively alter body composition and increase tissue size and tensile strength resulting in lower injury potential. The preparation phase should be used to increase soccer-specific fitness, with the phase typically being divided into general and specific parts. This process should enable players to become match fit prior to competition.

A guiding principle for all planning is that the programme of physiological preparation should develop from general to specific requirements and be coupled with the development of training duration towards and including specific intensity requirements (Maile, 1999). The practitioner must also allow for adequate rest and regeneration. The preparation phase should concentrate on four important aspects:

1   improving high-intensity exercise endurance;

2   changing body composition, especially increasing muscle mass;

3   decreasing injury potential;

4   increasing power.

The later portion of the preparation phase would include a lower volume of training, with an emphasis on high-intensity exercise. The length of time spent in the preparation phase depends upon the training status and the level of player.

## In-season phase

This phase is used to maintain optimal performance levels throughout the competitive period. The training load should not be reduced at the expense of training intensity during this phase. The management of training intensity is the key, as high-intensity exercise remains a critical component for maintenance or further enhancement of training-induced adaptations. It is fundamental that elite players continue to develop the ability to repeatedly perform high-intensity exercise during the maintenance phase. This outcome can be achieved by conducting frequent sessions of aerobic high-intensity and speed endurance training specific to the physical, movement, technical and tactical demands of the game (Iaia et al., 2009).

As a general guideline, Mujika (2010) outlined the following guidelines for practitioners.

1   High intensity training is associated with maximal physiological and performance adaptations during periods of intensive training in highly trained individual sports athletes.

2   Training intensity is key to maintaining and enhancing physiological and performance adaptations during the taper, so the training load should not be reduced at the expense of intensity.

346

3   Intense exercise is a critical component of team sport performance, and the optimisation of players' ability to perform this type of effort should be a training priority.

4   Team sport athletes could benefit from a high-intensity tapering programme to optimally prepare for the regular season and tournament-style competition.

A key principle during the in-season phase is to ensure that a balance is reached between training/match load and adequate rest and recovery. Continued high-intensity and high-volume training over extended periods of time may contribute to potentially long-term debilitating effects associated with overtraining and increased occurrence of injury events (Nimmo and Ekblom, 2007). Player performance parameters, together with actual physiological stress imposed on the athletes (Internal Training Load) need to be carefully monitored, and supplementary recovery sessions should be considered for players during heavy fixture periods. For squad players who do not play regularly, training load must be sufficient to cope with the physical requirements of a match. Pronounced mismatches between the demands of match-play compared with those of training, together with abrupt and severe increases in workload (due to switching from non-play to regular play) may enhance the risk of injury occurrence. Non-regular players, therefore, should perform additional field-based high-intensity training or engage in practice matches during such periods.

The summation of training stimuli plays a key role in the adaptation of each player. By monitoring the internal load in response to training, important information concerning the physiological status of the players can be ascertained (refer to section on systematic monitoring of work rates). Marked differences between internal and external training load over extended periods of time may contribute to detraining, underperformance or increased injury occurrence. To maximise training adaptation and reduce injury risk, it is important that players are exposed to different stimuli on a day-to-day basis, thus avoiding monotony. The inclusion of low-intensity and recovery sessions, together with high-intensity aerobic, speed and speed-endurance sessions will help to achieve this aim, and so each training week should be carefully planned. Table 18.6 provides guidelines for a weekly training template (1 x game per week) for elite soccer players. Note that the recommendations are based on a first team squad of 24 players that includes regular playing members, non-regular playing members and elite young players (U23 players training with the first team squad but non-playing).

Numerous authors have examined the effects of speed-endurance and repeated sprint training in soccer players (Dupont et al., 2004; Ferrari et al., 2008; Hill-Haas et al., 2009). The benefits of conducting frequent sessions of speed-endurance training have been well documented (Iaia and Bangsbo, 2010; Mujika, 2010), but systematic planning of these sessions must occur under the appropriate guidelines. This is particularly critical when planning the training programme around competition. Failure to follow these guidelines may result in a state of general exhaustion, leading to a decrease in performance and an increased risk of injury. Moreover, the period of regeneration is just as important as any training component and will allow time for compensation and, ultimately, overcompensation to be achieved.

The balance of work throughout the in-season phase necessitates the inclusion of peaking/maintenance periods where adequate attention is placed on rest and regeneration. The goals of this are twofold:

347

**Table 18.6** Guidelines for a weekly training template for elite soccer players.

| | Monday | Tuesday | Wednesday | Thursday | Friday | Saturday | Sunday |
|---|---|---|---|---|---|---|---|
| Playing squad | Aerobic low/ moderate | Leg strength<br><br>Aerobic moderate | Aerobic high | Injury prevention<br><br>Short speed<br><br>Aerobic moderate (short) | Quick feet/reaction | **GAME** | Recovery<br><br>Core/upper body |
| Non playing squad | Aerobic high | Leg strength<br><br>Aerobic moderate | Speed endurance | Injury prevention<br><br>Aerobic moderate/ high | Quick feet/ reaction<br><br>Short speed | **GAME** | Injury prevention<br><br>Aerobic moderate<br><br>Repeated sprints |
| Elite group | Short speed<br><br>Aerobic high | Leg strength<br><br>Aerobic moderate | Injury prevention<br><br>Speed endurance | Aerobic high | Quick feet/reaction<br><br>Short speed | Leg power<br><br>Aerobic high | Injury prevention<br><br>Aerobic moderate |

*Source*: Modified from F. M. Iaia (unpublished data).

1  reduction of overtraining potential;

2  peaking at the appropriate time or providing a maintenance programme during the competitive season.

These goals are met by appropriate variation of training volume and intensity factors and by appropriate exercise selection. The introduction of a taper facilitates these goals. The aim of the taper is to diminish residual fatigue induced by intensive training by reducing the training load during the final days leading up to competition (Bosquet et al., 2007). From a soccer perspective, the load reduction can be achieved by various modifications to the player's training programme, such as reducing the number of training sessions (frequency), reducing the duration of training sessions (volume) and making the training drills less demanding for a given period of time (intensity).

Because elite soccer players are expected to perform 40–60 times over a 42-week period, a taper phase is not always included during the competition phase. Nevertheless, frequent changes to the training programme in terms of volume, intensity and frequency assist in maximising physiological adaptations and performance throughout the annual competition phase. This concept of 'undulating periodisation' allows the player to adapt to new stimuli on a regular basis, thus avoiding training monotony or staleness. In addition, careful

A.J. Strudwick

manipulation of training load and exercise selection facilitates the maintenance of specific physiological parameters throughout the playing season, while at the same time raising the general levels of athletic abilities through a long-term development plan. Clearly, adherence to a weekly taper that occurs from match to match will assist in this process of managing load prescription.

## Transition

Following the competitive in-season phase, both physiological and psychological recovery are necessary. Thus, recovery from the in-season should take the form of 'Active Rest' (AR), in which the volume is kept low and the intensity of training is low to moderate.

## PROMOTION OF RECOVERY AFTER TRAINING AND COMPETITION

A chronic problem in high-performance sport remains the continual risk of an imbalance between the training, competition and recovery components (Budgett, 1990). Successful training must involve overload while avoiding the combination of excessive overload plus inadequate recovery (Meeusen et al., 2006). As a consequence of intense training and competition, players may experience acute feelings of fatigue which temporarily reduces functional capacity and performance. During the subsequent rest period, positive adaptations may follow. This process of overcompensation should be considered as the foundation of all functional increases in athletic efficiency. However, if the optimal balance between training stress and adequate recovery is miscalculated the adaptation process will lessen, leading to overtraining.

The continual challenge to the practitioner is to determine the appropriate type and volume of training/competition for players and to ensure that performance is optimal, while not eliciting any negative adaptations. Clearly, there is a boundary between optimal stimulus and overtraining, but this is not easily identifiable and therefore there is a need for the careful monitoring of training and the promotion of recovery following exercise to ensure that overtraining is prevented.

The principle of recovery relates to the encouragement of adaptive processes after the presentation of the stimulus. If there is sufficient recovery before the next workload the underlying system or fuel store stressed during training can improve its capacity to cope with the next stressor. An appropriate recovery results in the restoration of physiological and psychological processes, so that the player can compete or train again at a suitable level. Recovery from training and competition is complex and involves numerous factors and is typically dependent on the nature of the exercise performed and any other outside stressors to which the player may be exposed. Performance is affected by numerous factors and, as such, adequate recovery should consider such factors as training/competition, nutrition, psychological stress, lifestyle, health and the environment.

Planning appropriate recovery activities accelerates adaptation by reducing the time it takes for a player to reach the overcompensated state. Adaptation varies from one individual to another, so it is not always appropriate to prescribe the same workloads for all players, but it is essential to monitor their responses to training so that workloads can be varied accordingly.

Elite sport has provided the foundation for players to focus purely on training and competition. Furthermore, the importance of successful performances has led players and coaches alike to continually seek any advantage or edge that may improve performance. In this regard, optimal recovery from training and performance may provide numerous benefits during repetitive high-level training and competition; and the rate and quality of recovery in the elite player may be as important as the training itself. While further empirical evidence is required to support recovery practice at elite level, elements currently employed by elite players include:

1   active recovery;

2   compression;

3   contrast therapy;

4   ice therapy/cryotherapy/cold water immersion;

5   massage;

6   pool recovery;

7   stretching.

Following the completion of training/competition, there are three areas of importance in maximising training adaptation and reducing injury risk. Namely, intensive recovery programme, analysis of markers of fatigue and managing the physiological loads imposed on players. These areas, along with the appropriate strategies, are summarised in Table 18.7. Adopting these strategies can produce very positive effects on recovery from competitive

Table 18.7  Strategies for managing the recovery process following training and competition.

| Intensive recovery programme | Analysis of markers of fatigue | Managing physiological loads |
| --- | --- | --- |
| Nutrition programme | Performance (e.g. Jump tests) Daily Analysis of Lifestyle Demands (DALDA) | Internal load monitoring |
| Massage/physiotherapy | Training logs (Hooper et al., 1995) | External load monitoring |
| Hydrotherapy | Biochemical, immunological and hormonal markers | Matching training to individual requirements |
| Body weight/hydration status | Physiological markers (e.g. HR recovery and HR variability) | Modified session planning |
| Cryotherapy | | Subjective/objective assessment of players |
| Stretching/postural sessions | | |
| Reduced arousal following matches | | |

A.J. Strudwick

matches, significantly lowering incidence of illness, maintaining sprint capacity of players and increasing self-rating of daily wellness (Flanagan and Merrick, 2000).

## SYSTEMATIC MONITORING OF WORK RATES

To develop a successful training programme, the physical demands of training and competition need to be fully understood. The physiological requirements of match-play vary from match to match (Gregson et al., 2010) and depend upon playing position, tactical role and team success, amongst other factors (Bradley et al., 2009; Di Salvo et al., 2009; Rampinini et al., 2007). Consequently, the subsequent volume and intensity of training and/or recovery should be individually prescribed according to the player's previous loadings and future requirements in an attempt to optimise their readiness to perform in the next match.

A continual system of monitoring is essential to ensure that the correct decisions are made with regard to individual player requirements. The four methods frequently used to monitor elite training programmes include: the use of retrospective questionnaires; training diaries; physiological screening; and the direct observational method (Meeusen et al., 2006).

Recently, physiological assessment during training has been described in terms of its outcome and its process (Impellizzeri et al., 2004). The outcomes of training are anatomical, physiological, biomechanical and functional changes specific to the sport, while the training process is characterised by the quality, quantity and organisation of the physical exercises (Viru and Viru, 2000). Although physiological tests are commonly used to assess training outcome, the training process is often described as the external load (external TL), that is, the training prescribed by the coaches. According to Impellizzeri et al. (2004), this is inappropriate because the stimulus for training-induced adaptations is the actual physiological stress (the internal TL) imposed on the athletes by the external load (Viru and Viru, 2000). Moreover, despite the external load being the main determinant of the internal load, there are other factors (i.e. genetics, training level) that influence the internal load imposed on the athlete and, consequently, the outcome (Bouchard and Rankinen, 2001). Therefore, an integrated physiological assessment of both outcome and process (external TL and internal TL) is highly relevant to monitoring and controlling soccer-specific training (small-sided games/drills), due to the variability in group exercises (Rampinini et al., 2003).

The external TL refers to the external work imposed by the coach on his/her players and can be reported in terms of time (i.e., min.day$^{-1}$, hours.week$^{-1}$). However, it can also be reported in terms of distance covered (i.e., km.week$^{-1}$). Modern technological advancements in Global Positioning Systems and movement analysis provide the contemporary coach with a wealth of information pertaining to the external TL. This factor is of particular interest throughout the in-season, where external load reduction can be achieved during intense competition periods via reducing the number of training sessions, reducing the duration of training sessions and making the training drills less demanding by reducing the dimensions of the playing areas (Hill-Haas et al., 2011).

The assessment of internal TL requires quantification of the intensity of the physiological stress imposed on the player and can be determined by different methods, such as heart rate (HR), rate of perceived exertion (RPE) and blood lactate concentration. Many of the contemporary

351

methods used to quantify the internal TL during soccer are based on HR monitoring (Impellizzeri et al., 2004). HR is a useful indicator of physiological strain and intensity of effort during exercise (Reilly, 1997). In addition, subdivision of heart rate data expressed as a percentage of maximum heart rate can provide important information concerning time spent above, at or below critical exercise intensities. Such data offer valuable information in assessing, monitoring and adjusting training intensities in order to ensure an optimal training stimulus.

An alternative method to HR for quantifying internal TL has been proposed and validated by Foster (1998). This method consists of multiplying the rating of perceived exertion (RPE) of the whole session as measured by Borg's CR10 scale (Borg et al., 1987) and the total duration of the session expressed in minutes. For example, to calculate the training load for a 60-min training session with the athlete's RPE being 5 (Hard), the following calculation would be made:

$$\text{Training load (AU)} = 5 \times 60 = 300 \text{ units}$$

Recently, researchers have reported that the session-RPE method compares favourably with the more complicated methods of quantifying training loads in both endurance and team sports (Foster et al., 2001; Impellizzeri et al., 2004). The most value a practitioner can get from accurately monitoring the internal TL is a better understanding of each individual player's tolerance to training. This factor is of particular importance in team sports, as the physiological stress induced by the extensive use of group exercises often differs between individuals.

## GYM-BASED INJURY PREVENTION STRATEGIES

In the preparation of elite athletes, practitioners have a responsibility to implement a comprehensive and planned training programme that allows for gym-based injury prevention strategies. The athlete has to be trained in such a way that the body will be prepared for optimum response to the physical demands of competition. Strength training has been increasingly employed in the holistic management of contemporary soccer players. In simple terms, strength training involves increasing the ability of the athlete to apply force. The ultimate objectives of strength training are to develop the capacity to reproduce forceful bursts of energy and withstand the forces of physical impact, landing and deceleration. Following specific screening protocols for local muscles, as well as joints and lower back/pelvis, preventative gym-based programmes in the form of core stability, balance, proprioception, muscular strength and power should be implemented to address the increasing issues of muscle strains in contemporary elite soccer.

Training that prepares the muscle and muscle cells for the trauma and damage caused by repeated high force generation has become an area of increased attention in the training of elite soccer players. Friden and Leiber (1992) suggest that eccentric activity, given the relatively small amount required to induce muscle damage and adaptation, may have a valuable role to play in a training regime. It follows that eccentric training in the form of gym-based preventative exercises may be an effective way to promote resistance to muscular damage. Therefore, a well-planned training programme should include periodic and systematic exposure to activities involving the generation of large muscle forces to stimulate changes in

352

A.J. Strudwick

the cytoskeletal system. Clearly, for this type of adaptation to be transferable to soccer, one must ensure that the high-force activities fully exploit the muscles and motor units, the range of motion and the contraction velocity typical of movements performed.

While there are many components that need to be incorporated into gym-based injury prevention programmes, the following areas may be included in the physical preparation programme of elite players:

1    mobilisation/activation;

2    core stability and rotational strength;

3    power exercises;

4    eccentric exercises;

5    reactive exercises;

6    balance/proprioception;

7    strength exercises;

8    stretching.


## INDIVIDUALISED NUTRITIONAL SUPPORT

In order to maximise adaptations from training and enhance recovery after match-play it is essential that players follow an effective individual nutritional support strategy. Moreover, a systematic approach to providing the appropriate nutrition-based strategies will yield

Table 18.8 Critical components of performance nutrition strategy.

| Component | Application |
| --- | --- |
| Body composition analysis and monitoring | Valid and reliable fat and muscle mass measurements. |
| Menu planning | Liaising with catering staff for training and competition. |
| Recovery/muscular adaptation | Individualised strategies for training, resistance sessions and competitions. |
| Fat mass loss | Catabolic approaches to reduce fat mass quickly and safely without impairing immunity. |
| Pre-event fuelling | To support training/competition. |
| Supplementation | Specific, literature-supported recommendations from a reliable, batch-tested source. |
| Immunity | Strategies to support immune function (including gut health) during the domestic season. Cycling of key antioxidants, amino acids in extreme environments (e.g. pre-season training camps). |
| Diet coaching | To support positive lifestyle management. |

favourable results in terms of training adaptations, recovery and match performance. Table 18.8 provides critical components associated with the development of a performance nutrition strategy.

## SUMMARY

This chapter has considered the key issues that impact upon the physical preparation of elite soccer players. Contemporary match-play is physically demanding and players require elevated fitness levels to cope with these energy demands. With increased financial incentives, commitment to training and competition is, as a result, extremely high. In addition, coaches and players operating at an elite level are well aware that the small increments in performance standards that are possible at the highest level require training programmes that are extensive in scale and need to be conducted at a high intensity. For this reason, practitioners need to have an enhanced appreciation of the processes that are involved in the holistic management of elite players.

At the elite level of soccer, the next decade will see improved coach education, sports science knowledge and player management. Moreover, elite soccer teams will move towards high-performance environments where the development of systematic performance models and increased accountability are commonplace. Innovations in player preparation are more challenging by the year and expectations continue to rise. Therefore, player preparation has to be sharper and better informed. These factors call for superior sports science support models and deeper insights into issues relating to the management of elite performance.

## REFERENCES

Bangsbo, J. (1994). The physiology of soccer – with special reference to intense intermittent exercise. *Acta Physiologica Scandinavica* 151, Suppl. 619, 1–155.

Bangsbo, J. (2008). *Aerobic and Anaerobic Training in Soccer: With Special Emphasis on Training of Youth Players. Fitness Training in Soccer I.* Bagsvaerd, Denmark: HO+Storm.

Bloomfield, J., Polman, R., and O'Donoghue, P. (2007). Physical demands of different positions in FA Premier League soccer. *Journal of Sports Science and Medicine* 6, 63–70.

Borg, G., Hassmen, P., and Lagerstrom, M. (1987). Perceived exertion related to heart rate and blood lactate during arm and leg exercise. *European Journal of Applied Physiology and Occupational Physiology* 56, 679–685.

Bosquet, L., Montpetit, J., Arvisais, D., and Mujika, I. (2007). Effects of tapering on performance: a meta-analysis. *Medicine and Science in Sports and Exercise* 39, 1358–1365.

Bouchard, C., and Rankinen, T. (2001). Individual differences in response to regular physical activity. *Medicine and Science in Sports and Exercise* 33, S446–S451.

Bradley, P. S., Sheldon, W., Wooster, B., Olsen, P., Boanas, P., and Krustrup, P. (2009). High-intensity running in English FA Premier League soccer matches. *Journal of Sports Sciences* 27, 159–168.

Budgett, R. (1990). Overtraining syndrome. *British Journal of Sports Medicine* 24(4), 231–236.

## 354

Davenport, T, H., and Harris, J. G. (2007). *Competing on Analytics: The New Science of Winning.* Cambridge, MA: Harvard Business School Press.

Di Salvo, V., Gregson, W., Atkinson, G., Tordoff, P., and Drust, B. (2009). Analysis of high intensity activity in Premier League soccer. *International Journal of Sports Medicine* 30, 205–212.

Di Salvo, V., Baron, R., Tschan, H., Calderon Montero, F. J., Bachl, N., and Pigozzi, F. (2007). Performance characteristics according to playing position in elite soccer. *International Journal of Sports Medicine* 28, 222–227.

Dupont, G., Akakpo, K., and Berthoin, S. (2004). The effect of in-season, high-intensity interval training in soccer players. *Journal of Strength and Conditioning Research* 18, 584–589.

Ferrari, B. D., Impellizzeri, F. M., Rampinini, E., Castagna, C., Bishop, D., and Wisloff, U. (2008). Sprint vs. interval training in football. *International Journal of Sports Medicine* 29, 668–674.

Flanagan, T., and Merrick, E. (2000). The effects of tournament-play on elite youth soccer players. *Insight: The FA Coaches Association Journal* 3(4), 15–19.

Foster, C. (1998). Monitoring training in athletes with reference to overtraining syndrome. *Medicine and Science in Sports and Exercise* 30, 1164–1168.

Foster, C., Florhaug, J. A., Franklin, J., Gottschall, L., Hrovatin, L. A., Parker, S., Doleshal, P., and Dodge, C. (2001). A new approach to monitoring exercise training. *Journal of Strength and Conditioning Research* 22, 109–115.

Friden, J., and Leiber, R. L. (1992). Structural and mechanical basis of exercise-induced muscle injury. *Medicine and Science in Sports and Exercise* 24, 521–530.

Gregson, W., Drust, B., Atkinson, G., and Di Salvo, V. (2010). Match-to-match variability of high-speed activities in premier league soccer. *International Journal of Sports Medicine* 4, 237–242.

Hill-Haas, S. V., Dawson, B. T., and Coutts, A. J. (2011). Physiology of small-sided games training in football: a systematic review. *Sports Medicine* 41(3), 199–220.

Hill-Haas, S. V., Dawson, B. T., Coutts, A. J., and Rowsell, G. J. (2009). Physiological responses and time-motion characteristics of various small-sided soccer games in youth players. *Journal of Sports Sciences* 27, 1–8.

Hooper, S.L., Mackinnon, L.T., Howard, A., Gordon, R. and Bachmann, A. W. (1995). Markers for monitoring overtraining and recovery. *Medicine and Science in Sports and Exercise* 27, 106–112.

Iaia, F. M., and Bangsbo, J. (2010). Speed endurance training is a powerful stimulus for physiological adaptations and performance improvements of athletes. *Scandinavian Journal of Medicine and Science in Sports* 20 Suppl 2, 11–23.

Iaia, F. M., Rampinini, E., and Bangsbo, J. (2009). High-intensity training in football. *International Journal of Sports Physiology and Performance* 4(3), 291–306.

Impellizzeri, F. M., Rampinini, E., Coutts, A. J., Sassi, A., and Marcora, S. M. (2004). Use of RPE-based training load in soccer. *Medicine and Science in Sports and Exercise* 36, 1042–1047.

Kelly, D. M., and Drust, B. (2009). The effect of pitch dimensions on heart rate responses and technical demands of small-sided soccer games in elite players. *Journal of Science and Medicine in Sport* 12, 475–479.

Little, T., and Williams, A. G. (2006). Suitability of soccer training drills for endurance training. *Journal of Strength and Conditioning Research* 20, 16–319.

Maile, A. (1999). Applied physiology in sports coaching. In N. Cross and J. Lyle (eds), *The*

355

*Coaching Process. Principles and Practice for Sport* (pp. 91–112). Oxford: Butterworth Heinemann.

Meeusen, M., Duclos, M., Gleeson, M., Rietjens, G., Steinacker, J., and Urhausen, A. (2006). Prevention, diagnosis and treatment of the overtraining syndrome. *European Journal of Sports Science* 6(1), 1–14.

Mohr, M., Krustrup, P., and Bangsbo, J. (2003). Match performance of high-standard soccer players with special reference to development of fatigue. *Journal of Sports Sciences* 21, 519–528.

Mujika, I. (2010). Intense training: the key to optimal performance before and during the taper. *Scandinavian Journal of Medicine and Science in Sports* 20 Suppl 2, 24–31.

Nimmo, M. A., and Ekblom, B. (2007). Fatigue and illness in athletes. *Journal of Sports Sciences* 25, S93–S102.

Rampinini, E., Sassi, A., and Impellizzeri, F. M. (2003). Reliability of heart rate recorded during soccer training. Communication to the *Fifth World Congress of Science and Football, Lisbon, Portugal*. London & New York: Routledge.

Rampinini, E., Coutts, A. J., Castagna, C., Sassi, R., and Impellizzeri, F. M. (2007). Variation in top level soccer match performance. *International Journal of Sports Medicine* 28, 1018–1024.

Reilly, T. (1994). Physiological aspects of soccer. *Biology of Sport* 11, 3–20.

Reilly, T. (1997). Energetics of high-intensity exercise (soccer) with particular reference to fatigue. *Journal of Sports Sciences* 15, 257–263.

Strudwick, A. J. (2006). A profile of elite soccer players with special reference to the load imposed on players during training and match-play. PhD thesis, Liverpool John Moores University.

Viru, A., and Viru, M. (2000). Nature of training effects. In W. Garrett and D. Kirkendall (eds), *Exercise and Sport Science* (pp. 67–95). Philadelphia: Lippincott Williams and Williams.

Williams, A. M., and Hodges, N. J. (2005). Practice, instruction and skill acquisition: challenging tradition. *Journal of Sports Sciences* 23, 637–650.

# CHAPTER 19

## MENTAL PREPARATION OF ELITE PLAYERS

M. Nesti

## INTRODUCTION

This chapter focuses on a number of issues that are frequently encountered by players in professional soccer. Some of these are felt more keenly in the higher levels of the professional game, whilst others occur more frequently in the lives of lower league players. However, irrespective of the level of play, there are several common experiences associated with different stages of a player's career. In particular, there are critical moments (Nesti and Littlewood, 2011) that must be successfully negotiated to ensure continued success. Critical moments have been described by Nesti and Littlewood (2011) as being those frequently experienced moments in our lives where we must confront an important change in our identity.

Professional players often talk about focusing on one game at a time. This sound strategy is not just restricted to matches, but very often it is the way that players approach their careers. The desire to avoid 'getting ahead of yourself' can be easily understood in a profession where players can start off at a top club on an incredible salary, and finish the season being sold to a much lower-level team and earning a considerably reduced income. Facing up to a reality that often involves fear about suffering a career-ending injury, falling out with the manager, difficulties with the media and being considered as 'past it' means that professional players exist in a world of considerable uncertainty (Roderick, 2006). Nesti (2010) suggests that players will experience anxiety during these critical moments and that, whilst this is not a comfortable feeling, it can be a good sign. The existential approach (Nesti, 2004) describes normal anxiety as being the feeling that accompanies moments and events that we care about. Existential phenomenological psychology argues that this type of anxiety can be beneficial when we embrace it and, despite its presence, move forward to consider and act on our choices. This perspective, unfortunately, has been little studied in sport psychology, despite its pre-dating Freudian perspectives on anxiety and having emerged almost 100 years before cognitive psychology.

The experiences of new players at a club, especially those from overseas, can also provide a number of very unique challenges. These can relate to differences in language, communication style and culture. The progression of young professionals into the first-team environment represents another example where players are often confronted with unfamiliar psychological demands that must be met quickly to ensure survival and success (Parker, 1995).

Issues common to all players in professional soccer include the experience of de-selection, insufficient playing time, poor relationships with the manager and coaching staff, and contractual negotiations. Sometimes players are unable to play in their preferred position, due to tactical reasons or because of injury. They will often have to deal with seeing new players brought into the club as their possible replacements. In addition, there is a general requirement to maintain standards and intensity levels in training and matches throughout the entire ten and a half months of the campaign. This factor is especially the case at first-team levels in professional clubs. Psychological issues associated with these challenges may result in players losing focus and motivation.

It will be argued here that much of what is actually at stake is about the question of personal and professional identity. The topic of identity and how important this is in the work of the sport psychologist operating in elite-level professional soccer will be briefly addressed in the chapter. The role of sports psychologists in helping players to deal with these challenges and critical moments is considered. A very important topic centres on whether it is appropriate for the sports psychologist to assist players in enhancing performance, or whether their role should be, as Andersen (2009) has argued, exclusively one that involves providing emotional support and athlete care. The view taken here is that the performance-or-care debate (Brady and Maynard, 2010) represents yet another false dichotomy that seems very prevalent in academic sport psychology, and that does not stand up to scrutiny from an applied perspective.

In contrast, by drawing on holistic and in-depth approaches to psychology, and guided by work with players at the highest levels of the sport, this chapter is based on the idea that a caring perspective *and* a performance focus are equally essential. Quite simply, it is impossible to work with elite-level professional athletes if they think that your interest is not in helping them to improve or maintain their performance. Why should they waste time engaging with a sport psychologist if this is not an aim? Of course, to develop trust and be able to work with full confidentiality and deal with difficult issues that cannot usually be resolved by traditional mental skills training means that the athlete must know that the sport psychologist cares about them as a person. This factor does not mean that they become friends. However, it does mean that empathy is not merely a sophisticated technical term for attentive listening! It is argued that, although mental skills have been found to be effective in dealing with a number of psychological challenges in sport, there is increasing recognition (Lindsay et al., 2007) that these techniques cannot be usefully employed in all situations. This fact is especially likely to be the case with elite-level athletes, as we know from many years of research and applied practice that most at the highest levels already possess excellent mental skills (Fifer et al., 2008). It will be argued that, to assist players to deal with the types of issues commonly encountered in professional soccer, a more person-centred approach (Ravizza, 2002) that is much less focused on mental skills training is required. In addition, this chapter will briefly identify and discuss the skills and personal qualities needed by sports psychologists to carry out this work effectively.

The chapter draws partly on earlier work by Gilbourne and Richardson (2006), in that it is constructed to encourage readers to engage in critical reflection about their own practice and consider how this is underpinned by the literature. The theoretical approaches that are used here are included to suggest how particular issues and practice can be understood in ways that are quite different to the dominant perspectives in the discipline of sport psychology. It is hoped that, through use of creative vignettes (Sparkes, 2002), the reader will be able to gain a more authentic understanding of the topic being discussed. Three brief vignettes focusing on critical moments and the types of experiences that are common in elite-level professional soccer are provided. The examples used do not relate to any particular player or specific club.

# 358

However, they are based on confidential one-to-one counselling sessions carried out with many professional players during a 15-year period (1995–2010), including Premier League players at Bolton Wanderers, Newcastle United and Hull City during nine seasons of applied work inside these clubs.

In terms of structural characteristics for how clubs could organise the delivery of sport psychology within professional soccer, little has been written apart from the recent work of Nesti (2010). His work provides some suggestions about how sport psychology could be delivered alongside other sport science disciplines. However, it is not based on research and draws heavily on the author's experiences at a small number of elite clubs. Sport psychology provision in professional soccer could be divided into two discrete areas: organisational psychology and one-to-one performance-focused support for players (and staff). Because of the considerable differences between the aims and culture at first-team and youth levels, the optimum provision would be for there to be sport psychologists who worked exclusively with each of these parts of the club. It would also be important for all the sport psychologists to work closely together to ensure sharing of good practice and a common philosophy underpinning the work.

There should be one lead sport psychologist. This role could involve management of the interface between coaches and sports scientists, helping to shape and drive forward longer-term strategy for the team on matters such as player and staff recruitment, developing internal communication systems and co-ordinating staff training and development needs. In some ways, one could view this type of support as being similar to that provided by human resource managers and occupational psychologists in many business organisations. The work would be aimed at creating the conditions for a high-level performance culture by addressing systems, structures and organisational climate. A sport psychologist should be employed to deliver confidential, individually focused interventions for players and staff. This role could not be carried out as effectively by the club's organisational psychologist because of the scale of the task in terms of time commitments, and crucially, because individuals will not 'open up' easily or fully if they perceive that the psychologist is too close to the manager and other senior staff. This model can be extended to the Academy or youth section at the club. However, to ensure that players experience a constant and consistent message as they move up to the professional ranks, it is important that communication systems and opportunities for dialogue exist between all sport psychologists at the club.

## CRITICAL MOMENTS IN PROFESSIONAL SOCCER

### Vignette 1: Pre-season euphoria – meeting the person first, the player second

Player (P): I'm really up for it! Feeling good, focused and fit. Training is so much better, you know, variety and organised, than at my last club. Getting a real buzz from how everyone, the staff, gaffer, players and fans are reacting to me. It's just great to be respected again, after how it all ended last season.

Sport psychologist (SP): How are you settling in to the area? Are you out of the hotel yet? How have your wife and children found things here?

P: Great so far. We're used to it, you know. This has been my fourth or fifth time in this situation so we know how it goes. The hotel is fine – got our eye on an apartment near the town. We really fancy being able to live close to the stadium and get to feel part of this place. I hope to be here a long time. We'll see, but I'm really hoping that I can be a big part of this here. It's so good to be somewhere where I'm accepted just for being me – it's not always been like this in the past!

SP: Good stuff. I know you told me that the family was important to you, that it's important for it all to feel right, on and off the pitch.

P: Yeah, I'd say that knowing my wife and kids are sorted, you know, feel settled and happy, is maybe the biggest thing in my life. I'm experienced enough now to know what I need to do to prepare for games. To be fair, I've never really had any real problems with this for many years now. Used to worry a lot that I worried a bit too much about my mistakes in games, but now I know that's normal for me – it's probably just how I am, and it's because I have pride, you know, in doing stuff well. I suppose you could say I care a lot about doing myself justice. It's more for me – so I can look at myself in the mirror – never been as much bothered about others – gaffer, media and punters' views – although don't get me wrong – I do respect their views and they are important.

SP: Just to pick up on the last thing you said, as it ties in well with reminding you about how I work over the season. I'm not here to teach you to suck eggs – you know, tell you about mental skills techniques relating to confidence, motivation etc., as I know you can't get to your level without having most of these well sorted already . . . by the way, just to be a boring academic, we have loads of research in sport psychology that tells us this fact as well! But if a tough time comes, or I should really say, when it comes, we may need to make sure you're using your mental skills fully and maybe we can freshen these up or even add something small.

P: No problem. I'm always checking myself anyway to make sure I'm on top of my mental preparation. But yeah, of course it would be good to have someone on my case as well, especially as you say, there will be some tough moments ahead, as always . . .

The dialogue presented in Vignette 1 is intended to show that mental skills training and issues relating to more personal matters are often discussed by players during sessions with sport psychologists. This factor suggests that players understand the importance of good mental skills and they are aware that their performances can be affected by situations and challenges beyond matches and training. Additionally, the vignette is attempting to capture the idea that critical moments are sometimes very positive and enjoyable phases, and that they can impact on everything in the player's life. This notion is consistent with broader, more holistic approaches found in counselling psychology, where focus is on what the person feels is important to their success. These factors can range from narrow performance concerns to broader life issues.

## DE-SELECTION

One of the hardest parts of a professional player's life is the issue of de-selection. Most players want to feature at the highest level they can and to be given extensive playing time. It does

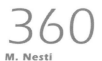

not require complex psychological reasoning to understand the motivation behind this! The motives can quite easily be described in relation to intrinsic and extrinsic rewards. For players as professional athletes, financial achievements are closely related to success on the field of play. Very few players can survive for a long period of time without appearing frequently in the starting 11. For those who are unable to break into the team, there is the threat of being moved on to another club, through either loan or sale. In addition, players who rarely feature over a season will find themselves in a much weaker position when the time comes to renegotiate contracts.

However, beyond the above issues and extrinsic motives, research confirms that intrinsic motives are very important to many elite performers in sport and in other areas of human endeavour. The seminal work of Deci and Ryan (1985) provides one of the most scholarly and clearest descriptions of intrinsic motivation. Their account, which is grounded in cognitive psychology, has been used by many researchers in sport psychology to examine the importance of intrinsic motivation in sport settings. Deci and Ryan's original work defined intrinsic motivation in terms of perceived competence and self-determination, which can easily be related to professional players. The desire to play in the team on match day can be understood because this gives players an opportunity to engage in something they believe they are good at (perceived competence) and which they have chosen to do in their lives (self-determined). Deci and Ryan's organismic perspective on intrinsic motivation is based on the idea that this is something that is innate. That is, they argue that all of us wish to enjoy the feelings that accompany doing something really well, and engaging in something we have freely chosen.

Although the extrinsic rewards available at the highest level within the sport are significant, players are fully aware of the importance of intrinsic motivation in their professional careers. Often a player will be de-selected with very little explanation given for this decision. Even where coaches, the manager and others provide some rationale for their decision, there will usually be a large and significant subjective element behind this action. This is unavoidable in a team sport where successful performance cannot be reduced to purely objective data around fitness levels, performance statistics and specific outputs. Team selection will usually be based on all of this quantifiable data and other, more informal and subjective assessments. For example, a manager may drop a player from the starting 11 because of poor attitude in training, or because they feel the player can be a bad influence on younger players in the squad. Conversely, a player who is unable or unwilling to train at the required intensity, but who brings a positive mood to the changing room prior to major games, may be selected for a period of crucial fixtures, despite being physically less than optimal. The complexity of decision making surrounding who will start , which players will be in the squad, and who will travel to away matches, makes these, arguably, the most important decisions the manager and coaching staff must make each week.

Where the player has had many previous experiences of these moments, the sport psychologist can draw on this material in meetings. This will allow discussion to consider how the player responded to a prolonged absence from the team in previous situations. The sport psychologist's role will be to get the player to describe in detail how they felt about this and identify the actions they took to try to resolve the issue. The sport psychologist's input could be to help the player in recognising where they have come up with constructive solutions in the past and in examining whether these could prove useful in their current critical moment. It might be that different circumstances will require an adaptation of previous actions and that a new solution should be proposed. This is not a straightforward and rational technique, such as goal setting. Sometimes the most effective plan may involve the player in adopting a different view of success and striving to develop greater patience, as opposed to taking a more action-oriented perspective. In other words, this deeper level of analysis could provide an opportunity for further development of a player's identity. Undoubtedly, there will be occasions where a more simple set of mental skills techniques, such as goal setting, could usefully assist the player to work towards re-selection for the team. However, often this is insufficient in professional soccer because the achievement of this particular goal is ultimately not within the player's control. An approach where the player is encouraged to focus on process goals can sometimes be a useful strategy, however; often players are already working towards these in a systematic and focused way.

In contrast to the 'technique driven' superficial approaches of mental skills training (Corlett, 1996a), a more 'in-depth psychology' perspective could be beneficial. For example, a humanistic, existential or other person-centred counselling approach could help the player to address the issues very differently. Using these approaches to deal with a prolonged period of de-selection, greater emphasis would be placed on guiding the player to take a step back so as to understand more clearly why they find this inevitable element of their professional life so psychologically demanding. A humanistic psychology approach might emphasise that the player must find their own reasons for why they need to succeed in their sport beyond important extrinsic rewards. An existential psychology approach would go one step further by emphasising that finding the reasons to continually strive to achieve in difficult circumstances is often an uncomfortable experience, and one that can be surrounded by doubt and anxiety. This view emphasises that deeper questions about pursuing one's goals and life choices are not always resolved by positive feelings. The aim is to pursue personal fulfilment and achievement despite difficulties. In this manner, existential psychology counselling differs from positive psychology (Seligman and Csikszentmihalyi, 2000), in that it contends that pursuing *achievement* and seeking *meaning* is the route to happiness. Or, to put it differently, the existential phenomenological approach sees happiness as a *by-product* rather than the aim of psychological work.

Players facing prolonged periods of de-selection and lack of playing time may be de-motivated and experience genuine despair. There can be a feeling that they have little control over events and therefore they can only rely upon luck (or injury to others or their lack of form). Sometimes a player may try too hard and attempt to do things they are not capable of, in an effort to force their way back into the side. The task facing the sport psychologist in these situations is to help the player to recover a more balanced response. Part of this can involve the player's winning back some self-respect.

However, before players can respect themselves they need to know themselves (i.e., to have self-knowledge) in the first place. This topic has been central to many of the most important writings relating to psychology, from antiquity to the present day. The subject of self-knowledge has been central to the work of some of the most influential psychologists of the last 150 years, such as Freud, Jung, Kelly, Maslow and May. It has also been considered in the more philosophical writings of Husserl and Heidegger on the phenomenology of authenticity.

Unfortunately, for the most part, the discipline of sport psychology remains unaware of the importance of such work, even though it has support from some of the most important thinkers and writers in the parent discipline of psychology. As Nesti (2004) has previously argued, applied sport psychology has been seriously held back by the tendency to conceive the subject exclusively in terms of cognitive, behavioural or trait psychology. Although a few perceptive practitioners and researchers have recently identified that something important is missing in our applied work (e.g., Friesen and Orlick, 2010), there seems to be a lack of awareness about the very different philosophical assumptions that underpin holistic approaches in psychology. Greater understanding of these approaches and increased knowledge in relation to counselling psychology (Lavallee and Cockerill, 2002) will enhance the work of sport psychologists in elite and professional sports, including soccer.

## Vignette 2: De-selection

P: What more do I have to do to get back in the side? It seems that no matter what I do in training and in the Reserves, the manager doesn't give me a chance! We are 12 games in and I've only started 3 and come on late in one 3 weeks ago. This is not what I've moved my family to another country for! No matter what I do, it doesn't seem that it gets noticed.

SP: Have you thought long and hard – you know, had a close look at all of your work, including on the mental side of things, to see if there is anything more you can do, or is there some important stuff you usually do but have not been doing recently?

P: No, as we've spoken about before, I am a bit of a worrier you could say, so I always make sure I attend to everything pretty consistently you know. I have noticed that I'm getting a lot more frustrated and reacting a bit in training, especially if things don't go well. Apart from that though, the hardest thing is how tough it is on my wife and the questions all the time from the media here, and especially at home, about what's wrong with me!

SP: Tell me a bit more about the frustration in training. Are you not performing as well as you can because of it? Are you trying to do anything about it to help?

P: Well, I maybe need to remind myself to anticipate this before I go out to train so that I won't over react as much. Maybe I need to talk to myself about this and make sure it's more contained – I know it doesn't help performance and isn't good for the gaffer and rest of the staff to see.

SP: OK good, but what about the effect of all of this on you and your wife? What does this feel like, you know, what would you say things are like for you with this day to day?

P: It's really not good! I feel that I can't do much more and don't have very much control over things, you know, getting back in the side. It's making it really stressful for me and I'm not about to talk about it really to anyone, even to my wife. It feels too raw, and it's difficult to be calm about it. It's not just that I'm not playing, but that it's been done in such a very poor way. No one, manager, coaches or anyone, speaks to me about why I'm not in the side. How can I know what they are looking for if they don't tell me? To be honest, I don't feel respected for who I am, you know, what I've done before, and why I came here to give it a go.

SP: How is this affecting you here at the club, training and matches in the Reserves?

P: It's making me think back to what I've done in situations like this before. It's just I didn't expect it to happen here after such a great pre-season!

SP: What did you do then, before I mean?

P: Spend time remembering about who I am! You know, what I'm about, what I stand for and my values and things. I know that this isn't right and I'm not getting a fair chance to show what I can do here. I know that the team are doing OK and it's hard to get back in, but I feel I could make a real impact, especially in the next 5 or 6 games when we are away from home at 3 top 6 sides in what's going to be a very tough period. I've spent quite a lot of time going back in my mind, seeing myself playing well in games, just to help keep me focused and confident. Also the performance analysis lads have been great with the DVDs they've given me of some of the best stuff from my first two games here and the pre-season match against Ajax. I keep on top of the fitness data – John always gives me a report regularly and it's good to know that my figures are strong.

SP: So, what more can you do to keep belief, focus and motivation up during this tough time?

P: All the stuff I've mentioned is good, but really though, it's about me reminding myself that this won't break me, that I'm strong enough to come through this and succeed again. This is who I am, you know, someone who stays true to who they are – it's really important to know you're being yourself in these moments. If I can't back myself, I can't expect others to do so! But to do this I must keep reminding myself of what I am all about – that doesn't mean ignoring advice from others – but it does mean that ultimately I am responsible for finding a way through this. It's important for me to keep on believing, battling, doing the right things, showing that I'm strong, up for it, and ready to give it everything, no matter what. This is for me, my wife and family. It's about who I am and what I'm all about – nothing more, nothing less!

Vignette 2 is included to highlight that during difficult and uncomfortable critical moments the main role for the sport psychologist is sometimes to help the player regain a sense of self. Theoretical perspectives in psychology, such as those based on Kelly, Maslow, Rogers and May, emphasise that when facing challenges it is important that individuals think about their identity, that is, who they are and what is most important to them. The rationale for this is that to be able to take back some control and begin to construct some choices the player must build themselves back up. This process is sometimes achieved by considering past achievements and what is important to the person in their professional and personal lives. When facing a very demanding and frustrating critical moment it is easy to feel that nothing can be done to change things, sometimes to over-react or, at other times, to look for a quick fix. Often these only make matters worse, since what is needed is to renew one's identity and sense of self so that any future decisions and actions can emerge from a solid and clarified base.

## COACH–ATHLETE COMMUNICATION

Another commonly experienced critical moment that provides an opportunity for the professional player to develop their identity is where coach–athlete relationships are dysfunctional or break down. In such a volatile, highly pressured and fast-paced culture as elite professional soccer there are many reasons why these important relationships can be fractured. Coaching staff may believe that a player is not preparing properly and professionally for training, or that they are not doing everything to fulfil the competitive process in matches. Beyond the match and training ground, considerable tension and communication problems can arise over media speculation about players' behaviours, rumours about moving clubs, activities of agents and communication with fans and the public via multimedia sources.

Within a team environment it can be very difficult for the manager and coaching team to find sufficient periods of time to communicate properly and fully with each player. This issue is exacerbated at elite levels, where the manager must work closely with sports science, sports medicine and coaching teams that can sometimes consist of over 25–30 individuals. Misunderstanding and suspicion can easily arise in these types of cultures, especially where a very informal and ad hoc approach to communication is the norm. In addition, there is often a reluctance to engage in personal dialogue, for fear of being viewed as weak within the aggressive and macho environment that is often encountered in professional soccer (Gilbourne and Richardson, 2006). In this type of culture, it may be very difficult to find acceptable mechanisms to allow sport psychologists to deal with critical moments where player–staff relationships break down. These do not just have an impact in a general way, but often they directly affect a player's performance.

Sometimes the solution to this may be unavailable to the player where the manager and senior staff are deliberately using communication as a tactic to punish a player. This issue is common in professional soccer and can be a very uncomfortable experience for the player concerned. Typically, this type of behaviour is used as a last resort, where staff feel that a player is behaving in an unprofessional way in relation either to their match performances, training, preparation, or off-field activities. However, inevitably there will be many examples where the player experiencing this 'cold shoulder' is being penalised unfairly. In those situations, where the player knows that they are being victimised or being scapegoated for other, wider problems with the team, there will frequently be deep resentment and a desire to withdraw from their responsibilities and roles. These situations can present an opportunity for the sport psychologist to help the player. However, this will be a difficult task from a practical and ethical dimension, where senior staff may wish that the player should be isolated and ignored.

## IDENTITY

The important topic of identity in the lives of professional players can be informed by considering work on the importance of identity development in psychology and psychotherapy. In a rather unfortunate continuation of the dualistic psychological approaches that have dominated research for over 40 years, the discipline of sport psychology has tended to explain identity in terms of athletic identity (Grove et al., 1997). This concept refers to the degree to which an individual sees themselves as an athlete. Recent research in professional soccer from a more sociological perspective (Brown and Potrac, 2009) suggests that young players can experience many problems where they have a narrowly focused self-identity based exclusively on their identity as players.

However, within the ranks of full-time professional soccer the situation is, arguably, somewhat different to that facing a young, amateur player. Although research on career transitions and retirement has helped sports psychologists to consider how this process can be dealt with more positively, there has been a failure to acknowledge that professional and elite sports performers, in particular, frequently face very significant challenges to their identity throughout their careers. The work concerned with identity in sport has provided a useful if somewhat limited account of this important psychological factor. Much of the research has concerned itself with the construct of athletic identity in relation to children and youth sports performers, with few researchers focusing on older athletes.

However, broader approaches to identity derived from the work of Erikson (1962) and existential psychologists, in particular, could provide a much more extensive and theoretically complex account that could be used to guide understanding and applied work in elite sport settings. For example, Erikson based his theory on many years of extensive applied work where he discovered that the ability to deal with crisis and critical moments depended upon an individual's self-identity. Elite professional players must be able to manage a situation where it is common for their professional identity to be undermined and challenged. This issue is much more demanding in elite professional soccer because media coverage can be extremely intrusive and personal.

All critical moments repeatedly encountered across an elite professional player's career, such as losing form, being sent on loan and being injured, can affect identity severely. Sometimes a player will be unable, at least initially, to move forward quickly. In these situations their sense of self, their identity, can be subject to an intense level of scrutiny. The theoretical perspectives embraced by Erikson and others in existential phenomenological psychology suggest that at these critical moments personal growth can occur by developing a stronger sense of self.

The sport psychologist could assist here by encouraging the player to examine their attitudes, beliefs and values. Arguably, these represent the most important parts of a person's identity. During critical moments, for example, when experiencing a prolonged period of de-selection, players will often feel unsure about themselves and what action should be taken. This factor can quickly turn into feelings of self-doubt and depression. According to May (1977), there will be an increase in feelings of anxiety and a sense of powerlessness at these moments. To avoid these distressing feelings and thoughts, players may 'give up the fight' and merge into the group. Others may go in the opposite direction and try to force the issue by publicly threatening to leave the club, or by criticising the manager in the media. According to the existential phenomenological approach, neither of these strategies will help the player. Sport psychologists may make this situation even worse by directing the player to use mental skills techniques. Corlett (1996a) has pointed out that these may be useful in addressing symptoms, but fail to deal with the underlying issues. From an existential psychology view the key issue here is that of identity. The sport psychologist must work with the player to confront and embrace the existential anxiety they are facing and support them to take responsibility to consider the choices they can make. In order to do this, the player must know who they are and what they stand for as an individual. This task can be achieved through encounters and dialogue between the sport psychologist and player. The aim is for the player to become authentic. That is, to become themselves again, so they can decide on what they must do next,

**M. Nesti**

rather than allowing others to do this for them. This is no easy or simple task, and usually takes some considerable time and effort. Renewal of self-identity in a culture like professional soccer, where there is often so much inauthenticity (Heidegger, 1962), requires courage (May, 1975), persistence and patience.

## Vignette 3: Moving on

SP: We are now getting towards the business end of the season but I know it's been a difficult last few months for you.

P: There's been some good moments, especially when I played those four matches back in December back to back, but since then it's not been easy. I've got some decisions to make.

SP: What has this felt like for you over this last phase?

P: I've felt really composed and calm, sort of relaxed but determined. I know it sounds strange, but knowing that I've kept my standards up all year, mentally and physically, I feel good about myself if not the situation I'm in. My wife and family, especially my brothers, have been fantastic support – always listening and standing by me. I think I've been able to give more to them during this period – you know, think of myself a bit less and regain some balance and hope again. They've been so important – their presence reminds me what I know but can sometimes forget – that I'm not just a footballer but equally lots of other very important things as well, like a dad, husband or brother.

SP: And how has this related to your performances at the club?

P: It's given me – no, that's wrong! – it's renewed my perspective – that I'm more than a footballer, I'm a person as well! It's helped me be able to give all I can in training and when I've played, knowing that not getting proper recognition is not the end of the world – which doesn't mean I don't care passionately about it of course! It's just that my whole life is not completely linked to my being a footballer. This sense of perspective did disappear early on in September and early October, especially when I was so angry about not making even the bench sometimes. But I realised this was something that was eating away at me – my motivation and confidence – and I managed to pull out of it. Our talks and stuff from my brothers were really important – got me to think again and start to accept my responsibilities and focus on the things I could control. It's so easy not to do this – so tempting to just let yourself be hurt, feel a victim and kind of give up. Sort of go through the motions.

SP: What more can you do to try to get back into the side? Are you using your mental skills as well as you could, and what about performance analysis data?

P: Yes, I am if anything, even more committed to being on top of my mental preparation. It's easier to do this anyway, once you feel good about yourself again, even if you are not achieving your goals here. And that has made me realise that I need to move on or get a loan for next season. So I'm working as hard as I can in training and Reserve games to make this happen.

SP: I'm sure this is good for both you and the club – and maybe you just might get back into the side here again with a bit of luck!

P: That of course would be good, but if not, I'm ready for new challenges and the chance to show what I'm about somewhere else . . .

Vignette 3 attempts to highlight that maintaining an identity that goes beyond one's professional role can be very important during challenging critical moments. The dialogue reveals that the support of the sport psychologist and other individuals close to the player has assisted them to regain some control, motivation and confidence. This change has happened through clarifying what is most important to them, which has helped them to regain a sense of perspective. From this process, the player has been more prepared to trust his/her own assessments more fully, rather than acting as a pawn or someone without much influence over their future. In essence, this captures one of the ideas contained within existential psychology: to choose well, you need to know yourself first. When someone is angry, frustrated and feels impotent, it is all too easy to abandon this freedom and resign oneself to the wishes of other people. This vignette is intended to show that only the player themselves can make this choice, although the guidance and help from others is often of vital importance.

## SPORT PSYCHOLOGIST APPROACH

To operate in a holistic way will involve the sport psychologist and players in taking a long, hard and deep look at who they really are, their achievements, motives, aspirations and dreams. For many individuals in difficult critical moments, this form of counselling can prove very beneficial. This process allows the individual to see that they have some measure of control over what choices they can make to deal with a situation or event. This issue often involves the player talking about their most important values and beliefs. According to Nesti (2007), it is these elements that define the self more fully than personality type, temperament or psychological skills. In fast-moving, volatile and incredibly pressured environments such as professional soccer, it is all too easy for players to forget or ignore who they really are and what they hope to achieve. It is often more comfortable and easier to abandon your individual identity and go with the flow.

An existential phenomenological psychology approach would suggest that this is a very dangerous, and ultimately ineffective and unproductive, strategy to adopt. Where this happens it is common to find that the player is unsure about who they really are. This in turn makes it difficult to know how they should respond to events and challenges. This issue can then undermine their capacity to face up to and make decisions about their future. This type of paralysis around identity impacts on their ability to learn and to meet new challenges. Rather than initiating change, players facing these anxiety-infused situations often act as though they are mere pawns in a game, and as if there is nothing they can do to influence those who control their lives. This feeling can eventually lead to self-disgust and, for some individuals, result in an aggressive reaction to everyone around them and destructive behaviours. For another player, the same failure to confront these issues could lead to complete acquiescence and over-compliance with the wishes of everyone else.

The above factor brings up one of the most important issues that impacts on how a player will be able to react to the difficult critical moments they encounter within their careers. As Nesti and Littlewood (2011) point out, these critical moments are experienced several times in a season, or sometimes on a weekly basis, and even daily in some very demanding environments. According to the holistic approaches to counselling in psychology, it is only by returning to the *self* that a player in these situations can start to become themselves again. It is only by becoming themselves again, referred to as *authenticity* in existential and humanistic coun-selling, that they will be able to make choices for themselves and construct a way forward. Without building up the self again, they will struggle to accept their responsibility for helping their own progress, and will be unable to accept that they can ever have more than partial control over what they hope to achieve. The sport psychologist in professional soccer can help this by encouraging the player through a process of self-analysis and clarification.

What, then, are the types of skills and personal qualities needed by the sport psychologist to work effectively in professional soccer? What knowledge do they need and what should the sport psychologist provide?

## SUMMARY

Cognitive and behavioural techniques such as visualisation, goal setting, relaxation training and others are not the most important for work in this environment. However, this does not mean that such techniques are of no use at all. For example, several very experienced practitioners working at elite and professional levels of sport (e.g., Ravizza, 2002) incorporate mental skills training into their work by locating these skills within broader, more humanistic, existential and other person-centred ways of working. The sport psychologist who hopes to work effectively in professional soccer must be able to use mental skills training when required, but this should always be adapted to the context and specific situations faced. This challenge will mean that the successful sport psychologist in professional soccer will be highly skilled in reading the culture. They must be sensitive to the organisational dynamics around such things as player hierarchies, the use of banter, and traditional informal communication styles. Beyond this, the sport psychologist will be welcomed into this challenging and often closed world if they possess personal qualities such as courage (Corlett, 1996b), integrity, authenticity and a sense of humour! It will be the existence of these qualities and others like them that ensures the survival and success of the sport psychologist in this environment.

However, there is another factor of equal importance for the sport psychologist that will impact on their professional confidence and likelihood of being accepted in the role; there is a need to know that their approach to practice (Lindsay et al., 2007) is grounded in an established, tried and tested body of underpinning work, rather than being derived only from personal reflections and a homespun philosophy. I would suggest that to meet some of these require-ments there is a great need to acquire more knowledge about *counselling psychology* rather than just counselling *skills*, useful though these often are (Katz and Hemmings, 2009). In this way, the concepts and theory from a long-established branch of psychology can be used in a way that helps to broaden the discipline of sport psychology and that, ultimately, will assist us in our work in the unique culture of professional soccer.

This chapter has argued that professional soccer players face critical moments throughout their careers and that these must be successfully negotiated to achieve success. The sport psychologist can assist the player during these moments to maintain motivation and accept that they always have some control over how they respond. To be effective, the response must belong to the player, rather than being based on direction given to them by the sport psychologist. The sport psychologist's role is to help guide the player as they wrestle with these choices. As has been discussed, the existential psychology approach contends that by facing up to and moving beyond the anxiety associated with choice, a person develops a stronger sense of self. This helps them to grow in confidence and be more prepared to think for themselves in the future.

The concept of identity is closely connected to the above issue; knowing who you are (i.e., self-knowledge) is vital to thriving in an environment like professional soccer. It has been suggested that the sport psychologist can help a player by getting them to clarify 'what they stand for' and what is important to them. Without this, it will be very difficult for a player to fulfil their potential in what is very often a transient, fickle and brutally volatile performance culture.

## REFERENCES

Andersen, M.B. (2009). Performance enhancement as a bad start and a dead end: a parenthetical comment on Mellalieu and Lane. *The Sport and Exercise Scientist* 20, 12–14.

Brady, A. and Maynard, I. (2010). At elite level the role of the sport psychologist is entirely about performance enhancement. *Sport and Exercise Psychology Review* 6, 59–66.

Brown, G. and Potrac, P. (2009). You've not made the grade son: de-selection and identity disruption in elite level youth football. *Soccer and Society* 10, 143–159.

Corlett, J. (1996a). Sophistry, Socrates and sport psychology. *The Sport Psychologist* 10, 84–94.

Corlett, J. (1996b). Virtues lost: courage in sport. *Journal of the Philosophy of Sport* 23, 45–57.

Deci, E.L. and Ryan, R.M. (1985). *Intrinsic Motivation and Self-Determination in Human Behaviour*. New York: Plenum Press.

Erikson, E. (1962). *Identity: Youth and Crises*. New York. W.W. Norton and Co.

Fifer, A., Henschen, K., Gould, D. and Ravizza, K. (2008). What works when working with athletes. *The Sport Psychologist* 22, 356–377.

Friesen, A. and Orlick, T. (2010). A qualitative analysis of holistic sport psychology consultants' professional philosophies. *The Sport Psychologist* 24, 227–244.

Gilbourne, D. and Richardson, D. (2006). Tales from the field: personal reflections on the provision of psychological support in professional soccer. *Psychology of Sport and Exercise* 7, 335–337.

Grove, R. J., Lavallee, D. and Gordon, S. (1997). Coping with retirement from sport: the influence of athletic identity. *Journal of Applied Sport Psychology* 9, 191–203.

Heidegger, M. (1962). *Being and Time*. New York: Harper and Row.

Katz, J. and Hemmings, B. (2009). *Counselling Skills Handbook for the Sport and Exercise Psychologist*. Leicester: DSEP, British Psychological Society.

Lavallee, D. and Cockerill, I. (eds) (2002). *Counselling in Sport and Exercise Contexts*. Leicester: The British Psychological Society, Sport and Exercise Psychology Section.

Lindsay, P., Breckon, J.D., Thomas, D. and Maynard, I. (2007). In pursuit of congruence: a personal reflection on methods and philosophy in applied practice. *The Sport Psychologist* 21, 335–352.

May, R. (1975). *The Courage to Create*. New York: Norton.

May, R. (1977). *The Meaning of Anxiety*. New York: Ronald Press.

Nesti, M. (2004). *Existential Psychology and Sport: Theory and Application*. London: Routledge.

**M. Nesti**

Nesti, M. (2007). Persons and players. In J. Parry, M.S. Nesti, S. Robinson and N. Watson (eds), *Sport and Spirituality: An Introduction* (pp.135–150). London: Routledge.

Nesti, M. (2010). *Psychology in Football: Working with Elite and Professional Players*. London: Routledge.

Nesti, M. and Littlewood, M. (2011). Making your way in the game: boundary situations within the world of professional football. In D. Gilbourne and M. Andersen (eds), *Critical Essays in Sport Psychology*. Champaign, IL: Human Kinetics.

Parker, A. (1995). Great expectations: grimness or glamour? The football apprentice in the 1990s. *The Sports Historian* 15, 107–126.

Ravizza, K. (2002). A philosophical construct: a framework for performance enhancement. *International Journal of Sport Psychology* 33, 4–18.

Roderick, M. (2006). *The Work of Professional Football: A Labour of Love*. London: Routledge.

Seligman, M. and Csikszentmihalyi, M. (2000). Positive psychology: an introduction. *American Psychologist* 55, 5–14.

Sparkes, A.C. (2002). *Telling Tales in Sport and Physical Activity: A Qualitative Journey*, Champaign, IL: Human Kinetics.

# CHAPTER 20

## DEVELOPING A PHYSIOLOGY-BASED SPORTS SCIENCE SUPPORT STRATEGY IN THE PROFESSIONAL GAME

D. Burgess and B. Drust

### INTRODUCTION

The majority of the world's professional soccer teams no longer rely solely on the influence of the team manager, coaching staff and a limited number of medical personnel to influence the outcome of competitive matches. It is now far more common for clubs to operate with a more diverse range of support staff who fulfil specialist roles related to the development of both the individual and the team. Although these individuals can fulfil relatively diverse roles depending upon the club in question, they are frequently categorised broadly as 'sports scientists'.

Sports scientists have become increasingly accepted by key stakeholders within professional teams over the last few decades. Behind every successful performance is a complex framework of principles and practices that have been developed to increase the likelihood that a given outcome will arise. Such frameworks have traditionally been based on the experience and practical skills developed by managers and coaches from a lifetime dedicated to the game. An increased pressure to win in contemporary competitions has resulted in greater awareness of the role that may be played by scientists in regard to both the importance of research and applied practice. The preparation and organisation of training as well as pre-game, within-game and post-game strategies are all possible areas that are open to scientific research.

Science can also inform the approaches used to develop young players within the sport. It may also have a role to play in operationalising the organisational strategies and frameworks within which all the individuals involved in the club operate. This chapter outlines a practical guide to the implementation of a physiology-based support strategy for players and coaches within a professional club. Such a strategy should, ideally, be one component of a holistic, multi-disciplinary support system that is implemented within the club. While the communication of such generic principles in developing a physiological support strategy may be of some use to the interested reader, it should be stated from the outset that all strategies should be tailored individually to the organisation to ensure that the chances of success are optimised.

### PERFORMANCE IN SOCCER

The starting-point for developing a sports science support strategy for any activity is an understanding of the factors that determine successful performance. Performance is especially

# 372

complicated in soccer, as a large number of factors related to both an individual player and a team's performance can influence the outcome of matches (Drust *et al.*, 2007). An individual's performance in a game is related to technical and tactical competency, physical fitness and psychological make-up. The technical and tactical competency of individuals is of obvious importance, as the ability to carry out game-specific actions (e.g., passing, tackling, shooting, heading) in relevant parts of the pitch is crucial to match outcome. These technical/ tactical abilities are partly dependent on the physiological characteristics of each player. The physiological requirements that are important are multi-factorial and include such elements as aerobic fitness, muscular strength, speed, power and flexibility. Such attributes enable players to perform the relevant movements and specific actions across the entire match as well as helping to ensure that players avoid the high incidences of injury that are common in the sport. A player's psychological make-up complements the other two areas. Important attributes in this area include aspects of cognitive functioning such as decision making, and individual characteristics such as personality.

It is very difficult to accurately determine the relative contribution of these three areas to an individual's overall performance, as the proportion will almost certainly vary between individuals as well as for a given player across a variety of games. Match outcome (the ultimate indicator of success) is very rarely a function of a specific individual player's performance, but rather a composite of the overall contribution of each individual player's tactical, technical and physical input to the team effort. This factor may be highly variable, depending upon the specific requirements of the match. When analysed together, these issues clearly demonstrate that a thorough understanding of performance in soccer is currently incredibly difficult to obtain, compared to sports that have much simpler performance requirements. A difficulty that arises is that frequently both scientists and applied practitioners within the sport are required to make use of a reductionist approach in understanding performance. They select potentially important variables in a given area(s) (see Figure 20.1) that are seen as important in their own right for performance or, in turn, provide some predictive capability for overall match outcome.

## IMPORTANT AREAS FOR CONSIDERATION IN APPLIED SPORTS SCIENCE SUPPORT PROGRAMMES

Effective sports science support programmes will frequently include a number of areas of specific focus in an attempt to improve performance. The three key areas that determine performance (technical and tactical skill, physical fitness and psychological attributes) are in turn influenced by considerations such as the nutritional support of players. The role of effective strategies for injury management and prevention is also vital, as these can influence both individual players and team selection. Figure 20.1 provides a representation of the major areas that are frequently included in sports science support programmes within professional clubs. The attention given to any one area will be highly dependent on the individual practitioner's characteristics (e.g., skill base, level of knowledge, personal philosophy) and the specific requirements of the individual players and the club. For example, successful teams at the highest level that face a large number of fixtures in short time scales may strategically target physiological and psychological recovery strategies, while teams with fewer competitive fixtures and poor fitness levels may concentrate on physiological development. The inter-ventions become a product of the practitioner's ability to take relevant scientific information and apply it within the environmental constraints. Such constraints are a function of a large number of factors that include the culture of the club, the philosophy of the coaches, attitude of the players and the available resources. The following sections outline the potential contribution that some of the areas highlighted in Figure 20.1 can make to the support of a club and its players. The most effective systems will integrate all these individual areas into a multi-disciplinary programme of player support.

Probably the most common single area of sports science that is utilised in professional soccer is physiology. This area of input is intrinsically linked to the strength and conditioning specialists that are now almost always employed as a key part of the coaching structure around the team at the highest level. Physiology can potentially impact on two broad areas of practice within soccer: the planning and delivery of training; and the evaluation of performance. An evaluation of the physiological aspects of performance is crucial, as an awareness of the demands of the sport provides a framework for the work that is required in training to address weaknesses that may exist or to rehabilitate players following injury (Reilly, 2007). Staff may also take responsibility for the nutritional advice given to players. Suitable dietary intake is important in ensuring that the energy requirements of the training load are met. The composition of foods and fluid and the timing of ingestion are important considerations in this context. The nutritional strategy used can also influence the adaptive process to the training that is com-pleted. Sports medicine is also important. The diagnosis and treatment of injury is clearly a crucial component of the performance plan of any athlete. Trained medical personnel such as team doctors and physiotherapists will provide the majority of the input into these areas. Where relevant, this will include support from independent consultants who possess specialist training in specific areas.

Technical and tactical support is provided in some shape or form to every soccer team. In a large number of cases this area is not significantly influenced by the traditional approaches associated with sports scientists, but is rather shaped by the experience and the philosophy of the manager and coaching staff. However, coaches are increasingly aware of the potential of robustly collected data to inform everyday activities within the club. Potential areas that may be influenced by science include the organisation of coaching and training sessions, approaches to match preparation and the overall strategy for management and development

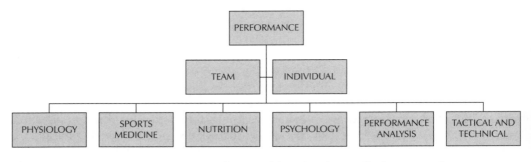

**Figure 20.1** Some important areas for consideration in applied sports science support programmes in soccer.

374

of the high-performance sport environment. Performance analysis can support the technical and tactical preparation by providing important information on the strengths and weaknesses of both a club's own team and the opposition. This information is crucial in providing objective feedback on the outcomes of the coaching process.

Few practitioners would argue against the importance of the psychological component of performance in soccer. This awareness does not, however, frequently translate into the integration of a full-time psychologist working within the club. Those individuals who do find involvement with teams can again fulfil a diverse range of roles. These include working with individuals in traditional areas of 'performance' psychology such as dealing with stress and arousal, goal setting and motivation. Potentially more important than these domains is the lifestyle support that can be provided to players across the age span.

## Physiology-based support in action: a case study

The remaining discussion in this chapter focuses on providing an example of a physiological scientific support programme for an elite team. The content provided should be viewed as a case study, as the specific nature of the application of sports science in a professional team environment is dependent on many factors. These factors can include the philosophy of the club, the manager/coach and the resources and facilities available. The philosophy of the manager/coach is perhaps the biggest influence on sports science delivery within a team. The sports scientist is fundamentally a component of the team that works with the manager to fulfil the objectives of the club. As such, the sports scientist is obligated to adhere to the instruction of the manager at all times. These directions can serve to either enhance or restrict delivery, depending on the specific nature of the situation. This balance of power is infrequently recognised outside of organisations, despite its being fundamental to the framework within which all support systems must work.

## Staffing and support structure

The nature of the performance requirements of the elite player may necessitate the involvement of a number of individuals in a scientific support programme. The extent of this staffing will be largely dependent on the funding available to the sports science department. Smaller clubs that may not be resource rich will frequently address their sports science requirements by employing a single individual. Large clubs with more financial capability will make use of a number of individuals. These individuals will fulfil specific roles within a complex organisational support structure aimed at the holistic support of the individuals within the team. An example of staffing structure encapsulating all the aspects of performance delivery relevant to sports medicine and sports physiology for a team is illustrated in Figure 20.2.

In the model presented in Figure 20.2, the Sports Science Director is responsible for overseeing all aspects of delivery of the scientific support programme. This role will focus not only upon the day-to-day management of the systems and processes that are incorporated into the players' daily activities but also on the management of the staff who directly interact with the players and coaches for specific activities/interventions. It is essential that this specific individual

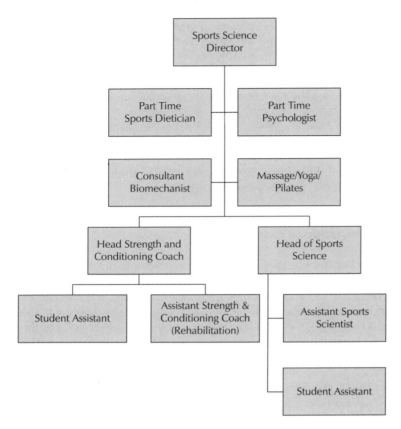

**Figure 20.2** Example of staffing structure for a well-resourced professional club.

possesses both a significant understanding of the available theoretical knowledge base (including contemporary research findings) within relevant subject areas and substantial practical experience within soccer. It is also advantageous if he/she has an awareness of fundamental concepts in organisational and management psychology.

The Head Strength and Conditioning Coach and the Head of Sports Science are fundamental to the day-to-day delivery of the sports science support programme. The Head Strength and Conditioning Coach is responsible for delivery of all physical training components of the programme with the players, including the pre-training warm-ups, the design and implementation of all on- and off-field training programmes and post-exercise recovery strategies. The Assistant Strength and Conditioning Coach provides vital support in these areas and may take control of specific aspects of the conditioning programme, such as the rehabilitation of players following injury. The Head of Sports Science complements the activity of these two individuals by taking responsibility for the monitoring of all training sessions. The accumulation, management and analysis of data provide important objective feedback as to the status and progress of players within their individual training programmes. This process helps to ensure that the balance between physiological stress and recovery is appropriately managed. The

**D. Burgess and B. Drust**

extent of these data can necessitate additional support in this area through employment of an Assistant Sports Scientist and the deployment of students on internship programmes (such students can also be valuable to support the activities of the strength and conditioning personnel within the club). Such internship programmes, especially when coupled with registration for a higher degree, are becoming increasingly important mechanisms for the training of future generations of practitioners.

The potential diversity of problems associated with players and their training and match performances may necessitate specialist help. The infrequency of specialist interventions may not make it financially viable to employ such specialists on a full-time basis. An alternative is to sub-contract such staff on a part-time or consultancy basis. Such areas of support may include a dietician, a biomechanist and a psychologist. A good source for recruiting such individuals can be the local university, especially if there is sport-specific subject expertise within the faculties. Other areas that may be beneficial are additional health service providers such as Pilates and Yoga instructors and massage therapists. These individuals can provide a valuable resource for both the recovery interventions used with players and any injury prevention programmes that may be included in the day-to-day activities of the squad.

## AREAS OF SCIENTIFIC SUPPORT

The potential areas of physiological support for players can be broadly defined. For the purposes of this chapter, two main areas will be identified and discussed. First, the strategies used for the preparation of players for competitive matches will be discussed, followed by a review of the approaches used to plan and support the training of individuals.

### Match preparation

The role of the sports science team on game day is to try to maximise the performance of the players. Typically, the Head Strength and Conditioning Coach is the only member of the extended team who travels with the squad, and therefore delivers the complete range of services to players during this time. The services provided by the sports science team on match day include:

Team warm-up

The specific timing of this activity typically depends on the manager's philosophy, as well as competition regulations. Ideally, 20–25 min should be used, particularly during winter matches, when body temperature may be lower and can take longer to increase to the required levels. The content of the warm-up is subject to individual and team preference, but a combination of dynamic flexibility and ball-work should be incorporated. Any heavy emphasis on static stretching and athletic preparation drills should be replaced with more soccer-specific movement patterns during this period (Perrier et al., 2011). It is also important to include some time for individual player preparation.

## Nutrition/hydration

The preparation and content of an appropriate pre-game meal is important (Williams and Serratosa, 2006). This meal should include a combination of complex and simple carbohydrates as well as protein. The content of meals/fluids in the 48 hours leading into the game is just as crucial to game-day performance as the food/drink consumed on match-day, so these should not be ignored in the preparation strategy (Reilly et al., 2008). All venues at which the team are staying should be contacted and provided with appropriate menus that have been pre-determined by the team dietician in conjunction with the players and other staff, ahead of the match. It is also important that all food is checked by the Head Strength and Conditioning Coach (or alternate member of the travelling team) for the quality and content of food provided before it is consumed by players. The pre-game meal should be consumed between 2.5 and 3 hours before the match (Williams and Serratosa, 2006). This period allows sufficient time for preliminary digestion to occur, thus avoiding any gastric distress during game play.

Player hydration status should be assessed on game day. This process typically involves assessment of each player's urine specific gravity or osmolarity (Shirreffs et al., 2006). Staff should assess this prior to the game, leaving enough time to effect any change necessary. For example, testing each player's urine upon arrival at the ground may be too late to change hydration status before the match. The implementation of such late re-hydration strategies may distract players from their pre-game preparation and could, in addition, increase the opportunity for gastric discomfort.

Prior to the players arriving at the venue, the sports scientist should ensure that all nutrition and hydration options are set out for the players. These can include sports drinks, special electrolyte replacement supplements and water for hydration, as well as salted snacks (pretzels, rice crackers), muesli bars, fruit and confectionery for nutrition. Players should try any fluid/food options during training, to avoid any gastric distress pre-game. It is important to remember that each individual player's taste preference should be an upmost consideration, maybe more so than the adherence to strict scientific principles of provision.

Unlike other field sports, there are limited opportunities for players to rehydrate or refuel during the match. Players should therefore be educated to re-hydrate/re-fuel during any stoppages for injuries or substitutions that may occur. This is particularly important during the second half, when players are starting to become dehydrated and low on fuel. Half time is an important opportunity to take on fluid and fuel.

Post-game nutrition plays a vital role in player recovery (Burke et al., 2006). It is crucial that the team provide players with optimal carbohydrate, electrolyte, fluid and protein to ensure that an optimal environment exists for muscle re-synthesis. Player compliance is important, so taste, consistency and product type should be considered and trialled extensively with each player. This process will provide the framework for the application of individual player-preferred drink/food combinations. Additional supplementation to assist recovery might be provided post game. For example, HMB, creatine monohydrate, beta alanine, and branched chain amino acids have all been shown to assist muscle recovery in athletic populations (Burke et al., 2009, Mujika et al., 2000, van Someren et al., 2005). Their use should therefore be considered at these times.

# 378

### Team cool-down

The team cool-down is often compromised, due to the space available, weather, time constraints when at an away game and player compliance. It is the responsibility of the sports science staff to ensure a cool-down is performed. Cool-down options can include light flexibility activities, mobility movements, ice or contrast baths and massage (Dawson *et al.*, 2005). Light activity could occur on the field after the game or, if space permits, in the dressing room. Additional recovery strategies may include the use of compression garments and portable massage/electrotherapy devices.

### Substitution conditioning

Conditioning for unused (or little-used) substitutes is the responsibility of the sports science team on a match day. Generally, substitutes are allowed 15–20 mins worth of training on the field after the completion of matches. Staff should utilise this small window of opportunity if they feel that players could benefit from the extra conditioning that would have come about as a consequence of playing in the match. However, this should occur only if no training is scheduled for the following day. Where training is scheduled for the following day, the substitutes from the game should be provided with match-specific training in order to try to prevent losses in fitness.

## TEAM TRAINING

The preparation of players for competition is clearly a vital aspect of any scientific support programme. If players are better prepared they are more likely to withstand the demands of competition, increasing their potential to be successful in important match fixtures. The preparation of players can be broadly split into two complementary areas: the planning of training and the subsequent implementation of these programmes within the confines of the week-to-week and day-to-day activity of the squad.

## Planning training

For the sports scientist, the two most important periods of training in the players' annual cycle are the pre-season and in-season training periods. Suitable preparation strategies at these times of the year will support the technical and tactical work delivered by the coaches in the build-up to games.

### Pre-season programming

For professional teams, the pre-season period typically lasts from 6 to 10 weeks. Often during this period teams are required to prepare for the coming season by completing a number of training sessions, play non-competitive games, travel to various locations to compete in sponsor-supported international tournaments and stage a 'team camp' in which a 7- to 14-day period of intense training combined with trial matches is completed. The main challenge

*developing a physiology-based support strategy*

is to plan and deliver a training programme that balances the stress of training with the need for recovery, as the exposure of players to high volumes of training during this time period can lead to fatigue and burn out of players either in the short term or during the season (Jeong et al., 2011). A gradual build-up in training load, with frequent squad rotation during pre-season games, is recommended in order to improve fitness and remain fresh for the length of the competitive season. It is important that sports science staff ensure that selected drills as well as entire sessions reach game intensities for each player at various stages throughout the pre-season period. This process makes sure that players are capable of playing at game intensities when the season commences. Fundamental to this approach to training provision is the monitoring and analysis of the total weekly training and match loads.

The sessions that are delivered in the pre-season programme are largely determined through a process of consultation with the appropriate sports science staff and the manager and the coaching team. Any plan that is developed needs to be flexible, in so far as it may need to be adapted at relatively short notice.

In-season programming

Periodised programming in professional soccer is a complex process. The ability to apply structure to training within a season is largely dependent on manager/coach preference, in addition to the philosophy of senior sports science staff. As a result, programming often strays from typical periodisation models, leading to the implementation of a different approach to that of individuals who deal with cyclical sports or athletic pursuits where competition structure tends to be more fixed and training can therefore be more easily periodised

In leagues where games occur once per week, it is possible to assign types of training to various days of the week. For example, Table 20.1 outlines three possible weekly training scenarios during a week where matches occur on Sundays. Options 1 and 3 allow for a recovery on Monday followed by a day off, whereas Option 2 provides a day off after the game, followed by a recovery/light tactical session. If the sports science team, in conjunction with the manager, feel that an additional day off is required during the week, then Options 2 or 3 might be preferable. If this is not the case, then Option 1 might be chosen.

**Table 20.1** Examples of a weekly in-season training schedule for a team that plays one game per week.

| Sunday | Monday | Tuesday | Wednesday | Thursday | Friday | Saturday |
|--------|--------|---------|-----------|----------|--------|----------|
| Game | Recovery | Off | Soccer-specific conditioning | Tactical training | Tactical training | Tactical training |
| Game | Off | Recovery/tactical training | Soccer-specific conditioning | Off | Tactical training | Tactical training |
| Game | Recovery | Off | Soccer-specific conditioning | Off | Tactical training | Tactical training |

**D. Burgess and B. Drust**

All three of the options outlined above involve specific conditioning sessions on Wednesday. The nature of this conditioning session is dependent on the philosophy of conditioning agreed upon by the manager, coaching team and sports scientist. Ideally, the session will contain activities specific to soccer that involve the ball. It is important that drills are carried out in competitive situations, though care must be taken not to either train players too vigorously during this session or allow the competitive nature of the drills to become unmanageable. Players who play each weekend may rarely need additional conditioning work, as the games probably provide ample stimulus for the maintenance of soccer-specific fitness.

When teams play mid-week fixtures sporadically throughout a season, the periodisation structure of the week becomes problematic. As player rotation is common during such game periods, it becomes very difficult to provide a common periodisation model for all of the squad. In these circumstances, it is essential to utilise the information from individual player monitoring programmes.

Table 20.2 provides some potential options that are available for training organisation when the team has a mid-week fixture. If squad rotation is an option for the specific team in question, two different training programmes can run simultaneously during the week, depending on the playing requirements of these individuals. Table 20.2 provides some options for weeks when fixtures are scheduled for Wednesday and Thursday.

## Day-to-day organisation

It is useful to consider processes and activities in relation to the planning, organisation and delivery of training that occur on a day-to-day basis within a club. An awareness of these provides an opportunity for the reader to understand the factors that shape the specific individual training stimulus that is delivered to each player.

For senior members of the sports science staff, the training day begins with a meeting with appropriate medical/physiotherapy staff to discuss the specific requirements of each player's training programmes for that day. As there are many factors that influence an individual's fitness and/or rehabilitation requirements, the communication between medical and sports science staff is essential. These discussions provide a platform for the smooth delivery of group

**Table 20.2** Options for training organisation when playing mid-week fixtures.

| Sunday | Monday | Tuesday | Wednesday | Thursday | Friday | Saturday |
|--------|--------|---------|-----------|----------|--------|----------|
| Game | Recovery | Tactical training | Game | Recovery | Tactical training | Tactical training |
| Game | Recovery | Tactical training | Game | Off | Recovery/ tactical training | Tactical training |
| Game | Off | Recovery/ tactical training | Tactical training | Game | Tactical training | Tactical training |

and individual training sessions for both fit players and those that are either rehabilitating or injured. This initial meeting is followed by a separate discussion with the technical coaching staff. Ideally, the Head Strength and Conditioning Coach and/or the Director of Sports Science should meet with the manager and his/her coaches each morning before training. This meeting should cover two main areas: (1) any relevant injury news from the previous medical meeting (including players who are available/unavailable for training, as well as status updates on all currently injured players); and (2) a discussion and confirmation of the general outline of training that the technical coaches have devised for the day. This meeting allows all parties to review the specifics of that day (i.e., player numbers, programme requirements, recovery of players) and adjust the training session if necessary.

In professional clubs, there may be occurrences where injuries or international duty dictate that training numbers are quite small. Coaches may need to call up additional players from other, more junior squads within the club (e.g., reserve team or junior players) in order to deliver a session that fits the weekly plan. This scenario highlights the need for senior sports science staff to have direct lines of communication with other support staff who may work with other squads. These lines of communication will ensure that staff members are aware of the individual programmes of players from different squads as well of specific players' injury/fatigue status. The development and operation of club-wide testing and monitoring procedures will simplify this process and ensure transferability of data.

## Training preparation

The sports science staff members need to ensure that all equipment and procedures that are required for training are in place prior to the start of the session. This preparation should include:

- set-up for the warm-up;
- setting up the gym areas for any pre-habilitation for injury activity or for the rehabilitation of injured players;
- organisation of monitoring equipment (e.g., HR belts, GPS vests and devices).

## Training warm-up

This warm-up should be soccer specific and, where possible, specific to the training session about to be carried out. For example, if the coaches wish to start the session with a small-sided game or small-sided possession drill with large changes in direction, then the staff administering the warm-up (typically the Head of Strength and Conditioning) should include specific preparation for this activity. A typical warm-up should begin with some injury prevention activities even if a dedicated pre-habilitation session has been completed (for example the 'FIFA 11Plus', http://f-marc.com/11plus/). Light activity in order to promote increases in blood flow should follow these exercises. This light activity could include dynamic flexibility work as well as a variety of movement patterns (e.g., jogging, lunging, carioca). Finally, some soccer-specific movements, possibly including the ball, should occur. Variety in warm-ups can be challenging throughout the season. Where appropriate, the use of different types of equipment such as cones, poles, ladders, balls, hurdles can assist in keeping warm-ups interesting and fresh. It may also be useful to use other staff to provide a change for the players. This variety is encouraged, providing the main function and structure of the warm-up are not compromised.

### During training

The sports science staff members can fulfil a number of functions during training. These may include the roles listed below.

- Observing specific players who may have had recent injuries. This should include the observation of movement patterns and/or unusual training habits that might indicate a player is fully recovered from injury.
- The monitoring of training load parameters in real time.
- Communicating with coaches with respect to drill time and session progression.
- Rehabilitating injured players.

### Cool-down

Team cool-down should be performed after each session (Twomey et al., 2009). Typically, this could include light activity followed by flexibility exercises. After heavy sessions, pool recovery, ice/contrast baths and massage may be added.

### Player/coach feedback

It is important that players and coaches are provided with any feedback on the training session as soon as possible after training. It is also important that training load information (if collected) is distributed in an appropriate format to players and coaches. Information should be simplified so as to ensure that players and coaches are not confused by scientific terminology (see Figure 20.3).

## PLAYER MONITORING

The previous sections have mentioned the importance of developing a comprehensive monitoring strategy in the sports science support programme. An awareness of the relative 'readiness' of each individual player within the squad for each given competitive fixture is probably the most crucial consideration for the sports scientist. This readiness is predominantly a function of the balance between the response to the physiological stress of training and the recovery from previous competitive matches and/or training sessions. Collecting and analysing objective data on these concepts should, hopefully, enable more informed judgements to be made about the relative status of a player. This process can, in theory, help to optimise team selection. These procedures become especially important when the team is required to play a large number of games within a short space of time and the rotation of the squad is essential. Effective data collection and analysis can assist staff in maintaining the fitness levels of players when they are not regularly starting in the team's competitive matches. It is likely that such strategies can help to inform the injury prevention strategies that may be in place within the club, as excessive loading is an important injury risk factor.

383

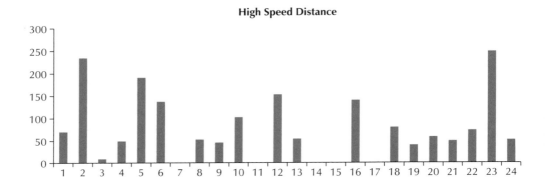

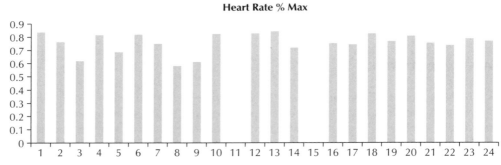

**Figure 20.3** An example feedback sheet for players on the training monitoring from a specific individual session. The figure illustrates individual player responses for both the total distance and the high-speed running distance covered during the training sessions. The heart rate response to the exercise is also illustrated as a percentage of the maximal heart rate recorded from each player during a standardised test.

**D. Burgess and B. Drust**

The nature of the sport and the varied training requirements for players make monitoring within professional soccer complicated. There is no one method that is universally accepted as the 'gold standard' for monitoring training and match loads. This demand frequently results in clubs using strategies that are determined by a delicate balance between the scientific rationale that supports a given approach and the practicality of applying the methodology in the real world. It is therefore common to see a number of different methods being employed in any given team to analyse the demands of training and matches (Alexiou and Coutts, 2008). Certain principles should be important to the sports scientist, irrespective of the method used. The principles of validity and reliability are clearly always important (Atkinson and Nevill, 1998). It is also essential to consider the demands placed on support staff in terms of analysis time for the data. A clear decision should be made to collect information only if it can be effectively utilised by staff to improve the decision-making process. Large amounts of superfluous data collection will only lead to player unrest, additional workloads on staff and poor decisions. It also should be noted that effective monitoring requires data collected over large periods of time. Such longitudinal information enables within-player comparisons to be made. These issues are undoubtedly the most sensitive for the detection of performance changes, player fatigue or injury predisposition.

The following section provides a very brief description of a monitoring strategy used by sports science staff in soccer. It should be noted that the available evidence for the majority of these approaches in real-world use in the sport of soccer is at best limited. The application of these procedures is therefore based on a combination of the applied experience of sports science staff and the available generic literature on these strategies.

## Blood and saliva monitoring

The collection and analysis of blood samples can provide an indication of the status of a variety of physiological systems within the body (e.g., metabolic, hormonal, muscular, immune). Obtaining such information at regular intervals (e.g., one to two days post game and following intense periods of training) may therefore give an indication of the status of the player. Markers such as creatine kinase have been associated with muscle damage and so may represent an indicator of game/training stress (Lazarim et al., 2009). Other parameters such as testosterone and cortisol may be associated with over-reaching/overtraining (Cormack et al., 2008). The availability of portable analysis equipment provides an option for immediate feedback, though such systems can be prohibitively expensive. Cheaper laboratory methods suffer the drawback of an unacceptable delay in the data being made available for the decision-making process. Collection and analysis of saliva provides an alternative method for parameters such as testosterone and cortisol. While such methods may lead to better player compliance, they still suffer from the difficulties of analysis time in most cases and high inter-individual variability.

## Heart rate monitoring

Heart rate is easily measurable using cost-effective electronic devices that do not interfere with players during training or competition. Heart rate provides an indication of the body's cardiovascular response to any given training load. The ease of use with multiple players and its physiological relevance make heart rate a valuable monitoring procedure for soccer (Drust et al., 2007), albeit the data can be misleading if used in isolation. For example, elevated heart rate responses without any objective quantification of training intensity could indicate either poor fitness or high activity levels during training. Similarly, a dampened heart rate response could indicate a lack of effort in training or superior fitness in comparison to the remainder of the squad. Assessing the sub-maximal heart rate response either to a standardised exercise protocol or following exercise during a standard period of recovery can allow the assessment of how quickly heart rate recovers. Changes in this recovery rate (RR) may indicate either improvements in the physiological capabilities of an individual or a temporary state of fatigue. The recording of heart rate at other times may provide other useful information on the relative fatigue of players (Bricout et al., 2010). Heart rate variability represents the variation in the RR intervals for an individual. This variation is a consequence of changes in the autonomic nervous system on the sinus node of the heart. Assessing the heart rate variability following an orthostatic challenge may help sports science staff to identify early signs of overtraining, as well as non-training-related life stressors placed on the player. Under such conditions, it may be relevant to alter the training load to which players are exposed to ensure that there are no increases in player susceptibility to injury.

## Subjective ratings

Asking players how hard they found the session, using a standard scale (e.g., Borg scale), upon completion of the session, is a simple but effective method of gauging perception of the training stimulus (Impellizzeri et al., 2004). This scale provides a subjective evaluation of the training load and may be one of the most sensitive indicators of within-player variation in physical status. For this monitoring tool to be effective, players need to be well educated on appropriate scoring ranges, which may necessitate the inclusion of more objective data at times to help support the player's decision-making. It is also important that scores are collected individually, to prevent peer pressure influencing the data. The individual ratings can be multiplied by the session duration to provide an indication of training load (Impellizzeri et al., 2004). This simple calculation provides sports science staff with a suggestion of both training volume (time) and intensity (Rate of Perceived Exertion). This procedure can provide a very quick representation of the total load placed on players. Once this figure is calculated, additional variables such as training monotony (weekly average training load/weekly standard deviation training load) and training strain (weekly training load x training monotony) can be calculated. Training monotony is a measure of daily training variability in the training stimulus. When elevated levels of this variable are combined with high training loads there may be an increased propensity for an onset of overtraining (Foster, 1998). Training strain provides a similar indication of low training variability combined with high training loads. Simplified ratings of sleep quality and muscle soreness, when taken daily, can provide useful supplementary information to these data.

D. Burgess and B. Drust

## Global Positioning Systems (GPS)

Monitoring training using GPS technology provides an estimation of the training stimulus for each player in a given session. GPS systems provide a range of variables related to the movement profiles of players during drills (e.g., total distance, high-speed distance, time in specific speed zones) (Harley et al., 2011). The inclusion of an accelerometer within the unit enables data to be collected on the types of movements completed (e.g., accelerations, decelerations, impacts). This detailed breakdown of an individual's response to a given training drill leads to clear understanding of the physical loads, facilitating the detection of players who may be under-/over-training. The interpretation of GPS information should be viewed in relation to the limitations associated with the level of technology that is in use (Aughey, 2011). These limitations include the sampling frequency of the units and the quality of the satellite coverage of the training environment.

## Physical screening and/or performance assessments

The completion of regular physical screening using recognised physiotherapy tests (e.g., ankle dorsi flexion range, Thomas test, adductor strength) or movement-based screens (e.g., functional movement screen) may facilitate the early detection of muscle weaknesses or imbalances that can lead to injury (Parchmann and McBride, 2011). Rigorous adherence to testing protocols is also important in this respect. Simple assessments of neuromuscular function, such as various jumping protocols, may provide useful supplementary information on the status of the neuromuscular system (Cormack et al., 2008). These tests can be carried out anywhere, as the equipment is highly portable. This makes such tests useful for training camps and competitions away from the usual training environment. Such tests should ideally be completed at similar times in the schedule, so as to prevent extraneous variables influencing the test outcome.

## SUMMARY

It is clear that scientific knowledge and process are playing an increasing role in the support of the modern soccer player. The application of this knowledge in professional soccer is the responsibility of the sports scientist(s). The application of science to performance is diverse and can cover areas such as the preparation and organisation of training as well as pre-game, within-game and post-game strategies. Science can inform the approaches used to develop young players within the sport as well as play a role in operationalising the organisational strategies and frameworks within which all the individuals involved in the club operate. The specific nature of the interventions developed for a given soccer club/organisation are a product of the ability of the applied practitioner(s) to take relevant scientific information and apply it within the environmental constraints. This process is dependent on the specific individual in question, as well as on a large number of factors that include the culture of the club, the philosophy of the coaches, the attitude of the players and the available resources. As a consequence, there is little consensus as to the specific nature of the operational processes used to support players and coaches at the elite level. The most effective programmes will therefore draw on the most relevant scientific evidence to inform activities and be highly specific to the environment in question.

# REFERENCES

Alexiou, H. and Coutts, A.J. (2008) A comparison of methods used for quantifying internal training load in women soccer players. *International Journal of Sports Physiology and Performance* 3, 320–330.

Atkinson, G. and Nevill, A.M. (1998) Statistical methods for assessing measurement error (reliability) in variables relevant to sports medicine. *Sports Medicine* 26, 217–238.

Aughey, R.J. (2011) Application of GPS technologies to field sports. *International Journal of Sports Physiology and Performance* 6, 295–310

Bricout, V.A., Dechenaud, S. and Favre-Juvin, A. (2010) Analysis of heart rate variability in young soccer players: the effects of sport activity. *Autonomic Neuroscience* 19, 112–116.

Burke, L.M., Loucks, A.B. and Broad, N. (2006) Energy and carbohydrate for training and recovery. *Journal of Sports Sciences* 24, 675–685.

Burke, L.M., Castell, L.M., Stear, S.J., *et al.* (2009) BJSM reviews: A–Z of nutritional supplements: dietary supplements, sports nutrition foods and ergogenic aids for health and performance Part 4. *British Journal of Sports Medicine* 43, 1088–1090.

Cormack, S.J., Newton, R.U. and McGuigan, M.R. (2008) Neuromuscular and endocrine responses to an Australian rules football match. *International Journal of Sports Physiology and Performance* 3, 359–374.

Dawson, B., Gow, S., Modra, S., Bishop, D. and Stewart, G. (2005) Effects of immediate post-game recovery procedures on muscle soreness, power and flexibility levels over the next 48 hours. *Journal of Science and Medicine in Sport* 8, 210–221.

Drust, B., Atkinson, G. and Reilly, T. (2007) Future perspectives in the evaluation of the physiological demands of soccer. *Sports Medicine* 37, 783–805.

FIFA 11plus http://f-marc.com/11plus/.

Foster, C. (1998) Monitoring training in athletes with reference to overtraining syndrome. *Medicine and Science in Sports and Exercise* 30, 7, 1164–1168.

Harley, J.A., Lovell, R.J., Barnes, C.A., Portas, M.D. and Weston, M. (2011) The interchangeability of global positioning system and semi-automated video-based performance data during elite soccer match play. *Journal of Strength and Conditioning Research* 25, 2334–2336.

Impellizzeri, F.M., Rampinnini, E. and Marcora, S.M. (2004) Use of RPE based training load in soccer. *Medicine and Science in Sports and Exercise* 36, 1042–1047.

Jeong, T.S., Reilly, T., Morton, J., Bae, S.W. and Drust, B. (2011) Quantification of the physiological loading of one week of pre-season and one week of in-season training in professional soccer players. *Journal of Sports Sciences* 29, 1161–1166.

Lazarim, F.L., Antunes-Neto, J.M.F., da Silva, F.O.C., Nunes, L.A.S., Bassini-Cameron, A., Cameron, L.C., Alves, A.A., Brenzikofer, R. and Vaz de Macedo, D. (2009) The upper values of plasma creatine kinase of professional soccer players during the Brazilian National Championship. *Journal of Science and Medicine in Sport* 12, 85–90.

Mujika, I., Padilla, S., Ibanez, J., Izquierdo, M. and Gorostiaga, E. (2000) Creatine supplementation and sprint performance in soccer players. *Medicine and Science in Sports and Exercise* 32, 518–525.

Parchmann, C.J. and McBride, J.M. (2011) Relationship between functional movement screen and athletic performance. *Journal of Strength and Conditioning Research*. EPub.

388

Perrier, E.T., Pavol, M.J. and Hoffman, M.A. (2011) The acute effects of a warm up including static and dynamic stretching on countermovement jump height, reaction time and flexibility. *Journal of Strength and Conditioning Research* 25, 1925–1931.

Reilly, T. (2007) The training process. In *The Science of Training – Soccer: A Scientific Approach to Developing Strength, Speed and Endurance* (pp. 1–19). London: Routledge.

Reilly, T., Drust, B. and Clarke, N. (2008) Muscle fatigue during football-match play. *Sports Medicine* 38, 357–367.

Shirreffs, S.M., Sawka, M.N. and Stone, M. (2006) Water and electrolyte needs for football training and match-play. *Journal of Sports Sciences* 24, 699–707.

Twomey, D., Finch, C., Roediger, E. and Lloyd, D.G. (2009) Preventing lower limb injuries: is the latest evidence being translated into the football field? *Journal of Science and Medicine in Sport* 12, 452–456.

van Someren, K.A., Edwards, A.J. and Howatson, G. (2005) Supplementation with beta-hydroxy-beta methylbutyrate (HMB) and alpha-ketoisocaproic acid (KIC) reduces signs and symptoms of exercise-induced muscle damage in man. *International Journal of Sport Nutrition and Exercise Metabolism* 15, 413–424.

Williams, C. and Serratosa, L. (2006) Nutrition on match-day. *Journal of Sports Sciences* 24, 687–697.

# INDEX

392

393

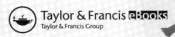